# Labor and Delivery Care

A Practical Guide

To pregnant women, with admiration and wonder
and
To Sharon and Judy

# Labor and Delivery Care

## A Practical Guide

**Wayne R. Cohen,** MD

Professor of Obstetrics & Gynecology and Women's Health
Albert Einstein College of Medicine
New York, NY, USA

**Emanuel A. Friedman,** MD, Med ScD

Emeritus Professor of Obstetrics, Gynecology and Reproductive Biology
Harvard Medical School
Boston, MA, USA

(W)WILEY-BLACKWELL

A John Wiley & Sons, Ltd., Publication

This edition first published 2011, © 2011 by John Wiley & Sons, Ltd

Wiley-Blackwell is an imprint of John Wiley & Sons, formed by the merger of Wiley's global Scientific, Technical and Medical business with Blackwell Publishing.

Registered office: John Wiley & Sons Ltd, The Atrium, Southern Gate, Chichester, West Sussex, PO19 8SQ, UK

Editorial offices:  9600 Garsington Road, Oxford, OX4 2DQ, UK
The Atrium, Southern Gate, Chichester, West Sussex, PO19 8SQ, UK
111 River Street, Hoboken, NJ 07030-5774, USA

For details of our global editorial offices, for customer services and for information about how to apply for permission to reuse the copyright material in this book please see our website at www.wiley.com/wiley-blackwell.

*Library of Congress Cataloging-in-Publication Data*

Cohen, Wayne R.
Labor and delivery care : a practical guide / Wayne R. Cohen, Emanuel A. Friedman.
    p. ; cm.
  Includes bibliographical references and index.
  ISBN 978-0-470-65459-0 (pbk. : alk. paper)  1. Labor (Obstetrics)   2. Delivery (Obstetrics)
3. Childbirth.  I. Friedman, Emanuel A., 1926–  II. Title.
  [DNLM:  1. Labor, Obstetric.  2. Birth Injuries—prevention & control.   3. Delivery, Obstetric—
methods.  4. Obstetric Labor Complications—prevention & control.  WQ 300]
    RG652.C63  2011
    618.4—dc23

                                                                                2011020592

A catalogue record for this book is available from the British Library.

This book is published in the following electronic formats: ePDF 9781119971535; Wiley Online Library 9781119971566; ePub 9781119971542; mobi 9781119971559

Set in 8/11pt StoneSerif by MPS Limited, a Macmillan Company, Chennai, India
Printed and bound in Malaysia by Vivar Printing Sdn Bhd

1  2011

# Contents

# Preface

The impetus for this book was born of satisfaction and lamentation. We celebrate the remarkable advances in obstetric care that have occurred over the span of our careers (encompassing 50 years). We are nevertheless troubled by the fact that the burgeoning medical technocracy has diverted attention from fundamental medical care skills in our specialty, and no doubt in others. The fall in maternal and fetal mortality and morbidity over the last half-century reflects in large measure gratifying advances in obstetric and neonatal technology. Surely the advent and increasing sophistication of ultrasonography, electronic fetal monitoring, prenatal diagnosis, antimicrobial therapy, molecular medicine, and advances in epidemiology have, among others, shaped the form and substance of obstetric care in ways that have done much to improve outcomes. Residents are now well versed in the complexities and subtleties of ultrasonography, molecular genetic diagnosis, and immunology; nevertheless, relatively few have mastered the essentials of clinical examination and decision making that can make obstetrics so satisfying to its practitioners and so much safer for its patients. The training of midwives and physician's assistants has in its way likewise tended away from the complexities of clinical assessment.

The recently awakened emphasis on patient safety initiatives in obstetrics puts this trend in high relief, as much of the focus of these performance improvement activities has been on improving basic clinical skills. Moreover, the majority of medical negligence litigation that has pestered our specialty for decades, reducing the happiness of its practitioners and its appeal to students, relates to alleged failures in application of fundamental clinical doctrine. So there is ample justification for a text that emphasizes our bedrock principles. Within them lie the solutions to many of our contemporary challenges.

Someday our medical heirs will use anatomic and functional imaging techniques and laboratory analyses now barely imaginable to evaluate and diagnose. Skillful physical examination and probing medical history may no longer be needed or taught. We have not yet, however, reached the crossroads leading to that brave new medical vale; rather we exist in a period of transition that requires attention to advanced technologic

approaches as well as to traditional techniques of diagnosis and problem solving. It is with reverence for the latter that we have directed this
volume.

Obstetrics, particularly the management of labor and delivery, has
always been a discipline that requires skilled physical diagnosis in order to
make the most refined diagnostic judgments. It demands the synthesis of
several simultaneously acquired lines of diagnostic evidence into a cohe-
sive probability matrix in order to balance the risks of intervention and
watchful expectancy. During labor, fetal information (e.g., state of oxygenation, lie, position, attitude, molding) must be integrated step by step
with facts about the mother (e.g., vital signs, medical condition, uterine
contractility, pelvic architecture) to determine changes in the probability
that a normal vaginal delivery will ensue or that some pharmacologic or
surgical intervention will be necessary to optimize safety. Decisions based
on these changing probabilities obviously require accurate and complete
clinical information to make them reliable. Ideally, that information
should have been demonstrated to be meaningful in appropriate investi-
gative studies.

We live in an era of the deification of "evidence-based" medicine. In
fact, evidence-based practice is not new. Good physicians have always
functioned by incorporating the best available scientific evidence into
their practice. They have, however, tempered the application of evidence
with sound clinical judgment and the wisdom born of experience and
sapient observation. We ourselves have always emphasized the importance of requiring objective proof whenever possible to justify clinical
interventions. We are, nevertheless, mindful of the fact that not everything can be studied with a randomized clinical trial. It is too often unac-
knowledged that most of what we do and think is right in medicine has
never been subjected to such investigation. This fact emphasizes the great
value of developing good clinical skills and an in-depth understanding
of the labor and delivery process. From those skills and understanding
derive the obstetric acumen and good clinical instincts that characterize
the best practitioners.

In this volume we have attempted to integrate science and clinical
evaluative arts. We have deemphasized issues related to the application
of electronic technology, such as ultrasound and electronic monitoring,
and focused on the application of good clinical skills and their interpretation. That is not to downplay the value of technology, which is of vital
importance to us; rather, it is done in the service of helping practitioners
establish first-rate clinical skills. We hope the result will prove useful to
anyone privileged to assist women in childbirth.

We are aware of the gender and other biases that tend to populate textbook writing, and equally conscious of (and appalled by) the solecisms, awkward syntax, and grammatical gymnastics often employed to avoid them. Throughout this book we have chosen certain default pronouns and nouns to promote easy reading and ensure uniformity of style. Thus, we use "she" and "her" when referring to the obstetric practitioner, and "attendant," "practitioner" or "provider" for any professional involved in patient care during labor. Similarly, we use masculine pronouns to refer to the parturient's partner in the birth process. Neither these choices nor the inevitable places in which we have strayed from our best intentions in this regard are meant to offend.

We are grateful to Martin Sugden and Michael Bevan, our editors at John Wiley & Sons and their team. Their professionalism, guidance, and confidence in the virtues of this project have been immeasurably helpful.

Wayne R. Cohen and Emanuel A. Friedman
*New York and Boston*

# How to Use This Book

*True obstetrics is a great art, and because it is a difficult art, it is easier to be a good "Caesarist" than a good obstetrician* (Archiv Gynäk 1955;186:41).

The sentiment conveyed by the eminent Austrian obstetrician Hans Zacherl in 1955 could very well have been expressed yesterday. While it is entirely appropriate that today's cesarean rate is considerably higher than in the 1950s, the frequency of cesarean delivery has reached alarming levels in many countries. This has occurred in part because many well-intentioned obstetricians believe that cesarean delivery usually serves the best interests of mother and fetus, a view that for the most part is not supported by available evidence. The cesarean delivery trend has also been nourished by the failure of our training system to teach the skills necessary for obstetric practitioners to make the complex clinical evaluations and judgments needed to identify and to manage cases in which vaginal delivery would be the safest alternative. This volume is devoted to helping you learn those skills. It will serve both the experienced clinician wishing to refresh her knowledge on a topic, and the novice.

The book consists of 15 chapters. A few readers will try to absorb it from cover to cover. That strategy will work for some, but may prove less profitable (if not soporific) for most. A piecemeal approach will work better.

The first five chapters cover basic principles, and set the stage for the ensuing chapters, which address specific obstetric issues. The last chapter provides a series of case studies with brief analyses that emphasize the principles advanced in the text. These cases can be used for self-study or as the basis for small group learning in a training program.

A glossary is provided for quick access to terms with which you may not be familiar.

You will best profit from the book by reading chapters in the context of your clinical experience. For example, if you read about face presentation right after you have seen one (or, better, while you are involved in the care of one during labor) it will do much to reinforce and expand your knowledge. Reviewing the chapter on evaluation of the pelvis before or during a tour on the labor floor will help you hone your examination skills. We hope you will use this as a handbook, and consult it frequently during your work with women in labor.

We have alluded only infrequently to ultrasonography, despite the fact that it has become part of daily obstetric practice for most of us. Imaging is a wonderful tool, but it is a mistake to use it in place of your hands, eyes, and ears. Rather, it should complement those senses. In fact, if you are a good sonographer, you can use those skills to reinforce your learning of physical examination skills. Verify with sonography, for example, your clinical determination of fetal presentation or position. With experience, you will find you will no longer need imaging very often. Clinical examination is faster, more efficient, less expensive, and available to everyone.

We hope that you will find this book to be a helpful companion. It is not easy to become a good obstetrician; but it is worth the effort.

# CHAPTER 1

# Communicating Effectively With Your Patient

Human labor and birth are remarkable events, imbued with wonder and beauty. They are, nevertheless, prone occasionally to challenges, infirmity, and even tragedy. Caring for women during these experiences is a remarkable privilege, often exhilarating, but not without its perils and trials. To meet the demands of this task as a labor attendant—whether obstetrician, family practitioner, midwife, or labor room nurse—you must be equipped with the necessary clinical skills, judgment, empathy, and emotional insight to deal with all possible events and outcomes. While many of the physiologic aspects of the birth process are familiar and predictable, each woman will experience them in her own way.

A woman's emotional and physical response to her labor and delivery is conditioned by many factors. These include her cultural background, personality traits, religious beliefs, and other aspects of her personal psychosocial context and history. You may have little ability to influence these factors, but it is important for you to understand them and to recognize how they influence the patient's expectations and coping mechanisms during times of stress. This insight should always inform the content and style of any communications you have with your patient.

Other influences on the parturient's ability to contend with labor are under more direct control. These relate to her physical and emotional comfort during the process of labor and birth. In that respect, the approach of the obstetric team is of great importance and can make the difference between an experience marked by satisfaction and contentment (even if there have been complications) and one that leaves a residue of resentment, regret, unhappiness, and unanswered questions. Not every labor and delivery experience can be idyllic, comfortable, and unencumbered by complications or missteps. We should, nevertheless, always aspire to that goal. Patients do value our endeavor and attitude. They expect and deserve our best efforts, even when they occasionally do not succeed.

*Labor and Delivery Care: A Practical Guide*, First Edition. Wayne R. Cohen and Emanuel A. Friedman. © 2011 John Wiley & Sons, Ltd. Published 2011 by John Wiley & Sons, Ltd.

## Special aspects of parturition

Labor and delivery can be extremely stressful for even the healthiest of women. It is a time when feelings of fragility, vulnerability, and defenselessness are common, as are apprehension and a sense of physical and emotional discomfort. The reasons for these feelings are obvious. Consider that the parturient is likely to be in unfamiliar surroundings. She is wearing a hospital garment that leaves her nearly naked. She is bombarded with attention, surrounded by strangers whom she has just met. This applies even if hospital personnel have properly introduced themselves, which is sometimes not the case. She may be besieged by nurses, students, residents, and laboratory technicians. All of them want things from her that she may be in no mood to provide. Labor, especially once contractions are strong and frequent, is physically and emotionally demanding. It is not, in short, the perfect context for thoughtful reflection and objective decision making.

Things happen unexpectedly during labor and may surprise even the best prepared patient. If you have not had the opportunity to get to know your patient during her prenatal course, your ability to address such events is especially challenged. This is becoming more of an issue as medicine moves to reduced work hours for physicians and the need for more frequent turnover of care to colleagues at personnel changes. It is a problem well recognized by nurses and other healthcare providers who have always worked in shifts, and one that requires the development of new skills to address well.

Much has changed in recent decades concerning the nature of the interaction between healthcare providers and patients. Previously, we (especially physicians) were considered omniscient leaders of the patient care team whose opinions and pronouncements were law, not to be questioned by professional subordinates nor, especially, by patients. That paternalism has given way to a more interactive collegiality that, ideally, values the feelings and opinions of all members of the healthcare team and of the patient. That approach has, in fact, been shown to improve patient safety. It certainly adds dignity and civility to the professional interactions that surround decision making during labor, and respects the needs and wishes of the parturient.

### The value of prenatal care

One of the best places to begin to assuage anxiety provoked by labor is during your patient's prenatal course. In addition to discussing what to expect during normal labor, it is important for you to talk to her about potential adversities, including cesarean or instrumental vaginal delivery or oxytocin administration, should the need arise. You should also address the possibility of shoulder dystocia as well as of postpartum hemorrhage. While some practitioners would prefer not to bring up such potential calamities because of their relative rarity, it is important for you to give your patient at least a general idea of what would be done if any of them should occur. With good communication skills you can accomplish this without alarming her.

Most important, prenatal care provides opportunities to forge a bond of trust with the patient. In that way you can learn to understand the nature of her fears, educate her about potential risks, and have her understand what to anticipate during her labor. She, in turn, will learn more about you and become comfortable with your communication style. Trust is vital because not every peril or need for intervention can be foreseen. When something unexpected does arise, it is the previously established trust and confidence in you as the practitioner that will help sustain the patient's composure and equanimity.

Establishing trust can be elusive and difficult for the patient because it requires her to relax her defenses and accept some vulnerability. She is seldom able to give it lightly because it ultimately requires exposure of the most private domains of her mind and body. One of the great virtues of prenatal care that extends for so long over the course of pregnancy is that your repeated meetings and discussions with the patient will serve to enhance her security and facilitate rapport. Needless to say, standards of professionalism require that you honor complete confidentiality in this respect.

Sometimes you may be called upon to form a bond of trust with the patient in a very short period of time. This occurs when you are covering for another physician or midwife, or have taken over at the beginning of a shift, or are functioning strictly as an inpatient "laborist" with no prenatal care responsibilities. As difficult as that process may be for you, it is even more of a problem for the patient, whose anxiety may be heightened by an unfamiliar face and manner. Establishing instant faith in these settings is not easy, but you, with experience, will learn to do so with success.

The key to establishing rapport with your patient involves your clear demonstration of empathy, respect, confidence, and availability. Openly acknowledge that this is a difficult situation for you both, but that you are committed to her comfort and good care. Let her know that you have every confidence in your ability to help manage her labor, that you are interested in her opinions and expectations, and that you will make every effort to meet them. Be approachable and available to answer her questions and those of her companion. Solicit questions from the patient rather than waiting for her to raise them, and be sure she understands that you will take the time to address them. Every woman in labor should feel that she is the most important person in your world at that time. This is only appropriate, because you are indeed filling that role in hers.

## Communication skills

### Use your powers of observation

Understanding the patient's needs and responding to her concerns require your rapt attention. It should be clear to her that you are interested in and concentrating on what she has to say. Listen carefully to her concerns and observe her body language as well. A great deal is conveyed by facial expressions and other forms of nonverbal communication. Interviewing the patient while focusing your eyes on the chart or computer screen can be perilous. Not only is your inattention an affront to the patient, but you may miss many vital clues to her medical condition and emotional state.

Try to avoid confrontational or judgmental interactions, even if the patient appears to be challenging you. Make the effort to understand what underlies her obdurate or hostile feelings. They are likely to have arisen out of fear, anxiety, frustration, personal conflicts, or other distress. Remember that your relationship with the patient is bidirectional, and learning to see things from her perspective is vital in developing good communication skills. Part of that process involves recognizing your own reactions to various kinds of patients, especially the difficult ones. Enhancing your sensitivity to the special emotional needs of every patient as a unique individual is crucial to your role as a complete healthcare provider.

With experience, you will learn to tailor the style and content of your discussions with a patient so as to provide a clear explanation of the situation in a manner appropriate to her ability to understand it. The content and nature of such discussions may vary depending upon the patient's level of education, what you perceive as her style of emotional defense or adaptation, and her interest in participating in the process. It is, under all circumstances, your responsibility to ensure that the patient understands the clinical situation clearly. Remember that, while a patient's level of education may influence her vocabulary or her scientific sophistication and comprehension, education does not necessarily correlate with intelligence. When you use appropriate language, patients of all educational levels can understand and make reasonable and informed decisions about even very complex clinical issues. This is a difficult skill, but one well worth cultivating.

### Disclosure of adversity

One of the things we have learned from the medical malpractice thorn of the past few decades is that patients are often driven to sue because they feel they have been abandoned by their doctor or by the medical system at a time of exceptional vulnerability and need. The residual burden of anger or resentment that spawns a lawsuit is more often born of the desperation and frustration at having been left with doubt and suspicion rather than of a conviction that harm has occurred because of an error in management. Often the search for answers is initially more important to the plaintiff than financial compensation, but that goal becomes subsumed in the legal quagmire of a formally filed tort action.

You can dissipate many of these concerns by frank and open communication with your patient during labor and afterwards, regardless of the outcome. It is regrettable that this does not always occur, particularly when there have been complications—the very time when discussion is most important.

Good communication includes involvement of the patient and, when appropriate, her family in decision making. It is vital for you to explain what is happening at every step of the process, even if there are complications or uncertainty. To repeat, you should tailor the timing, content, and tenor of these discussions to each patient and situation. As a general guiding principle, full disclosure of events is almost always the best path. As noted, explanations need to be individualized to comport with the patient's educational level, language abilities, and most importantly, her coping style.

Many of us who care for women through their pregnancies tend to be especially poor conveyers of bad news. Perhaps one thing that appeals to some of us is that the vast majority of our cases have happy outcomes. Students who are uncomfortable discussing grave complications or prognoses with patients may for that reason be attracted to obstetrics. This is understandable but unfortunate, as bad outcomes in obstetrics are experienced with singular pain and are given special significance by families. The primary source of such pain probably arises from primal psychological forces, and is aggravated because adverse results are uncommon and because expectations are high. Moreover, the grief-averse practitioner may have a tendency (real or simply perceived by the patient) to ignore the problem or, worse, to trivialize obstetric loss.

Some of us tend to dismiss fetal deaths, whether through early miscarriage or even late pregnancy stillbirth, as insignificant life losses because the patient has an opportunity to redress them with another (presumably more successful) pregnancy. This is a regrettable, self-serving, and ultimately destructive attitude that serves mainly to absolve us from dealing with the emotional consequences of the loss. While the death or injury of a fetus is certainly felt and coped with differently than, say, the unexpected illness or death of a child or of an ailing aged parent, the loss of each may be felt with equal intensity. There is thus a special need for you to develop keen skills for communicating adversity. Fortunately, this can be learned, and practiced. It is an ability as important as communicating and sharing joy in response to a good outcome.

## Dealing with family or companions

If your patient has a partner present during her labor, he can often be very helpful in providing emotional support and helping to communicate with you and the rest of the staff. Occasionally, however, the partner acts just like another patient, requiring his own support and reassurance. This may tax the patience of the staff. It will sometimes even divert personnel from their primary goal of serving the parturient. Always discuss with the patient when she is alone what her desires are regarding the role of her labor companion. This discussion helps avoid ambiguity, conflict, and confusion later as the labor progresses.

Sometimes, a large cadre of family and friends is allowed or even encouraged to attend the birth, a norm in some cultures. Under these circumstances you must ensure that the patient's best interests and wishes are fulfilled, regardless of who is present with her. It is also useful for you to set ground rules and expectations at the very outset. Determine with clarity directly from the patient whom she wants present in the room during the actual delivery. You should also come to an agreement with her in advance as to when and under what circumstances guests may be asked to leave. In the latter regard, the staff may sometimes have to serve as the patient's strong advocates, even acting forcefully against the contrary wishes of the guests.

Maintaining patient confidentiality in the context of a busy labor unit, especially when there are friends or relatives in the room, can be difficult, but must be honored as a basic priority and right. Bring family members into the discussions only with the direct consent of the patient, and be sure to obtain this consent from her when none of the other observers is present, lest she feel coerced into something with which she is not really comfortable.

## Know your limits

Pregnancy is a time of remarkable stability and optimism for some women, and one of emotional upheaval and apprehension for others. The latter may take the form of common anxieties shared by most women: Will the baby be normal? Will labor be too painful? Will I be able to care for a child? Such fears can usually be allayed or modulated by calm explanation, reassurance that they are common if not universal, and by having the patient understand that you will be there during the labor to help her deal with her concerns. Beware, however, the occasional patient whose level of apprehension, ambivalence, and conflict breach the normal envelope.

You need an astute eye and a discerning ear to recognize these often subtle manifestations. You should also recognize when the patient's need for counseling extends beyond your capabilities to handle professionally, and make appropriate referrals. This need to ensure prompt referrals to experts applies, of course, as well to instances in which you are confronted by perplexing medical and obstetric issues that lie beyond your expertise. No one, no matter how experienced or skilled, can be knowledgeable and proficient in all aspects of medicine. A fundamental aspect of caring for patients is, therefore, knowing your limitations and avoiding the temptation to try to exceed them. You are not only being prudent in adhering to this principle, you are serving your patients' best interests.

## Continuity of care

There are important virtues to ensuring continuity of intrapartum care, particularly over the course of a long labor. The benefit of serial observations and interactions with the patient is invaluable in decision making. It arguably outweighs the potential addling and dispiriting effects of fatigue in the competent practitioner (although the latter is hotly debated). That being said, it is increasingly uncommon for an individual provider to manage a patient during the entirety of a lengthy labor.

The recent trend to reduced work hours has led to the need to hand over the care of parturients frequently. As a consequence, care during a labor can sometimes span three or more obstetric teams. These changes can be offputting and disorienting to the patient. The ability of the new team to establish a sense of comfort and confidence quickly is important, but seldom easy and sometimes not able to be accomplished within the time constraints. When taking over the care of the patient, therefore, you should be sure to meet with her and her family promptly. Introduce yourself appropriately. Make eye contact with her and answer her questions directly. Avoid being judgmental and be sure you have had a thorough discussion beforehand with the team going off service about every aspect of the labor, no matter how minor it may appear at the time. Let the patient know that you are up-to-date on her situation.

## Ethics and maternal–fetal conflict

It is obvious that you and the rest of the obstetric team should always act ethically toward the parturient. This means observing and balancing the principles of beneficence and respect for patient autonomy. Honest and open communication with respect for the patient's opinions and values are the most important channels through which ethical treatment is driven.

Under most circumstances, the goals of the mother and her obstetric team are coincident, namely, to do what is possible to ensure a healthy outcome for mother and baby. Occasionally, however, there will be conflicts between you and the patient over medical or ethical issues. (These may in a sense be conflicts between mother and fetus.)

For example, a patient might refuse an intervention such as cesarean delivery that you deem to be in the best interests of the fetus. She might refuse blood products because of religious convictions. She might be using illicit drugs that place the fetus at risk, and persist in this behavior despite your admonitions to the contrary. These are challenging ethical dilemmas. Resolving them requires you to have finely honed communication skills. You will need to respect the patient's autonomy and to balance it against what you perceive to be your beneficence-based obligations to serve the best medical interests of mother and fetus.

Most ethical conflicts are related to clashes of values. In general, it is important not to impose your own values on the patient. Ideally, you have an obligation to understand her value system and to know whether it conflicts with your own. This cannot be accomplished in a short time, emphasizing another virtue of the continuity afforded when prenatal care is provided by the delivering practitioner. Assessment of values through many encounters during gestation and discussions of the patient's perspectives on challenging issues can avoid difficult contretemps during labor.

Do not expect a resolution of ethical conflicts during labor to make all parties completely comfortable. Despite your differences, remember that you and your patient remain partners in this process. Your role is to address potential conflicts and competing views unhesitatingly so that a satisfactory resolution can be achieved. In so doing, the moral autonomy and personal dignity of the patient will be best preserved and your moral obligations to her best fulfilled. You should expect no more and should abide no less.

## Violence

Nothing so defiles the dignity of women as does domestic violence. Be aware that psychological or physical abuse of pregnant women can arise or be exacerbated by the stress of pregnancy. This regrettable fact is true at all levels of society. It is vital that you ask appropriate questions to uncover abusive situations. Obviously, this would be difficult to accomplish unless you have already established the aforementioned trust and confidentiality with your patient. Ideally, the obstetric unit should be a sanctuary for women who have been victims of emotional or physical battering during their pregnancy. The anxiety brought to bear on the labor process in the presence of an abusive partner can be debilitating, taint an otherwise satisfying experience, and even potentially interfere with the normal course of the labor.

Dealing with a person who accompanies your patient and who is known to have abused her can be difficult, to say the least. First, ensure that the patient desires that he be present. If so, he should be carefully observed. Rarely will physical abuse occur during labor, but subtle or overt psychological abuse in the form of unsupportive or denigrating comments is common. Be alert for these and provide extra support to the parturient to try to neutralize his disparagement. A more delicate situation presents itself if your patient does not want the abuser present. Polite entreaties for him to do what is in the patient's best interest and to leave the premises sometimes work, but may heighten his anger. He may become abusive toward you as well. Avoid getting into a loud (or worse, physical) confrontation. Retain your own dignity and use hospital security in situations in which you feel the patient or staff may be in danger. These interactions are distressing in the extreme to all involved. Most important, they may compromise patient safety, so they cannot be ignored. A departmental meeting to develop a policy for dealing with these situations can be helpful. At the very least, it gets everyone thinking about how to identify and react when a problem is encountered. Having a mental health professional present at these discussions to explain abusive behavior and to suggest ways to cope with it can be helpful.

## Boundaries

An important aspect of medical care relates to the maintenance of appropriate boundaries to ensure that the provider–patient relationship remains professional and not unacceptably personal. The practitioner (or patient) who crosses that frontier does so at great hazard for both parties. That is not to imply that you must be distant, impersonal, or avoid sensitive and potentially disturbing issues. Quite to the contrary, a meaningful professional relationship should be one of sensitivity, compassion, and emotional closeness.

The boundary of appropriate behavior shifts with the prevailing social mores. It may be difficult to identify, and is today often approached with trepidation because of fears that your words or actions will be misinterpreted. To our thinking, the professional nature of your relationship with a patient can be preserved while its empathetic and emotional qualities are drawn upon to advantage. To do this properly requires skill and experience, but in doing so, you will enhance the richness of your relationship with the patient, a benefit for both parties.

## Does gender matter?

Midwifery and obstetric nursing have always been professions comprised overwhelmingly of female practitioners, whereas, until recently, physicians were mostly men. In recent decades, women have increasingly entered medicine in general and obstetrics and gynecology in particular. A field previously dominated by male physicians has now changed so that half of practicing obstetricians and upwards of 80% of residents are women. This has changed the culture of the specialty in many unexpected and interesting ways. One often-asked question is whether men should even enter the discipline.

There is in fact a general perception that women prefer obstetric practitioners of their own sex, although this has not been supported by objective studies of the issue. In truth, men and women are generally skillful empathetic practitioners, and an equivalent (fortunately small) proportion of each group is insensitive, unfeeling, and callous. Sensible patients avoid the latter, regardless of their sex, and choose doctors based on their medical skills, professionalism, and compatibility.

If a patient, for personal, cultural, or other reasons prefers a female to provide her care, that wish should be respected when possible. That advice notwithstanding, allowing a patient to reject a provider based on sex may leave you (and your institution) on a slippery moral slope if a patient desires to shun a caretaker because of some other demographic feature. Most women's choices are, fortunately, quality- and compassion-based, and tend to be gender-independent.

## Goals

Labor endows a unique emotional amalgam of fear and hope, anxiety and high expectations, in an admixture unique to each patient's experience. A woman's attitude toward and expectations concerning pregnancy are influenced by her social, psychological, and cultural background and by her experiences during gestation. No universal formula exists for the provision of emotional support; rather, you as the practitioner must respond to the patient's needs, encouraging her to express her questions, fears or concerns, and discussing them in an honest and reassuring manner. Sensitivity to her emotional and physical needs is foremost in a nurturing, supporting relationship that avoids paternalism.

You cannot promise a perfect outcome or an emotionally enriching birth experience in every case. You can, however, pledge to seek the best outcome possible for mother and fetus in the safest available manner. This will always involve your treating the laboring mother with the requisite gentleness, dignity, and compassion she warrants in the birth process.

## Key points

- A woman's emotional and physical response to labor and delivery is conditioned by her cultural and religious background, personality traits, and other aspects of her psychosocial context and history.
- Labor and delivery can provoke feelings of vulnerability, apprehension, and physical and emotional discomfort.
- Begin to assuage anxiety about labor during the prenatal course, when there are opportunities for you to forge a bond of trust with the patient. Learn about her concerns and educate her about what to anticipate during labor.
- The key to establishing patient rapport involves showing empathy, respect, confidence, and availability.
- Listen carefully to the parturient and also observe her body language. A great deal is conveyed by nonverbal communication.
- Modify the style and content of your discussions with patients to provide clear explanations in a manner appropriate to their ability to understand and to interpret the information.
- There is a special need for obstetric practitioners to develop keen skills for communicating adversity.
- Be aware that psychological or physical abuse of women by family members or others can arise or be exacerbated during pregnancy.
- Always act ethically toward the parturient, balancing the principles of beneficence and respect for patient autonomy. Open communication that shows due regard for the patient's opinions and personal views is most important.
- Most ethical conflicts are related to clashes of values. Do not impose your values on the patient. Help her to make decisions in the context of her own mores.

## Further Reading

### Books and reviews

Charles C, Gafni A, Whelan T, O'Brien MA. Cultural influences on the physician–patient encounter: The case of shared treatment decision-making. Patient Educ Couns 2006;63:262–7.

Chervenak FA, McCullough LB. Clinical guide to preventing ethical conflicts between pregnant women and their physicians. Am J Obstet Gynecol 1990;162:303–7.

Cohen WR. Maternal–fetal conflict I. In: Goldworth A, Silverman W, Stevenson DK, Young EWD (eds) *Ethics and Perinatology*. Oxford University Press, New York, 1995: 10–28.

Dattel JD, Chez RA. Battering. In: Cohen WR (ed) *Complications of Pregnancy*. Lippincott Williams & Wilkins, Philadelphia, 2000: 171–5.

Danziger S. The uses of expertise in doctor–patient encounters during pregnancy. Soc Sci Med 1978;12:356–67.

Fauci AS, Braunwald E, Kasper DL, Hauser SL, Longo DL, Jameson JL, Loscalzo J. The practice of medicine. In: Fauci AS et al. (eds) *Harrison's Principles of Internal Medicine*, 17th edition. McGraw Hill, New York, 2008: 1–6.

Harpham WS. *Only 10 Seconds to Care: Help and Hope for Busy Clinicians*. ACP Press, Philadelphia, 2009.

Karnieli-Miller O, Eisikovits Z. Physician as partner or salesman? Shared decision-making in real-time encounters. Soc Sci Med 2009;69:1–8.

Macklin R. Maternal–Fetal Conflict II. In: Goldworth A, Silverman W, Stevenson DK, Young EWD (eds) *Ethics and Perinatology*. Oxford University Press, New York, 1995: 29–46.

Nadelson CC. Ethics, empathy, and gender in health care. Am J Psychiatry 1993;150: 1309–14.

Pellegrino ED, Thomasma DC. *The Virtues in Medical Practice*. Oxford University Press, New York, 1993.

Woods JR, Rozovsky F. *What Do I Say? Communicating Intended or Unanticipated Outcomes in Obstetrics*. John Wiley & Sons, Hoboken, NJ, 2003.

## Primary sources

Cuttini M, Habiba M, Nilstun T, Donfrancesco S, Garel M, Arnaud C, et al. Patient refusal of emergency cesarean delivery. Obstet Gynecol 2006;108:1121–9.

Harris LH. Rethinking maternal–fetal conflict: gender and equality in perinatal ethics. Obstet Gynecol 2000;96:786–91.

Olson DP, Windish DM. Communication discrepancies between physicians and hospitalized patients. Arch Int Med 2010;170:1302–7.

Schnatz PF, Murphy JL, O'Sullivan DM, Sorosky JI. Patient choice: comparing criteria for selecting an obstetrician-gynecologist based on image, gender, and professional attributes. Am J Obstet Gynecol 2007;197:548.e1–7.

Zuckerman M, Navizedeh N, Feldman J, McCalla S, Minkoff H. Determinants of women's choice of obstetrician/gynecologist. J Womens Health Gend Based Med 2002;11:175–80.

# CHAPTER 2

# Examining Your Patient

The examination of women during labor shares many skills in common with medical evaluation in general, and also brings some special requirements to the fore. Pregnancy alters physical findings in most organ systems, sometimes in a manner that would be considered pathologic in the nonpregnant state. A full discussion of these changes is beyond the scope of this volume. Suffice it to say that in order for you to become a skilled examiner, you should become thoroughly familiar with the variations in physical findings attributable to pregnancy.

Physical examination skills are acquired slowly, requiring much practice and repetition. Be patient and devote the necessary time and effort to achieve proficiency. It will prove one of your most valuable assets.

## General principles

As with all medical examinations, there are several central principles that apply:

1 Always wash your hands prior to the examination. Preferably, do this in view of the patient so that she will have no doubt that your hands have been cleaned.
2 Before touching the patient, warm and dry your hands. Similarly, be sure that all instruments that contact the patient (stethoscope, speculum, etc.) have been warmed whenever possible before use.
3 A cordial greeting of patients whom you already know is essential. If you have not met the patient previously, introduce yourself directly by name and status. Tell her why you are there and what your role will be in her care. The content of what you convey to her and your demeanor during this introduction are important. First impressions count. Those first moments in the relationship are central to establishing the basis for trust in new patients.

*Labor and Delivery Care: A Practical Guide*, First Edition. Wayne R. Cohen and Emanuel A. Friedman. © 2011 John Wiley & Sons, Ltd. Published 2011 by John Wiley & Sons, Ltd.

4 Address the patient by her last name, unless she gives you permission to do otherwise.

5 Maintain eye contact whenever possible. Never discuss anything when standing behind the patient so that she is unable to see you. Avoid standing towering over her at the bedside, particularly when something important is being discussed. Sitting is better. However, do not sit on the patient's bed. Some patients find this an emotionally intrusive invasion of their personal space. Use a bedside chair instead. Doing so is both prudent and professional.

6 While you are taking a patient's history and examining her, be sure to listen to her carefully and observe her body language in response to your questions and physical assessments. You will learn to recognize that body language can sometimes reveal more important clues to her feelings than what she says.

7 Be truthful about what is happening, but always supportive and reassuring regardless of the situation. Be confident in your knowledge—within the limits of your knowledge—and your decisions. (Showing confidence, however, does not mean being paternalistic or haughty. Never demean your patient's lack of knowledge, misconceptions, or failure to understand what you are saying.) If you do not appear poised and secure or, worse, look frightened, the patient will quickly lose confidence in you. At the same time, remember that we are all fallible and have limitations. Thus, if you recognize that advice or formal consultation or referral is required before a decision is taken or a plan of action determined, acknowledge that need openly as in the best interests of mother and fetus. Your patient will appreciate this and thank you for it.

Your hands are your most important tool and their proper use should be cultivated. Suitable contact, whether it is an initial handshake or part of the physical examination, can convey a sense of composure and confidence to the patient that will serve both of you well as the labor progresses. All of your examinations should be done gently but not tentatively. When it may be necessary to probe deeply, warn the patient ahead of time that she may feel some pressure or even pain, and assure her that it is necessary—and why it is necessary—and that it will be transient. If you have done something, advertently or not, that has caused her discomfort, apologize promptly and explain why she felt tenderness. Your hands should transmit your own calmness and poise. Always demonstrate respect for the patient's privacy, for the intimate nature of the examination, and for her dignity.

Experienced practitioners may become jaded, dispassionate, or even indifferent over time about some of the normal events of labor. It is nonetheless important for you to remember that the patient may be experiencing these things for the first time. Even women who have had several children have minimal familiarity with labor and delivery compared to your own. Furthermore, no two labors are alike in all their essential features. Therefore, your comments to your patient should express reassurance about the normality of ordinary events. This is particularly true when discussing things that in another context might be embarrassing or humiliating, such as crying out loudly or losing sphincter control with urinary or fecal incontinence.

Always be sensitive to your patient's feeling about using medications for pain. Be sure this is not seen by her or by members of the staff as a failure or weakness on her part. This is sometimes the case in women who had decided in advance that they would eschew such aids. The mistaken notion that medications are always dangerous to the fetus is prevalent and you should gently repudiate it.

When you visit the patient periodically during labor, you should always inquire about how she is feeling and about how she is coping. There is a tendency among some practitioners to enter a room and focus on the fetal monitor or the electronic record screen or the medical chart rather than to address the patient directly. This is not only uncivil and disrespectful; it deprives you of important clues to the patient's state of mind and physical well-being. Avoid it.

## General examination

Most healthy patients who arrive in labor and who received prenatal care from you do not require an exhaustively thorough general physical examination. Everyone, however, needs at least an assessment of vital signs and an examination of the heart, lungs, abdomen, and extremities. Obviously, those with a known underlying medical problem (hypertensive, cardiac, pulmonary, etc.) should have a careful evaluation of pertinent areas. Doing a good review of systems during the history-taking will help focus the subsequent physical examination. For example, recent development of dyspnea or cough in a previously asymptomatic patient should prompt a careful exploration to determine its cause. A comprehensive history and physical examination are especially important if you are meeting the patient for the first time.

## Abdominal examination

You can glean a wealth of important clinical information from a methodical examination of the parturient's abdomen. Initially, with the patient supine or in some lateral tilt, observe the contour of the abdomen. Examine for skin lesions and surgical scars. Note the degree of obesity and whether the abdomen is pendulous or has hernias. Rule out hepatomegaly or splenomegaly. Search for tenderness arising from areas not occupied by the uterus. Then, turn your attention to the pregnancy.

## Presentation and position

There is considerable confusion concerning the terms *lie, presentation, presenting part,* and *position. Fetal lie* refers to the relationship that the long axis of the fetus bears to that of the mother. There are two basic lies: longitudinal and transverse. Longitudinal lies occur in about 99% of all labors. Most often the fetal head presents itself to the pelvic inlet; infrequently (<4%), the breech does. When the head presents, it is a *cephalic presentation*; when the breech or the lower limbs present, it is a *breech presentation.* When the lie is transverse, it is a *shoulder presentation.* In an *oblique lie*—a variant of a transverse lie—the head or breech occupies an iliac fossa.

Three general divisions of presentations are recognized:

1 Cephalic presentations include vertex, sincipital, brow, and face. The vertex presentation is normal; the others are not. They result from deflexion of the head and are, therefore, collectively called *deflexion attitudes.*

2 Breech presentations include frank, complete, and incomplete. All refer to various orientations of the lower extremities (Chapter 8).

3 Shoulder presentation or transverse lie includes shoulder, arm, and any other part of the trunk.

The portion of the fetus lowermost in the birth canal during labor is the *presenting part.* It is determined by the *attitude* (degree of flexion) of the head or the exact orientation of the breech or trunk. For example, in a cephalic presentation with the fetal head well flexed, it is the vertex of the head that is the leading part. This is considered a *vertex presentation.* If the head were quite extended, with the bregma lowermost, it would be a *brow presentation.*

*Fetal position* relates to the orientation of an arbitrary reference point on the presenting part to the four quadrants of the maternal pelvis. In most cephalic presentations, the occiput is the reference point; in breech presentations, the sacrum; in shoulder presentations, the scapula or acromial process; in face presentations, the chin (mentum); and in brow presentations, the bregma.

All terms concerned with direction (that is, position) of the fetus refer to the mother: anterior, the direction to the front of the mother; right, the right side of the mother, and so on. These terms have no relation to the examiner and they are not changed by any position the mother may assume. Keep this rule in mind to avoid confusion.

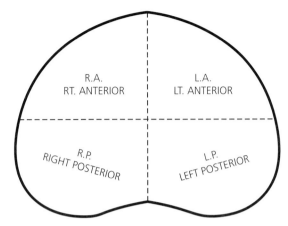

**Figure 2.1** The four quadrants of the pelvis used to describe fetal position, viewed as encountered during a vaginal examination with the patient in lithotomy position.

For easy description, the pelvis is divided into four quadrants; a left and a right anterior and a left and a right posterior. The position of the presenting part is defined according to that quadrant in which its reference point lies (Fig. 2.1). For example, if the occiput in a vertex presentation is in the left anterior quadrant of the pelvis, the position is left occiput anterior (LOA). If the occiput is in the axis dividing the right anterior from the right posterior quadrant, the position is right occiput transverse (ROT); if the occiput is found in the midline of the posterior portion of the pelvis, it is said to be in a direct occiput posterior position (OP).

## Approach to the examination

You should cultivate a uniform approach to the abdominal examination and follow it in each case. That is the best way to obtain accurate results and prevent omissions (Fig. 2.2).

First determine the fundal height by placing the hypothenar eminence of the upper hand (left hand if you are at the patient's right side) against the mother's abdomen. With gentle pressure, you will be able to perceive where the upper margin of the fundus is located. Uterine height can be quantitated by means of a centimeter tape measure. Lay the tape along the abdominal contour from the upper border of the symphysis pubis to the top of the fundus. In the course of a normal pregnancy with a fetus in longitudinal lie, among women who are not markedly obese, you can expect the fundal height, in centimeters, to be equivalent to the number of weeks from the beginning of the last menstrual period from about 20 to 36 weeks. Examine the surface of the uterus for tenderness or abnormal masses, and note if there is uterine enlargement suggesting polyhydramnios or multiple gestation.

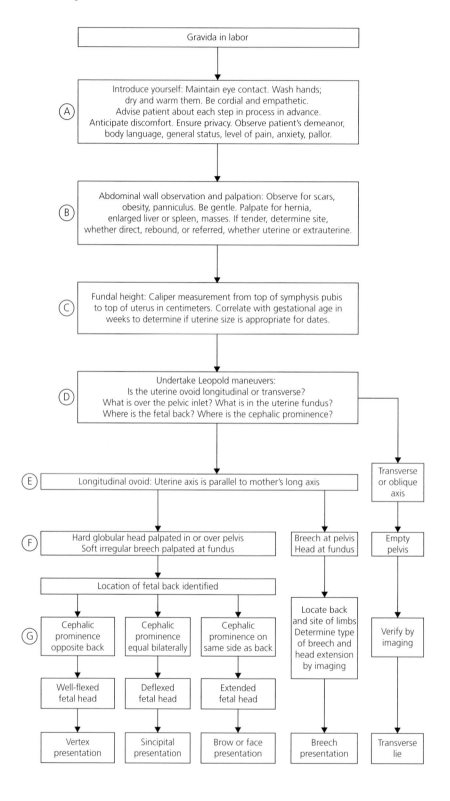

## Leopold maneuvers

After the size and the shape of the uterus have been determined, the following five questions should be answered. The series of evaluations you undertake to seek answers to these queries constitute the Leopold maneuvers.

1 Is the uterine ovoid longitudinal or transverse?
2 What is over the inlet?
3 What is in the fundus?
4 Where is the fetal back?
5 Where is the cephalic prominence?

**1.** To determine the orientation of the ovoid, face the patient's head while standing alongside her bed. Place your hands on either side of her abdomen, and palpate the uterine mass between them. In this way you can easily determine whether the fetal ovoid lies parallel with the long axis of the mother (i.e., the fetus is in a longitudinal lie) (Fig. 2.3). If the fetal ovoid is not parallel, the fetus is in an oblique or transverse lie.

**2.** To establish what is over the inlet, stand facing the patient's feet and place your palms down laterally over the lowermost aspect of the uterus. Gently press both hands into the inlet of the pelvis from the iliac fossas

**Figure 2.2** Algorithm for abdominal examination in labor.
**A**. Basic principles applicable to physical examination include activities aimed at putting the patient at ease, ensuring her privacy, and maintaining her dignity. Your attention to being cordial, civil, and empathetic is fundamental.
**B**. Observe for evidence of medical, surgical, or obstetric conditions on or in the abdomen that may be relevant to your patient's care.
**C**. Assess uterine size by measuring the fundal height, using a tape measure, from the top of the symphy is pubis to the top of the uterus. The number of cm of fundal height should correlate closely with the weeks of gestational age from about weeks 20 to 36. Consider reduced fetal growth or dating error if the uterus is too small; consider macrosomia, multiple pregnancy, hydramnios or dating error if the uterus is too large.
**D**. Carry out Leopold maneuvers to identify the fetal presentation, position, engagement, and flexion.
**E**. If the long axis of the fetus is parallel with that of the mother, the presentation is either cephalic or breech. If the fetal axis is perpendicular or oblique to the mother's long axis, you are dealing with a transverse or oblique lie, respectively.
**F**. Palpation of the fetal breech in the uterine fundus and head over the pelvic inlet tells you the presentation is cephalic. If the head is in the fundus and the breech over the inlet, it is a breech presentation. An empty pelvis confirms a transverse lie.
**G**. The relation of the cephalic prominence, palpated suprapubically, to the fetal back is important for determining head flexion or extension. Most often, the cephalic prominence is found on the side opposite the back, a sign that the head is well flexed in the common vertex presentation. Less often, the prominence is opposite the back, representing head extension, which is encountered if the head is in brow or face presentation. If the head is only slightly deflexed, as in a sincipital presentation, the cephalic prominence will be equal on both sides.

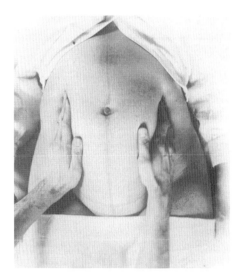

**Figure 2.3** Is the ovoid longitudinal or transverse? Facing the patient's head, apply your hands to the sides of the uterus to determine fetal lie.

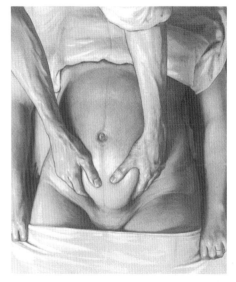

**Figure 2.4** What is over the inlet? Press deeply into the pelvis on either side of the lower abdomen to determine whether the hard head or relatively soft breech presents.

(Fig. 2.4). If a hard, ball-shaped mass is felt, you can reliably assume it is the fetal head. If your fingers encounter a soft irregular mass, the presenting part is likely the breech. If your hands almost meet above the inlet, it might mean that the head or breech is very high. Alternatively, there is no part over the inlet, indicating the shoulder is presenting and not engaged.

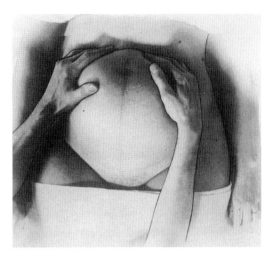

**Figure 2.5** What is in the fundus? Palpate the fundus to reveal the presence of the head or breech.

**3.** To reveal what occupies the upper region of the uterus, face the patient's head again and place both hands on the uterine fundus (Fig. 2.5). Attempt to grasp the object in the fundus between your hands, determining its hardness and shape. With experience you will be able to differentiate between the hard, round head and the softer, irregular breech. Remember, however, that the sacral side of the breech can feel quite as hard as the skull. To help you differentiate between breech and head, move the part laterally. When you move the fetal head, you will feel it move independently of the body, whereas moving the breech will bring the fetal body along with it.

**4.** To locate the fetal back, place your hands on the abdomen as for the first maneuver and press first one hand and then the other medially toward the umbilicus. You will appreciate the back as being smoother and offering more resistance. Moreover, the examining hand cannot be pressed in as much on the side occupied by the fetal back as on the opposite side with the fetal limbs. Unless the patient is quite obese, you ought to be able to palpate the small extremities on the ventral side of the fetus through the abdominal wall and the uterus. This side feels more irregular and more indentable than that encasing the fetal back. To complement these observations, try placing both of your hands on one side of the abdomen and palpating toward the midline. Comparing the resistance, regularity, and convexity of the underlying fetus will help you to identify the fetal back.

**5.** Having thus mapped out the general orientation of the fetus, you can next determine its position and attitude by abdominal examination. Study the head first. Facing the patient's feet once again, press both hands

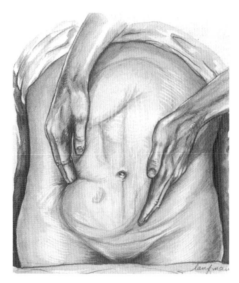

**Figure 2.6** Where is the cephalic prominence? Pass both hands along the lower abdomen, advancing your fingers suprapubically into the pelvis. The fetal forehead impedes one hand and the other descends until the occiput is reached. The forehead (shown here on the mother's right side) is the greater cephalic prominence in a well-flexed vertex presentation. In face and brow presentations, by contrast, the occiput is the greater cephalic prominence because the head is deflexed. In sincipital presentation, both are equally palpable.

downward suprapubically toward the true inlet. From the abdominal perspective, the occiput of a normally flexed head lies deeper (that is, more caudad) in the pelvis than the forehead. The occiput is flatter than the forehead, nearer the midline, and more difficult to outline. The forehead is reached sooner by the suprapubic hand, is farther from the midline, and easier to outline (Fig. 2.6). Distinguishing these two points will clarify the position of the head for you. In flexion, the forehead forms the cephalic prominence. You will reach the forehead first when your two parallel hands are thrust simultaneously into the inlet from above. You will be able to recognize that it is the forehead because you will find it on the side opposite the fetal back, which you found in the prior step. When the head is deflexed, the occiput is more prominent. In partial deflexion (so-called military attitude or sincipital presentation), the two portions of the head stand out equally and are reached simultaneously by your examining fingers insinuated suprapubically. Another method, which uses a single-handed grasp to palpate the head, is illustrated in Fig. 2.7.

You can ascertain the position of the fetal head by palpating the relation of the occiput and the forehead to the inlet. If you feel the forehead to the posterior right side, and when you attempt to reach the occiput your hand sinks deeply behind the left pubic ramus, the position is LOA.

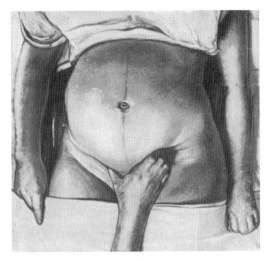

**Figure 2.7** Palpating the fetal head. Grasp the head with one hand. In ROP positions (shown here), the thumb sinks deep to the occiput, whereas the fingers strike the forehead over the left pubic ramus. Sometimes the chin can be distinctly felt.

If you palpate the forehead or chin over the left pubic ramus and the occiput is deep on the right side, the position is ROP.

A further method of determining position is facilitated by locating the shoulder. Pass one of your hands upward on the abdomen from the rounded head until you reach the soft prominence of the shoulder. If the shoulder is to the right of the midline when the back is on the left side, the position is LOA. If the shoulder is to the left of the midline, the position is LOP. A midline shoulder indicates a LOT position. Passing your hand upward from the shoulder, you will encounter a triangular space bordered by the side of the fetal trunk medially (the fetal flank), the thigh above, and the arm below (Fig. 2.8).

Another helpful technique can be used to help identify fetal position from the orientation of the back. First, identify which side the fetal back occupies, as above. Then form the hand into a C-shape. Place your thumb into the mother's umbilicus and your fingers over the lateral aspect of the uterus in which the back lies. Press down and note where your hand encounters the fetal back maximally. You will usually be able to recognize the lateral aspect of the back by this means. This can give you useful clues to determine fetal position. If you feel the lateral aspect of the back in the mother's ventral midline, the position is OT. If the back is anteriorly oblique, the fetus is likely LOA or ROA; if obliquely posterior, the position is ROP or LOP. If the lateral aspect of the back is in the maternal midline, the fetal position is OT; if the midline of the fetal back is in the mother's ventral midline, the fetal position is OA; and if the back is not palpable, the fetus is OP.

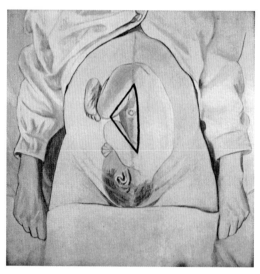

**Figure 2.8** The fetal triangle. Place the palm and fingers of one hand against the broad base of the triangle to feel the side of the fetus. Slide the hand toward the ventral aspect of the fetus and push upward to feel the thigh and downward to encounter the arm.

The breech and trunk closely follow the movements of the head. This means that, if you can outline the position of the breech well, you can readily deduce the position of the head. For example, if the breech is in the position it would occupy in LOP, the head can be expected to lie in this position. Just as the maternal pelvis is divisible into four quadrants, so is the fundus. If you find the breech in the left anterior quadrant, the position of the head is probably LOA; if the breech is in the right posterior quadrant, the position is likely to be LOP. The position of the back will offer similar information with regard to the position of the head.

The fetal weight should now be estimated. This is a difficult skill to learn. It is acquired through frequent practice and systematic comparison of actual birth weights with physical findings. It is most useful at the extremes of birth weight, i.e., you should be able to recognize when a fetus is unusually small or large by assessing its weight by abdominal palpation.

### Determining engagement

It is also important to determine the fetal station or degree of engagement. This important observation must be done frequently in every labor to evaluate the progress of fetal descent. First, place your two hands on the fetal head as done when determining what is over the inlet. Try to move the head from side to side. If it is movable, it is not engaged. Second, determine how much of the head can be felt above the inlet

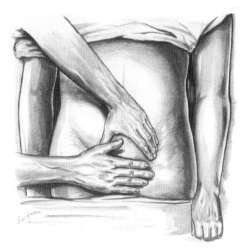

**Figure 2.9** Crichton maneuver. Use both hands to determine how much of the fetal head remains above the upper plane of the symphysis pubis. This will prove especially useful to you for distinguishing true descent from molding, especially when repeated serially in late labor.

using the pubis as a landmark (Fig. 2.9). This is the Crichton maneuver. When used serially in late labor, you will find this maneuver to be very helpful in distinguishing molding (when the palpable part of the fetal head remains above the inlet) from true descent (when the base of the skull that is palpated suprapubically progressively diminishes). If the forehead is palpable but not the occiput, even on deep pressure, and the head is fixed in the inlet, the head is engaged. You will acquire other information in this regard on the pelvic examination (see below).

## The pelvic examination

To obtain an accurate assessment of trends in cervical dilatation and fetal descent, and for determining fetopelvic relationships, you need to carry out periodic pelvic examinations during labor. You will get the best possible information and maximize your patient's comfort if you carry out each examination with gentleness and care. The frequency with which you examine your laboring patient will depend on the progress of labor and the presence of any complications. In general, unnecessary examinations should be avoided because of the risk of promoting ascending infection in the uterus, but a sufficient number will be necessary to monitor progress accurately and to recognize aberrant labor promptly. During the active phase of labor an examination should be done at least every 2 hours. The second stage requires more frequent evaluations, generally every 30 minutes.

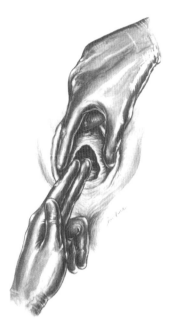

**Figure 2.10** Separate the labia so your fingers do not touch the surrounding vulvar or perianal structures. This minimizes bacterial contamination during a vaginal examination.

Maintenance of the patient's modesty and privacy is often quite a challenge during labor. Further, you should bear in mind that each pelvic examination has the potential to be uncomfortable and intrusive, particularly if not performed optimally. For you to obtain the most useful information, be sure to have the patient as relaxed and cooperative as possible. To this end, you should reassure her from the outset that you will treat her with appropriate thoughtfulness and respect.

Generally, the examination can be done with the patient supine in the labor bed and her thighs flexed somewhat. A "frog leg" position is comfortable for many people, with the knees flexed and abducted and the plantar surfaces of the feet meeting in the midline. Alternatively, the knees can be flexed and the feet separated with as much space as possible between them as they rest on the surface of the bed.

Sterile gloves should be used, and adequate lubricant. Some advocate pouring antiseptic solution (such as povidone iodine or chlorhexidine) over the vulva or gloves before the examination. The benefits of such practices are uncertain.

If you are right handed, position yourself at the patient's right side. Gently separate the labia using the thumb and the index finger of your left hand. Then slowly insert the index and middle fingers of the right hand into the vagina (Fig. 2.10), pressing them deeply and without undue pressure into the vaginal canal. Release the fingers of your left hand from the labia and allow them to close around your internal fingers. Take special care to avoid contact with the perianal area, which is heavily contaminated with bacteria.

Six items of information should be determined—and documented in the patient's record—during every vaginal examination performed during labor: (1) condition of the cervix, specifically its dilatation, effacement, consistency, and position; (2) status of the membranes; (3) fetal presentation and position; (4) station of the presenting part; (5) spatial relationship between fetal presenting part and maternal pelvis; (6) presence of any abnormalities.

## Condition of the cervix

Advance your fingers to the cervix. Note its consistency, length, position in relation to the pelvic axis, and degree of dilatation of the external os. As the cervix ripens prior to or in early labor, its consistency changes from firm to quite soft. This palpable change can take place over a period of weeks, but sometimes occurs in hours. It reflects the breakdown of collagen and changes in the connective tissue matrix of the cervix. Generally, the cervix will not dilate appreciably until the cervix has softened. Prior to labor, and in early labor, you will often find that the cervix is palpable quite posteriorly in the pelvis. It may be difficult to reach with your examining fingers. As labor evolves, you will feel the cervix rotating anteriorly until it is in the midcoronal (axial) plane of the pelvis. This anterior movement is generally completed before the active phase of dilatation begins.

The cervical os is measured in centimeters of dilatation, with a maximum of about 10 cm representing complete dilatation. In fact, the cervix will not dilate more widely than the presenting part passing through it. Therefore, complete dilatation will vary considerably according to the size of the fetal head.

Cervical effacement is often estimated as a percentage according to what one estimates the uneffaced cervix to have been (e.g., 70% effaced), even though this is seldom actually known. Alternatively, you can report the actual length of the cervix (e.g., 1.5 cm). You will find the latter to be a more objective measure—and therefore, we think, preferable—for following progressive cervical effacement as labor advances.

## Membrane status

If the membranes are felt a short distance below the head during a uterine contraction, this will confirm that they are unruptured. An experienced examiner can distinguish the smooth chorion from a rough, hairy fetal scalp. The discharge of amniotic fluid, vernix caseosa, or flakes of meconium will obviously confirm the diagnosis of ruptured membranes. If you suspect membrane rupture from the patient's description but you see no leaking amniotic fluid, you may find it helpful to determine whether the fluid found in the posterior fornix or the endocervix is alkaline. A form of pH paper (usually containing nitrazine as an indicator) is effective for this purpose. A neutral or alkaline pH with blue discoloration of the nitrazine paper indicates that the membranes have probably ruptured. False-positive readings can occur when there is an unusual amount of bloody show or the vaginal secretions are contaminated with alkaline urine or semen. Checking the sample for a microscopic ferning pattern on an air-dried slide can provide further information. Amniotic fluid will produce a typical arborizing pattern; cervical or vaginal fluid derived from other sources will not. Because ferning has greater sensitivity than pH as an indicator of membrane rupture, it can therefore be preferentially relied upon when the test results are disparate.

## Presentation and position

It is usually impossible to outline the sutures and fontanels through the lower uterine segment or cervix. Some degree of cervical dilatation is, therefore, necessary to allow you to determine fetal position vaginally. You should identify fetal position, among other pertinent observations, each time you examine your patient during labor. Intact membranes will not generally hinder your ability to palpate the sutures and fontanels. If the presenting part is the fetal head, feel for the fontanels and identify them and their orientation in the pelvis. In this manner, you should almost always be able to determine the position of the head with ease. In doubtful cases, especially when a caput succedaneum interferes with clear recognition of the landmarks, you may find it useful to search for an ear. This requires complete cervical dilatation. The position of the ear will disclose the position of the head, the tragus indicating the direction of the face.

## Fetal station

By a combination of external and pelvic examinations, you can accurately determine the degree of engagement or station of the head. The head is *floating* when it is freely movable above the inlet. It is *dipping* when it has entered the inlet but is still somewhat mobile. The head is *engaged* when its greatest presenting horizontal plane has passed the pelvic inlet. In vertex presentation, the widest part of the fetal head is the biparietal plane.

Engagement is usually assumed clinically when, on vaginal examination, you feel the lowest part of the skull has reached or passed the interspinous plane (i.e., the referent plane or station 0). This is a useful generalization, but applies only to anterior positions with well-flexed unmolded heads in normal size fetuses. The leading edge of the molded skull in a large fetus in an extended occiput posterior position may even

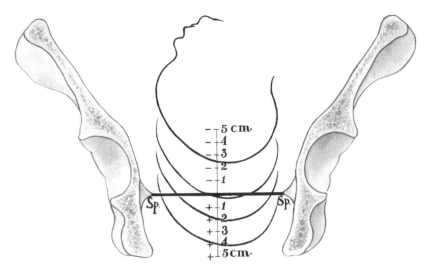

**Figure 2.11** Fetal stations, coronal view. Representation of the station, or degree of descent, of the fetal head. The location of the leading edge of the presenting part (here the vertex of the head) is designated by centimeters (stations) above or below the interspinous plane.

reach the pelvic floor without engagement having occurred, i.e., without the biparietal plane having yet reached the plane of the pelvic inlet.

An engaged fetal head is said to occupy the midpelvis when the biparietal plane has entered the inlet and the lowest part of the cranium lies below the plane of the ischial spines (usually no more than station +2), but the biparietal plane is still above the ischial spines. After the two parietal bossas have passed the ischial spines, the head is at the pelvic outlet when its lowermost part comes well down onto the perineum, lying in the distended vagina.

To express the station of the head exactly, imagine a coronal reference plane (designated station 0) passing through the ischial spines. By first touching the top of the fetal head and then passing the fingers to the ischial spines, you can easily determine the relation of one to the other. Parallel planes at 1 cm intervals above and below the reference plane are numbered, as shown in Figs 2.11 and 2.12. The centimeters above the ischial spine plane are designated as negative stations and those below as positive stations. If the lowest part of the head has reached the spines (i.e., just engaged for a flexed vertex presentation) the head is at station 0. If it is at station −2, its forward leading edge has descended to a plane just 2 cm above the spines. At station +2, the leading edge of the head lies 2 cm below the interspinous plane.

We cannot overemphasize the importance of accurately and repeatedly defining the station of the head in the birth canal during the course

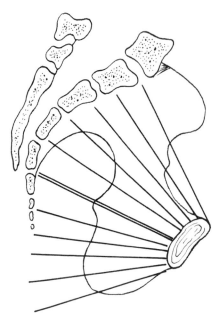

**Figure 2.12** Fetal stations, lateral sagittal view. Station lines are spaced 1 cm apart at their midpoints. The double line designates the interspinous plane (station 0).

of labor. Following the descent pattern can be most useful in uncovering serious labor disorders. In addition, before you even consider whether to perform a forceps or vacuum extractor operation to effect delivery, this information is absolutely essential.

### Spatial relations

Use your fingers to determine the size of the pelvic cavity, its capacity to accommodate the fetus, and its architecture. The relations of the fetal head to the maternal pelvis, as detailed in Chapter 4, have to be elicited as well. The aggregate of this information, used in conjunction with the labor progression curves, is necessary to guide you in your decision making about optimal labor care and intervention.

### Abnormalities

Determine the presence of the umbilical cord or fetal parts in the vagina, vulvar or vaginal neoplasms, excessive rigidity of the perineum, and other conditions that might affect delivery.

## Documentation

If you have done a thorough initial examination, you may have detected conditions that could adversely affect the course of labor or alter your management. In addition, you have made many important observations that can serve as baseline data against which to judge changes that occur during the labor. It is important for you to enter information in the patient's hospital record at each encounter with her, entering all relevant features of your examination. After all the information has been obtained and recorded, you are then in a position to weigh and consider all aspects of the various pieces of information you have gathered. The notes you write in the record should indicate not only what your observations were about cervical dilatation, fetal station, etc., but how these fragmentary bits of information were synthesized to make it possible for you to arrive at a substantive assessment and, flowing from that assessment, a logical plan for further evaluation and management.

## Key points

- Hands should always be freshly washed, warm, and dry.
- Greet your patient warmly. If you have not met her previously, introduce yourself and indicate what your role will be in her care.
- Address the patient by her last name, unless she gives you permission to do otherwise.
- Maintain eye contact whenever possible. Never discuss anything when standing behind the patient, and avoid standing over her bedside. Sitting is better, but avoid sitting on her bed.
- Listen carefully and also observe her body language. The latter can sometimes reveal more important clues to her feelings than what she says.
- Be truthful about what is happening, but always supportive and reassuring regardless of the situation.
- Seek referral for advice or formal consultation before making a decision or formulating a plan of action if you feel it is needed. The patient will appreciate this and thank you for it.
- A uniform approach to physical examination should be cultivated by every practitioner and followed in each case.
- Six points should be determined during vaginal examinations: (1) condition of the cervix; (2) status of the membranes; (3) presentation and position; (4) station of the presenting part; (5) evaluation of spatial relations; (6) presence of any abnormalities.

## Further Reading

### Books and reviews
Cole SA. *The Medical Interview*, 2nd edition. Mosby, St Louis, MO, 2000.
Elkayam U, Gleicher N. Cardiac evaluation during pregnancy. In: Elkayam U, Gleicher N (eds) *Cardiac Problems in Pregnancy*, 3rd edition. Wiley-Liss, New York, 1998: 23–32.
Swartz MH. *Textbook of Physical Diagnosis*, 5th edition. Saunders Elsevier, Philadelphia, 2008.

# CHAPTER 3

# Normal Labor and Delivery

Normal labor is the physiologic process by which the gravid uterus evacuates its contents at or near term. It requires a coordinated sequence of periodic myometrial contractions, which cause progressive cervical dilatation and fetal descent through the birth canal. This simple descriptive definition is accurate, but belies the complexity of the labor process, which is a biochemical, physiologic, and mechanical masterwork that, despite centuries of investigation, we understand incompletely. In this chapter you will first learn what clinical events occur during the course of labor and delivery. Then we will introduce the concept of graphic evaluation of labor, and explain how it should be integrated with other means of assessment.

Your clinical appraisal of labor should be assembled from observations that are readily made at the bedside and are quantifiable. These include intensity, duration, and frequency of contractions; dilatation and effacement of the cervix; and descent of the fetus. You can assess each of these variables, which serve as the primary database for evaluating labors in progress, accurately and reproducibly during labor by periodic abdominal and vaginal examinations. They provide you with the most useful and reliable means for determining whether or not your patient's labor is normal.

## Terminology

A review of basic definitions is in order, because these terms are often misused, leading to confusion that can affect decision making. *Gravidity* refers to a pregnancy regardless of its duration. A *gravida* is a pregnant woman. She is *gravid*, i.e., pregnant. A *primigravida* is pregnant for the first time; a *nulligravida* has never been pregnant. A *multigravida* has been pregnant more than once.

*Labor and Delivery Care: A Practical Guide*, First Edition. Wayne R. Cohen and Emanuel A. Friedman. © 2011 John Wiley & Sons, Ltd. Published 2011 by John Wiley & Sons, Ltd.

*Parity* refers to the completion of viable pregnancy. *Viability* is defined for obstetric purposes as one of sufficient duration to deliver a fetus weighing at least 500 g or one of gestational age of 20 weeks or more. A *primipara* is a woman who has had one pregnancy that resulted in a viable child. Although the terms *primigravida* and *primipara* are not synonymous, they are often erroneously used as if they were interchangeable. A *nullipara* is a primigravida or multigravida who has not yet delivered a viable infant. A *multipara* is a woman who has had two or more viable deliveries.

Parity involves delivery by any route. Thus, a woman who has had three term cesarean deliveries is a multipara. Nevertheless, the labors of parous women who have never had a vaginal delivery tend to conform to criteria established for nulliparas. That is to say, they behave functionally in terms of the course of labor as if they were nulliparas. Moreover, the number of infants carried during any given pregnancy is not a relevant factor in determining parity (or gravidity). A woman who delivers twins or triplets in her first pregnancy, for example, is still considered a primipara.

## Uterine contractility

Uterine contractions are obviously necessary for normal labor. However, despite extensive knowledge about the biochemistry and physiology of uterine smooth muscle contraction, we are as yet unable to use that information clinically to distinguish when labor has begun or to determine whether it is normal.

Similarly, although we often use electronic devices to register the contractility pattern of the uterus during labor, interpretation of that information cannot be used to establish reliably whether the labor is normal, or even whether it is true or false labor. Even when objective pressure measurement techniques are used and quantified to yield uterine work units (e.g., Montevideo units), their applicability to identifying dysfunctional labor is quite limited. Bedside recordings obtained from women in false labor have shown essentially the same wide range of uterine contractility patterns as those in normal labor. Further, there is enormous variation in such patterns in normal labor.

Thus, while various electronic approaches to monitoring uterine activity can be helpful to you in guiding the administration of oxytocin, they fall short in determining dependably whether labor is progressing normally. This is so, at least in part, because clinically measured contractile intensity is not always directly related to the effect it is expected to achieve, namely, timely cervical dilatation and fetal descent.

## Clinical course of labor

### Prodrome and labor stages

In most nulliparas and many multiparas there is a *prodromal stage* preceding labor, but its manifestations may be so slight that neither you nor the patient will notice them. When they are not recognized, labor seems to begin abruptly. The prodromal signs and symptoms may include *lightening* of the fetal presenting part into the true pelvis, with relief of pressure in the upper part of the abdomen and an increase in pressure in the pelvis and bladder; increasing recognition of Braxton-Hicks contractions; a discharge of mucus mixed with blood appearing from the vagina; and softening of the cervix.

The transition into labor is usually gradual, but for clinical purposes you should consider that labor has begun when the uterine contractions are perceived, usually painfully, and are recurring at regular intervals. Labor is not assumed merely because there is a bloody show or the membranes have ruptured. Remember that the diagnosis of labor made prospectively on the basis of regular contractions can be wrong. The diagnosis of false labor is made when these contractions abate without leading to progress in cervical dilatation.

We divide the process of parturition classically into three stages. The *first stage* extends from the beginning of regular uterine contractions until the external os is completely dilated and flush with the vagina, thus completing the continuous channel of the parturient canal. Fetal descent through the birth canal generally begins near the end of the first stage. The *second stage* extends from the end of the first stage until the expulsion of the baby is completed, and encompasses most of fetal descent. The *third stage* is the interval from delivery of the child until the placenta and membranes are expelled. Some recognize a *fourth stage* of labor, which includes the first hour or two after placental delivery. During this time, recovery of uterine tone occurs so that serious bleeding is averted, and maternal–neonatal bonding begins.

At the onset of labor in nulliparas, you will commonly find the external os dilated about 1–1.5 cm. In multiparas, prelabor dilatation of as much as 3 cm is common. Occasionally, the cervix is dilated to a greater degree, perhaps as much as 4 or 5 cm, even in nulliparas. The presence of some dilatation and effacement at the beginning of labor in many women is the consequence of prelabor *cervical ripening* or *maturation*. These changes often occur gradually during the last two or three weeks of pregnancy. They are the consequence of collagen and ground substance degradation in the cervix. Exceptionally, the external and internal os remain tightly closed until labor begins. In such cases, the entire process of cervical ripening occurs during the early portion of the first stage of labor.

Effacement is often complete or nearly so in nulliparas well before labor begins, sometimes days or weeks earlier. In multiparas, by contrast, most effacement takes place in the last portion of the first stage. Sometimes, complete effacement in nulliparas is reached only after considerable time in the latent phase of labor, signifying that the active phase will soon begin (see below).

## Cervical dilatation

The essential components of labor that you will measure to determine its normality are cervical dilatation and fetal descent. Assessing cervical effacement to determine labor progress is of little clinical value.

We measure dilatation clinically as if it were occurring parallel to the transverse plane of the mother, but the cervical rim is actually travelling in a curvilinear fashion along the surface of the fetal presenting part. Nevertheless, the clinical appraisal of dilatation is an effective and time-tested tool for the assessment of the first stage. With practice, your measurements of cervical dilatation will be made quite accurately and reproducibly.

While the time required for cervical dilatation varies considerably among individuals, the cervix dilates in a predictable and quantifiable pattern in all normal labors. It initially opens tentatively and gradually (the *latent phase*), and then much more rapidly as the *active phase* of the first stage evolves. At complete dilatation, the cervix has been retracted to the widest plane of the presenting part. Then as the cervix is taken up— i.e., retracted upward—and incorporated into the lower uterine segment, it can no longer be palpated as a discrete structure.

## Fetal descent

Cervical dilatation removes the barrier that acted so effectively to prevent spontaneous uterine evacuation prematurely. Once this hurdle is breached, fetal descent can follow in an unimpeded manner and lead to birth of the baby. The mechanical forces producing dilatation are entirely uterine in origin, whereas those effecting descent are a combination of myometrial contractions and voluntary expulsive efforts by the mother using her diaphragmatic and abdominal muscles. During descent, the fetus undergoes a series of changes in position and orientation (the *cardinal movements*), the characteristics of which (the *mechanism of labor*) are guided primarily by the bony and soft tissue architecture of the birth canal. Like cervical dilatation, fetal descent follows a predictable pattern during normal labors.

## The first stage

When labor begins, uterine contractions are usually 5–15 minutes apart. As labor progresses, they generally become stronger and more frequent,

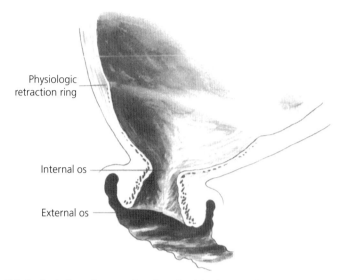

Physiologic
retraction ring

Internal os

External os

**Figure 3.1** Sagittal view of uterus showing physiologic retraction ring.

often occurring at intervals of 2–3 minutes by the late first stage. Each contraction begins before the patient perceives pain. During a contraction, the uterus rises forward in the abdomen, pushing against the anterior abdominal wall. (As a consequence, in a very thin patient you may sometimes see the round ligaments stand out sharply.) The movement of the uterine wall—and overlying abdominal wall—allows assessment of contractions using an external tocodynamometer, an electromechanical device that detects changes in the abdominal contour.

You should learn to palpate contractions and to judge their intensity by the hardness of the fully contracted uterine wall. During contractions, the uterus becomes rigid. On vaginal examination, you can often feel the cervix tensing, in response to the force imposed upon it by the fetal head countering the tension applied to the passive fibrous connective tissue of the lower uterine segment and cervix by the powerful contractions of the upper uterus. If the membranes are still intact, you may feel them bulging tensely toward, or even beyond, the external os.

The uterus may be considered to have two functionally distinct parts, an upper or contracting portion and a lower or dilating portion. The anatomic delineation of these parts is the physiologic retraction ring (Fig. 3.1). When a contraction occurs, the amniotic fluid and the fetal head are pressed down toward the cervix. At the same time the membranes (if intact) are impelled pouch-like into the cervical canal, pushing out the plug of mucus that had occupied it during the pregnancy. Once the cervix is completely effaced only the external os remains. Dilatation continues (Fig. 3.2) until

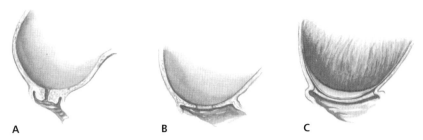

A                              B                              C

**Figure 3.2 A**. Cervix near end of pregnancy showing little effacement or dilatation.
**B**. Cervix during first stage of labor with complete effacement, but only partial
dilatation. **C**. Cervix at end of first stage illustrating complete effacement and
dilatation, and intact membranes.

the external os is opened so wide that it is flush, or nearly so, with the
vagina. Dilatation is now complete, the cervix having retracted around to
the widest diameter of the presenting part. From this point on, descent
is unimpeded and the fetus is able to pass into the vagina and ultimately
deliver.

Once the cervix is completely dilated, it is pulled up or retracted in
response to the force exerted by the active upper segment until it is often
out of reach of your examining fingers. Effacement of the cervix and dilatation occasionally occur simultaneously, especially in multiparas. After
the cervix is fully opened, the first stage of labor has ended and the second
stage begins. Coincident with these changes toward the end of the first
stage, you will observe the fetal head begin its descent through the pelvis.

## The second stage

After full cervical dilatation has been reached, descent begins in earnest
(if it has not already begun late in the first stage). Contractions tend to
grow stronger and become quite frequent, usually recurring every 2–3
minutes, occasionally more frequently. Because the cervical end of the
uterus is moored to the pelvis by the cardinal (Mackinrodt) and uterosacral ligaments, shortening of the contracting myometrium—in conjunction
with diaphragmatic and abdominal wall expulsive efforts and simultaneous thinning of the lower uterine segment—pushes the fetus downward
into the pelvis until it is born. Contractions of the round ligaments, which
occur synchronously with those of the upper uterine segment, may contribute to fetal descent.

As the vagina is distended by the descending presenting part, your
patient will have the sensation that there is something in the pelvis she
must expel. While this urge to bear down usually heralds the onset of the
second stage, it may be delayed for some time, particularly if the head
remains relatively high in the pelvis. Conversely, it may occur prior to

full dilatation if the head is deep in the pelvis toward the end of the first stage. The urge to bear down should be actively discouraged until the cervix has dilated completely, to avoid the risk of a cervical laceration. Not only does bearing down before full cervical dilatation offer no benefit in advancing labor, it will only serve to exhaust the gravida in the process. Remember, with epidural anesthesia women may not experience the urge to push out the fetus.

In most circumstances, to bear down, the parturient fixes her chest in inspiration, closes the glottis, braces her feet, and by powerful action of the abdominal and diaphragmatic muscles drives the fetal head toward the perineum. During the contraction the uterine wall is felt to be board-like, and may be tender. The maternal pulse becomes rapid, not infrequently in the 120–140 bpm (beats per minute) range, and sometimes higher.

The descending fetal head sometimes presses on the sacral and obturator nerves, explaining the pains radiating into the legs and back that your patient may experience. These are more likely to occur when the head is descending in an occiput posterior position.

As descent progresses (Figs 3.3 to 3.6), generally pressure is felt on the rectum. Feces in the lower bowel are forced down by the advancing head and may be evacuated. As the head reaches the pelvic floor, you will observe the perineum distend with each contraction as the fetal head is forced against it. Eventually, the anus begins to open and hemorrhoids, if present, swell. The perineum lengthens and thins out. Soon the labia are seen to part during the height of a contraction, exposing the wrinkled scalp of the fetus. As the contraction subsides, the elastic pelvic floor forces the head back.

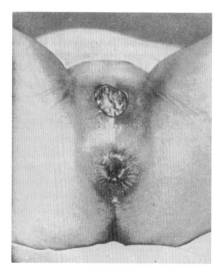

**Figure 3.3** Head beginning to distend the perineum, a process called *crowning*.

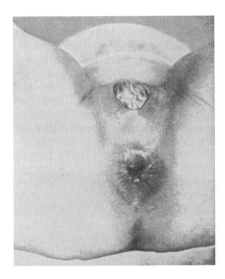

**Figure 3.4** Perineum much distended and thinned. The anterior wall of the rectum is visible through the dilated anus.

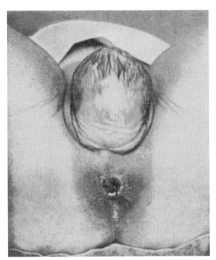

**Figure 3.5** Fetal head delivering by extension as the perineum slips back over the face of the fetus.

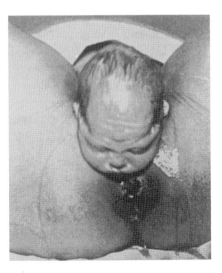

**Figure 3.6** Fetal head is delivered and the perineum is retracted under the chin.

With each succeeding contraction you will observe the perineum bulge more expansively. The anus opens wider, the labia separate further, and a larger segment of the scalp becomes visible. The introitus becomes a tense ring around the presenting part as it further distends the perineum, a situation called *crowning* (Fig. 3.3). As the contraction disappears, the head will recede somewhat. In the intervals between contractions, the woman lies back exhausted, resting.

Once the pelvic floor has relaxed sufficiently, the head rests persistently on the vulva. The patient often feels a burning or tearing sensation (even if there is no visible tissue damage) and feels an overwhelming urge to expel the fetus. Now, by supreme exertion, coupled with great emotional effort and powerful muscular contractions, the head is forced out, the occiput emerging from behind the pubis, followed in succession by the forehead, face, and chin rolling over the perineum. The nape of the fetal neck stems beneath the symphysis pubis. After this, there may be a pause for a few seconds or even minutes. Then the contractions are renewed. The shoulders are delivered, generally the anterior shoulder emerging first under the symphysis pubis if the mother is sitting or lying with her abdomen uppermost. If she is in the lateral position, the posterior fetal shoulder usually delivers first. After the shoulders, the trunk and lower extremities emerge in one long hard expulsive effort. A little blood and the rest of the amniotic fluid are discharged. Abdominally, the uterus rapidly contracts so that you can palpate its fundus at the level of the umbilicus. The second stage has ended. The uterus must still expel the placenta and the membranes.

## The third stage

The contractions of the third stage of labor help separate the placenta and promote its descent (Fig. 3.7). Your patient may feel regular contractions every few minutes. Occasionally, these are perceived as quite strong. Within several minutes to a half hour you will feel the uterine corpus rise higher in the abdomen and change in shape from discoid to globular. At the same time, you will observe the cord advance a few centimeters from the introitus. Some increase in vaginal bleeding occurs at this time. These signs indicate that the placenta has become separated from the uterine wall.

After this occurs, the placenta is usually expelled spontaneously in a few minutes by the combined efforts of abdominal and uterine muscles. The placenta usually emerges like an everted umbrella and draws the membranes after it, peeling them off the uterine wall. Sometimes it slides out without doubling up, the lower portion appearing first. Some blood is discharged with the placenta. Once it delivers, you will feel the uterus contract promptly into a hard mass.

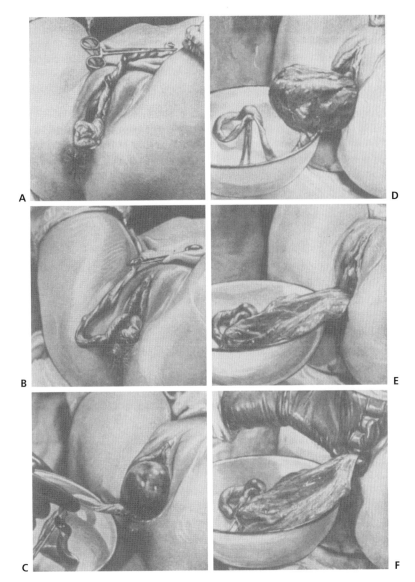

**Figure 3.7** Delivery of the placenta. **A**. The cord has been clamped and cut. A gauze sponge has been placed in the episiotomy wound. **B**. Cord advancing, showing that placenta has separated. **C**. Placenta, with blood behind it, appears. **D**. Placenta partially delivered. Little or no traction on the cord has been used. **E**. Only membranes still attached. Basin placed so weight of placenta pulls on the membranes to effect their separation. **F**. Last part of membranes can be aided with a finger or a Kelly clamp. Twisting the membranes with a clamp can encourage their final separation.

## The fourth stage

The uterus, emptied of its contents, now contracts powerfully, a mechanism that reduces postpartum blood loss. These contractions are sometimes quite painful for the first 30–60 minutes after delivery. Uterine contraction also squeezes venous blood from the uterus into the maternal circulation, where it helps compensate for the blood volume lost at delivery, which is commonly 300–500 mL. You should carefully inspect the perineum, vagina, and cervix after delivery. Repair of lacerations or episiotomy should be accomplished at this time.

Some women begin nursing their newborn right after delivery. This process releases oxytocin, which enhances uterine contractions that serve further to reduce blood loss. Nursing and handling the newborn also helps initiate the complex process of parent–infant bonding. This is an important time for you to see your patient. You will wish to ensure that the uterus is well contracted, that ongoing blood loss is appropriately small, and that she has no troublesome symptoms. It is also an opportunity to encourage and assist with attempts to nurse the baby, and a time to review the events of labor with the new mother. The latter is especially important if there have been any complications that require explanation, but even normal events and procedures deserve clarification.

## Graphic analysis of labor

Your evaluation of cervical dilatation and fetal descent can be facilitated by graphing the changes that occur against the time elapsed from the onset of labor using a simple square-ruled grid (Fig. 3.8). Thus plotted, normal cervical dilatation will always trace a sigmoid-shaped curve. Descent will describe a pattern that is nearly the mirror image of that of dilatation. To standardize nomenclature, certain terms have been applied to the several components of the pattern thus formed (Fig. 3.9).

### Curve of dilatation

The initial arm or *latent phase* of cervical dilatation extends from the inception of labor to the beginning of the *active phase*, characteristically marked by a detectable upswing in the curve. The pattern is seldom symmetrical in that the latent phase usually occupies most of the first stage, leaving a relatively minor period for the active phase. Nevertheless, most of the dilatation that will occur takes place during the active phase, which can be further divided into an initial brief *acceleration phase*, a midportion *phase of maximum slope*, and a terminal *deceleration phase*.

While most women can identify the onset of labor on the basis of their recognition of the discomfort associated with contractions that occur with

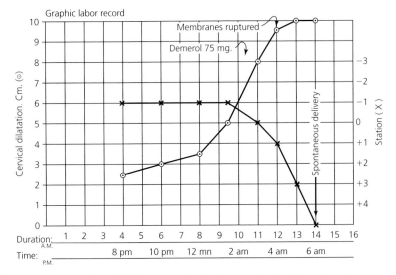

**Figure 3.8** A typical graphic labor record with elapsed time in labor along the horizontal axis and cervical dilatation (left) and station of the fetal presenting part (right) on the vertical axes. Each observation of dilatation (circle) and of station (X) is entered sequentially to trace the course of labor. Information about other events (medications, anesthesia, rupture of membranes, etc.) can also be entered on the graph to aid in assessment.

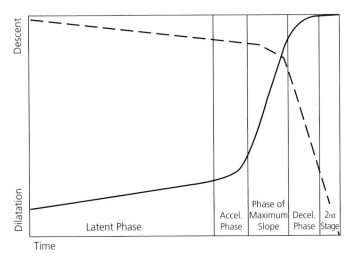

**Figure 3.9** Graphic illustration of the composite dilatation time and descent time functions in normal labor. The first stage is divisible into a latent and an active phase; the active phase is composed of the acceleration phase, the phase of maximum slope, and the deceleration phase combined. Descent begins concurrently with the onset of the phase of maximum slope of dilatation; descent reaches its maximum rate in the deceleration phase of dilatation.

predictable regularity, it is sometimes difficult to determine with precision when the labor began. This makes assessment of latent phase duration sometimes difficult. We pragmatically use the time when contractions were perceived as regular and strong to mark labor onset. This works quite well clinically.

As noted previously, a wide range of dilatation may be achieved before labor onset. Some labors begin with a closed, minimally prepared cervix and others with advanced dilatation, even in the occasional nullipara. The duration of the latent phase is inversely correlated with the degree of dilatation at the time labor begins; that is to say, the greater the dilatation at labor onset, the shorter the latent phase. In essence, one of the principal functions (speaking teleologically) of the latent phase is to accomplish the final biochemical and biophysical changes required to enhance the compliance of the cervix so it can accomplish the rapid dilatation of the ensuing active phase.

The transition from latent phase to active phase is not usually signaled by any recognizable objective change in the uterine contractility pattern or by alteration in the patient's subjective perception of her status. To identify it requires periodic assessment of cervical dilatation and graphic portrayal to show enhancement in the rate of dilatation from that of the latent phase. Dilatation during the latent phase is usually very slow or nonexistent. During the phase of maximum slope of the active phase, dilatation advances at its most rapid pace.

Do not attempt to identify the onset of the active phase on the basis of the attained degree of cervical dilatation. This is not useful, and may be misleading. While on average women enter the active phase with a cervix dilated about 4.5 cm, the actual range is considerable, and fully half of parturients may be in the active phase prior to that time. While it is logical to consider that a parturient whose cervix is 5 cm dilated is probably in the active phase, there is a high degree of error inherent in that assumption unless the active phase is confirmed as well by demonstrating the increase in the rate of dilatation expected of it.

During the phase of maximum slope, the graphic plot of dilatation against time is linear—that is, a straight line—under normal circumstances. In effect, the inclination of the line reflects the efficiency of the uterine contractions in producing dilatation. The stronger the contractile forces and the less resistive the soft tissues, the more rapid the dilatation will be.

The graphic appearance of the deceleration phase, which concludes the active phase and the first stage of labor, may seem surprising. Neither the contractile forces nor the patient's subjective reaction to them are reduced (if anything, they tend to be enhanced at this time), yet the rate of dilatation seems to be slowing. This results from the cervix being retracted in a cephalad direction (relative to the mother) around and alongside the fetal

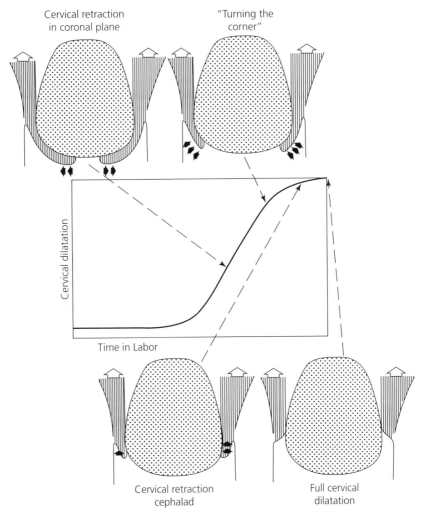

**Figure 3.10** Graphic explanation for the development of the deceleration phase. (From: Friedman EA. *Labor: Clinical Evaluation and Management,* 2nd edition. Appleton-Century-Crofts, New York, 1978: 35.)

head (Fig. 3.10). As it nears full dilatation, the cervix is no longer being dilated in a primarily transverse plane relative to the mother's pelvis. Because your examining fingers are only capable of assessing dilatation accurately in that plane, the rapid rate of dilatation you observed in the phase of maximum slope appears to decelerate, even though the cervical rim is still being retracted at about the same speed as before. The deceleration portion of the labor is often quite short in normal labors and is easily missed if examinations are not done with sufficient frequency. Despite the artifactual nature of the deceleration phase of the dilatation curve, it reflects a critically important time in labor. Deceleration generally marks the beginning of fetal descent, and its prolongation portends significant problems for the labor. Careful examinations during this portion of labor can yield important prognostic insights.

## Curve of descent

Just as the relation of cervical dilatation to time can be used to assess the course of the first stage of labor, the function of fetal descent with time serves a similar purpose, particularly in the second stage. Some descent often precedes labor. Engagement of the fetal presenting part deeply into the pelvis several weeks before term (so-called lightening) occurs in many nulliparas, but, in fact, most nulliparas begin labor with a fetal head that is not fully engaged in the pelvis. A degree of prelabor descent may also occur in some multiparas, but it is much less dramatic.

Once labor begins, little if any further descent will generally be detectable until late in the first stage. An exception is some descent that may occur in association with rupture of the membranes and loss of forewaters, permitting the presenting part to more closely adapt to the lower uterine segment and cervix. Also, when labor begins with a very unripe cervix, considerable effacement and thinning of the lower uterine segment occurs during the latent phase. These processes are often accompanied by some descent.

The static condition of the descent process will generally prevail during the entire course of the latent phase of cervical dilatation. That is to say, it is perfectly normal for fetal descent not to occur until late in the active phase. Not until dilatation accelerates well into the active phase will descent begin. It begins gradually, typically reaching its maximum slope at about the time the dilatation curve enters the deceleration phase. From this point on, descent tends to be linear as the fetal presenting part accommodates itself to the pelvic architecture (by the classical cardinal movements of flexion and internal rotation) and advances downward at a constant rate through the birth canal until the leading edge of the presenting part abuts the perineum. This straight-line descent normally progresses without interruption or deviation, beginning in the deceleration phase and continuing for most of the second stage. Descent slows a bit in the very late second stage when the head must distend the pelvic floor and finally undergo extension over the slowly stretching perineal tissues to deliver.

For consistency and uniformity in graphing the descent pattern, we recommend you use a centimeter scale to designate fetal station. Measure and record the distance of the lowermost advancing edge of the presenting part cephalad (negative values) or caudad (positive values) relative to the plane of the ischial spines (the referent plane, designated station 0) as determined by careful vaginal examination. The fetus thus traverses the normal size pelvis from about –5 station at the true inlet to +5 station at the outlet, when the perineum is bulging (Figs 2.11 and 2.12).

A potential problem with this system is that formation of the caput succedaneum or deformational molding of the head can introduce error in the determination of station. Thus, you will obtain a false impression of descent. This shortcoming can be overcome by periodically verifying that the presumed descent—based on advancing fetal station—is actually occurring; you do this by means of suprapubic palpation of the base of the fetal skull. The base of the skull is easily identified in the fourth maneuver of Leopold. When repeated serially over time (called the Crichton maneuver), it will reveal whether the skull is actually descending as the forward leading edge advances. Your external examining hands should be able to confirm that the fetal head is becoming progressively more deeply engaged as the forward leading edge advances. If not, you should strongly suspect that the lower station reflects molding rather than real descent, a sign of probable cephalopelvic disproportion.

The descent of the fetal head is not uniform, but is rather an oscillating phenomenon. The head progresses during each contraction, distending the birth canal and later the perineum. When the uterus relaxes and expulsive efforts subside, the fetal head regresses somewhat because of the elastic retraction of the vagina and perineum. Each of these progression–regression cycles leaves a positive balance so that the head remains a little lower in the pelvis and the birth canal after each uterine contraction.

The same stepwise progress occurs with cervical dilatation. Each contraction pulls the cervix open, only to have it regress between contractions. Yet, there is a positive increment in dilatation with each myometrial effort.

## Normal limits

To minimize confusion from the oscillatory nature of dilatation and descent in constructing labor graphs, always record measurements consistently either in the interval between contractions or at their peak. You may gather meaningful information about descent by examining your patient during the peak of a contraction, although such examinations tend to be more uncomfortable and distracting for her.

The elucidation of labor curves has had two great virtues. They have furnished remarkable insights into the mechanisms of normal labor, and they have provided the capacity to quantify the events of cervical dilatation and fetal descent in a manner that can be applied clinically with ease. Once normal limits for various definable aspects of labor progress were

**Table 3.1** Normal limits for labor divisions

|  | Nullipara | Multipara |
|---|---|---|
| Latent phase | 20 h[§] | 14 h[§] |
| Active phase* | 1.2 cm/h[†] | 1.5 cm/h[†] |
|  | 5.0 cm/h[§] | 10.0 cm/h[§] |
| Deceleration phase | 3 h[§] | 1 h[§] |
| Descent* | 1.0 cm/h[†] | 2.0 cm/h[†] |
|  | 5.0 cm/h[§] | 10.0 cm/h[§] |

*Maximum slope of dilatation or descent
[†]Minimal acceptable limit
[§]Maximal acceptable limit

established, it became possible to characterize abnormal labor events with precision (Chapter 5).

Norms for labor have been determined in the same manner as for other quantifiable factors or events we encounter in medicine. Labor graphs from large samples of women have been analyzed and the distributions of various aspects of labor characterized. Analysis of these distribution curves, stratified by parity, yields useful information that can be translated into clinically applicable signals for identifying abnormalities. Based on convention, the 5% of the population that falls into the extremes of the distributions are considered likely abnormal. Using these cut-points defines a subset of patients that warrant clinical attention. Thus, for example, in 95% of nulliparas the cervix dilates at least 1.2 cm/h during the linear portion of the active phase. A slower rate of dilatation is considered abnormal, and requires assessment. Similarly, dilatation at a rate above 5 cm/h in nullipara is considered abnormally rapid, or precipitate.

Several investigators have validated this approach, which defines normality in practical terms. The norms, listed in Table 3.1, are influenced considerably by parity, requiring partitioning into nulliparous and multiparous labors. Other factors (race, age, level of parity) affect these norms little or not at all. They can for practical purposes, therefore, be applied to any population.

## Key points
- In most nulliparas and many multiparas there is a *prodromal stage* preceding labor.
- For clinical purposes, consider that labor has begun when uterine contractions are perceived by the mother at regular intervals.

- The *first stage* extends from the beginning of regular uterine contractions until the external cervical os is completely dilated.
- Fetal descent through the birth canal generally begins near the end of the first stage.
- The first stage includes the *latent* and the *active phases*.
- The *second stage* extends from the end of the first stage until the expulsion of the baby is completed.
- The *third stage* is the interval from delivery of the baby until the placenta and membranes are expelled.
- While the time required for cervical dilatation varies considerably among individuals, the cervix dilates in a predictable and quantifiable pattern in all normal labors.
- Like cervical dilatation, fetal descent follows a predictable pattern during normal labors.
- Evaluation of cervical dilatation and fetal descent can be facilitated by graphing the changes that occur against the time elapsed from the onset of labor.
- In constructing labor graphs, be sure to be consistent in obtaining measurements either in the interval between contractions or at the peak of contractions, but not both.
- Normal limits for various aspects of the labor curves are derived from their distribution curves. Parturients whose labor characteristics fall below the 5th or above the 95th percentile limits are considered abnormal and require thorough evaluation.

## Further Reading

### Books and reviews

Al-Azzawi F. *Color Atlas of Childbirth and Obstetric Techniques*. Mosby Yearbook, St Louis, MO, 1990.

Cohen WR, Brennan J. Using and archiving the labor curves. Clin Perinatol 1995;22:855–74.

Cohen WR. Normal and abnormal labor. In: Reece EA, Hobbins J (eds) *Clinical Obstetrics: The Fetus and Mother*, 3rd edition. Blackwell Publishing, London, 2007: 1065–76.

Cohen WR, Friedman EA. The assessment of labor. In: Kurjak A, Chervenak FA (eds) *Textbook of Perinatal Medicine*, 2nd edition. Informa UK, London, 2006: 1821–30.

Cohen WR. Controversies in the assessment of labor. In: Studd J, Tan SL, Chervenak FA. *Progress in Obstetrics and Gynaecology*. Churchill Livingstone, London, 2006; 17: 231–44.

Friedman EA. *Labor: Clinical Evaluation and Management*, 2nd edition. Appleton-Century-Crofts, New York, 1978.

Oxorn H. *Human Labor and Birth*, 4th edition. Appleton-Century-Crofts, New York, 1980.

Schifrin BS, Cohen WR. Labor's dysfunctional lexicon. Obstet Gynecol 1989;74:121–4.

Shipp TD, Repke JT. Normal labor and delivery. In: Repke JT (ed) *Intrapartum Obstetrics*. Churchill Livingstone, New York, 1996: 67–108.

## Primary sources

Chazotte C, Madden R, Cohen WR. Labor patterns in women with previous cesareans. Obstet Gynecol 1990;75:350–5.

Mahon T, Chazotte C, Cohen WR. Short labor: characteristics and outcome. Obstet Gynecol 1994; 84:47–51.

Murphy K, Shah L, Cohen WR. Labor and delivery in nulliparas who present with an unengaged fetal head. J Perinatol 1998;18:122–5.

Friedman EA. The graphic analysis of labor. Am J Obstet Gynecol 1954;68:1568–75.

Friedman EA. The functional divisions of labor. Am J Obstet Gynecol 1971;109:274–80.

Jacobson JD, Gregerson GN, Dale S, Valenzuela GJ. Real-time computer-based analysis of spontaneous and augmented labor. Obstet Gynecol 1990;76:755–8.

Peisner DB, Rosen MG. Latent phase of labor in normal patients: a reassessment. Obstet Gynecol 1985;66:644–8.

Philpott RH, Castle WM. Cervicographs in the management of labour in primigravidae: II. The action line and treatment of abnormal labour. J Obstet Gynecol Br Commonw 1972:79:599–602.

Schauberger CW. False labor. Obstet Gynecol 1986;68:770–2.

Schulman H, Romney S. Variability of uterine contractions in normal human parturition. Obstet Gynecol 1970;36:215–21.

Studd J. Partograms and nomograms of cervical dilatation in management of primigravid labour. BMJ 1973;4:451–5.

# CHAPTER 4

# Evaluating the Pelvis

Anatomic characteristics of the bony pelvis have been shown to influence progress in labor. Many other factors, of course, affect the pattern of labor. Not the least of them is the size of the fetus. To understand what transpires in each case, you must consider all such factors. Most relevant among them is a thorough understanding of the dynamics of the structural concordance between fetus and pelvis. Thorough comprehension of these relationships is fundamental to your practice of safe obstetrics.

Our clinical concepts about human pelvic architecture were crystallized by the methodical and comprehensive observations of Caldwell and Moloy in the 1930s. Their work, and the widespread availability of pelvic radiography at the time, spawned a generation of obstetricians who regarded knowledge of the mechanical fundamentals of obstetrics and interpretation of x-ray pelvimetry to be essential for the management of labor.

Focus on the importance of such knowledge has changed for several reasons. They include liberal use of cesarean delivery, dissatisfaction with and concerns about the safety of x-ray pelvimetry, deemphasis on the importance of operative vaginal delivery, and a focus on more esoteric and technologic issues in training, especially for obstetricians. The change has served to reduce our collective understanding of fetopelvic relationships for optimal obstetric management. Some contemporary recommendations for the treatment of dystocia even emphasize liberal use of oxytocin without regard for evaluation of pelvic characteristics. This is regrettable, in part because it denies the obstetric attendant the satisfaction that comes with an understanding of the beauty and logic of the mechanism of labor. More important, ill-considered use of uterotonic agents or labor prolonged unnecessarily may be hazardous for mother and fetus, particularly when there is disproportion between the fetus and the pelvis.

*Labor and Delivery Care: A Practical Guide*, First Edition. Wayne R. Cohen and Emanuel A. Friedman. © 2011 John Wiley & Sons, Ltd. Published 2011 by John Wiley & Sons, Ltd.

Fetal exposure to diagnostic abdominal or pelvic x-rays in late pregnancy has been shown, although not consistently, to increase the risk of childhood cancer. As a result, radiographic pelvimetry is rarely used today. Fortunately, much information can be obtained from clinical cephalopelvimetry. The most lamentable loss from abandoning x-ray pelvimetry is that there is no longer any visual standard by which you can judge the accuracy of your manual assessment. You can, however, overcome this by disciplined self-education.

Perform clinical pelvimetry after every delivery. Relate your findings to the mechanism of labor you have just observed in your patient. Doing so will help you accumulate a library of information in your mind's eye to serve as a source for future examinations. For the beginner, these postpartum examinations are best done in women with epidural anesthesia. The patient will experience no discomfort, and soft tissues are maximally relaxed. It is an exceptional opportunity to accomplish a remarkably thorough anatomic assessment. With practice, details that seemed at first subtle even in the anesthetized woman will become readily discernible in an awake patient. The aggregate of information ascertainable by this technique regarding cephalopelvic relationships is an essential component of the dynamic evaluation of labor.

## Clinical anatomy of the bony pelvis

To deliver vaginally, the fetus must traverse a curved passage that is partly bony and partly fibrous and muscular. The bony pelvis is the compound structure made up of the confluence of ilium, ischium, and pubis laterally and anteriorly, and the sacrum and coccyx posteriorly (Fig. 4.1). The pelvis is divided into two parts by a ridge, the linea terminalis or iliopectineal line. Above this is the *false pelvis*, of little obstetric interest. It is made up of the flaring wings of the ilia laterally and of the lower lumbar spine posteriorly; the abdominal wall completes the circle anteriorly.

The size and the shape of the false pelvis have no relation to the characteristics of the *true pelvis*, which lies below the linea terminalis and is of immense obstetric importance. The true pelvis supports the muscles and fasciae of the pelvic floor and gives shape and direction to the birth canal. The true pelvis can be considered a cylinder with a lower end that curves anteriorly (Fig. 4.2). The entrance (inlet) and the exit (outlet) of the true pelvis are smaller in their anterior-posterior dimension than the middle portion (midpelvis), and have therefore been referred to as the *superior strait* and the *inferior strait*, respectively. The contour of the pelvic canal varies at different levels. It is customary to describe these variations by

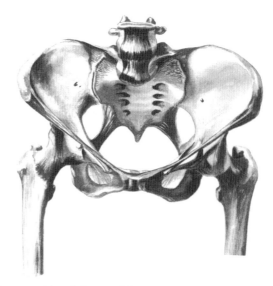

**Figure 4.1** The normal female bony pelvis.

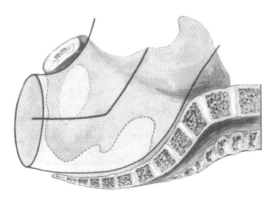

**Figure 4.2** Normal sacrum and pelvic outlet giving proper curve to the parturient canal.

reference to planes imagined at critical levels in the pelvis, i.e., the planes of inlet, midpelvis, and outlet.

Normal locomotion requires the support of a solidly fixed bony pelvic structure. During gestation, however, relaxation of pelvic ligaments occurs. This accounts for the waddling gait of many women in late pregnancy. Occasionally, this relaxation of the pelvic joints becomes extreme and pathologic. During labor, a modest widening of the symphysis pubis normally occurs, along with comparable changes in the sacroiliac joints. In addition, the mobile coccyx is easily pressed back by the descending fetal head, enlarging the outlet. These adaptations are presumed to help the passage of the fetus through the birth canal by enlarging the capacity of the pelvis.

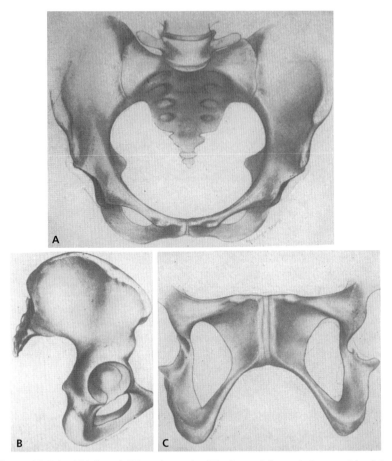

**Figure 4.3** Inlet (**A**), lateral (**B**), and anterior (**C**) views of the typical gynecoid pelvis showing well-rounded inlet, average inclination of the sacrum, ample sacrosciatic notch, rounded subpubic arch, and parallel sidewalls. (From Steer CM. *Moloy's Evaluation of the Pelvis in Obstetrics*. WB Saunders, Philadelphia, 1959.)

## The three planes

The plane of the *inlet* or *superior strait* is bounded by the upper border of the pubis in front, the linea terminalis at the sides, and the sacral promontory behind. The shape of the superior strait varies according to pelvic type as follows: rounded or *gynecoid* (Fig. 4.3); heart-shaped or *android* (Fig. 4.4); anteroposteriorly elongated ellipse or *anthropoid* (Fig. 4.5); flattened ellipse with transverse elongation or *platypelloid* (Fig. 4.6).

The inlet is an extremely important area of the pelvis. It plays a determinant role in normal labor (Fig. 4.7). The *true conjugate* is a critical diameter (Fig. 4.8). It extends from the top of the symphysis pubis to the top of the sacral promontory and normally measures 11–13 cm. This diameter

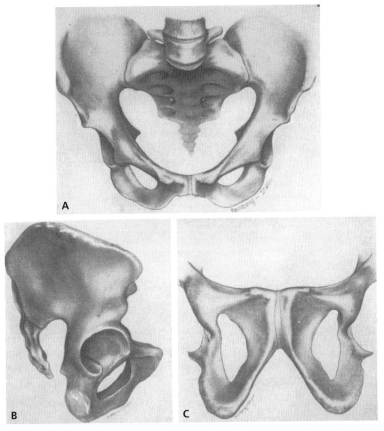

**Figure 4.4** Comparable views of a typical android pelvis illustrating heart-shaped inlet with narrow forepelvis and widest transverse diameter located close to the sacrum, which is angled forward with a narrow sacrosciatic notch and short sacrospinous ligament. The subpubic arch is narrow and the sidewalls converge. (From Steer CM. *Moloy's Evaluation of the Pelvis in Obstetrics*. WB Saunders, Philadelphia, 1959.)

cannot be measured directly by clinical examination. You can, however, obtain a useful approximation of the length of the true conjugate by first measuring the distance from the inferior margin of the pubis to the sacral promontory (Fig. 4.9) by means of a vaginal examination. This gives you the *diagonal conjugate*, which normally measures about 12.5 cm or more in a gynecoid pelvis. By subtracting 1.5 cm from the diagonal conjugate you will have a good approximation of the length of the true conjugate. Transversely, the inlet measures about 13–14 cm in the gynecoid pelvis. It cannot be measured clinically.

The anterior region of the inlet plane, or *forepelvis*, varies in its contour, tending to be broad in gynecoid and flat pelves and narrow in android and anthropoid types. The shape of the inlet determines the position of

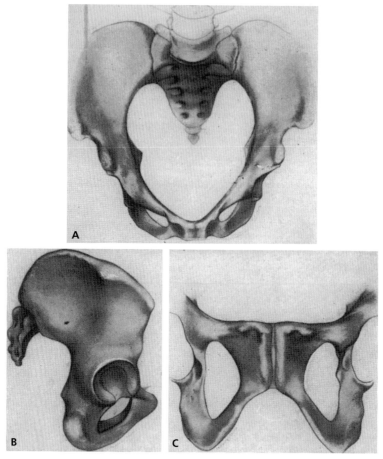

**Figure 4.5** A pelvis showing typical anthropoid features including elongated anteroposterior diameter and narrowed forepelvis. The sacrum has deep concavity with a wide sacrosciatic notch and elongated sacrospinous ligament. The subpubic arch is rounded and the ischial spines are prominent. (From Steer CM. *Moloy's Evaluation of the Pelvis in Obstetrics*. WB Saunders, Philadelphia, 1959.)

the fetal head at engagement and during the initial portion of descent. An inlet with a wide transverse diameter and a broad forepelvis, such as you will find in a gynecoid or platypelloid pelvis, favors engagement in a transverse or oblique position.

In the anthropoid or android pelvis, the narrow transverse dimension will accept the fetal biparietal diameter. The forepelvis will not accommodate the broad occiput, which will be found in the more ample posterior segment of the inlet. Therefore, occiput posterior positions are expected in the course of labor.

The *midpelvic plane* (also called the *midplane* or *midcavity*) passes through the apex of the subpubic arch, the ischial spines, and the inferior end

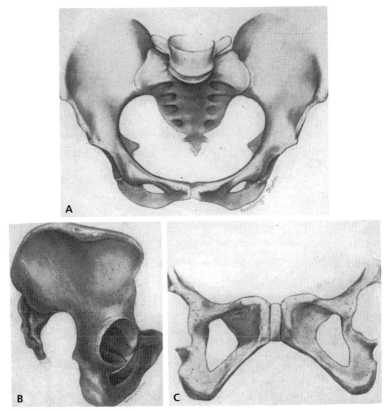

**Figure 4.6** Typical platypelloid (flat) pelvis with wide transverse diameter, foreshortening of the anteroposterior diameter, wide forepelvis, widening of the sacrosciatic notch, straight sacrum with forward inclination and J-projection at lower end, and broadening of the subpubic arch. (From Steer CM. *Moloy's Evaluation of the Pelvis in Obstetrics*. WB Saunders, Philadelphia, 1959.)

of the sacrum (Fig. 4.10). This area of the pelvis is frequently the site of clinically relevant pelvic contraction. The shape of its plane is generally ovoid, although it tends to be larger anteriorly. Its smaller posterior portion is bounded by the sacrospinous ligaments.

The most important midpelvic diameter runs transversely between the ischial spines (the interspinous diameter), and normally measures 10–11 cm in a gynecoid pelvis. You use the plane through the spines to determine the *station* of the fetal head in the pelvis. Fetal station reflects how far the forward leading edge of the fetal skull has advanced in labor in relation to the plane of the ischial spines. You will find it to be an important means for assessing progressive descent during labor.

Other clinically important features of the midpelvis are the sacrum and the sacrosciatic notch. The notch subtends an arc between the lateral border of the sacrum and the posterior border of the ischium. The sacrospinous

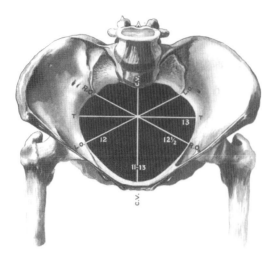

**Figure 4.7** View of the superior strait demonstrating its widest transverse (T), left and right oblique (LO, RO), and anteroposterior (true conjugate) diameters.

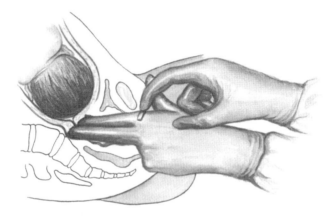

**Figure 4.8** Determining the diagonal conjugate.

ligament traverses the notch as it passes from the ischial spine to the lower portion of the lateral sacrum. The ligament is easily palpable in most women, and its length is a useful reflection of the width of the notch and the spaciousness of the posterior midpelvis.

The plane of the *outlet* or *inferior strait* passes through the arch and rami of the pubis, the ischial tuberosities, and the top of the coccyx, which is normally mobile (Fig. 4.11). This plane is the lower boundary of the bony outlet. Although it is rarely the site of contraction, it is important for you to evaluate the outlet. Its anteroposterior diameter is generally about 12 cm when the coccyx is extended, and it measures 10–11 cm transversely. You can measure the distance between the ischial tuberosities (it averages 10.5 cm in a gynecoid pelvis) by placing your fist against

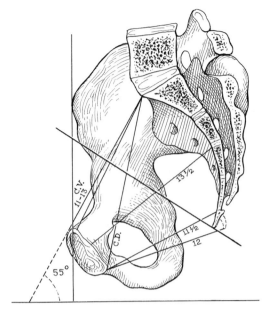

**Figure 4.9** Sagittal view of the erect pelvis showing anteroposterior diameters. CV, true conjugate; CD, diagonal conjugate. The pelvic inclination is shown as 55 degrees. (After Hodge HL. *The Principles and Practice of Obstetrics*. Blanchard & Lea, Philadelphia, 1864.)

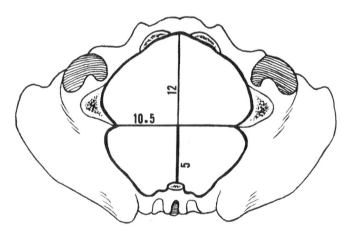

**Figure 4.10** The plane of the midpelvis.

the perineum. You can feel the tuberosities laterally, and if you know the diameter of your closed fist, you can estimate the intertuberous diameter. We have not found this measurement especially helpful clinically, except insofar as it may contribute information useful for constructing a mind's

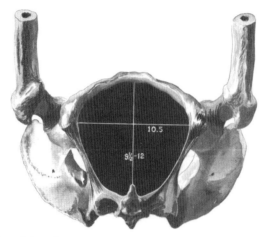

**Figure 4.11** The pelvic outlet, viewed from below. It passes through the arch of the pubic rami, the ischial tuberosities, and the tip of the coccyx.

eye view of the pelvic type. The intertuberous diameter will be narrow in the android and anthropoid pelvis and relatively wide in the gynecoid and flat pelvis.

## Changes in the fetal head

Evaluation of the fetal head is a critical component of the cephalopelvi-metric examination. Normal features of the skull are shown in Figs. 4.12 and 4.13. The shape of the head undergoes definite changes in labor. They vary with the presentation of the fetus. They are caused by pressures exerted by the maternal structures (Fig. 4.14). In ordinary cephalic presentations, with a moderately snug birth canal, the face and the forehead are flattened, the occiput is drawn out and the cranial bones overlap. Usually, the occipital bone is pressed under the two parietals; the frontal bone also somewhat underlies them. One parietal bone overlaps the other; the one that lies against the sacral promontory is the one that is prevented from advancing.

The head thus offers a long narrow cylinder to the birth canal instead of a globular form. These changes in shape, called *molding*, are possible because of the malleability of the bones and the loose connections they have with one another at the sutures. If this molding does not take place, labor may prove to be difficult.

A soft, boggy, circumscribed swelling, the *caput succedaneum* (often shortened to *caput*), appears on the area of the head that is most dependent and least subjected to pressure, particularly in long labors. In vertex

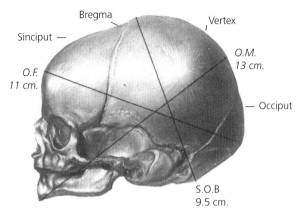

**Figure 4.12** Lateral view of fetal skull showing regional designations (reference points) and main diameters. OF, occipitofrontal; OM, occipitomental; SOB, suboccipitobregmatic

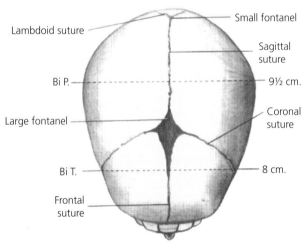

**Figure 4.13** Top view of the fetal skull, showing cranial bones, anterior and posterior fontanels, and sutures. The two important diameters (BiP, biparietal; BiT, bitemporal) are shown.

presentation, the caput is formed on one of the parietal bones. It is caused by venous and lymphatic stasis at the place where the ring of resistance (the opening of the cervix, vagina, or even the vulva) is pressed against the fetal head in response to uterine contractile pressure. This results in congestion of the scalp with edema formation. Small hemorrhages persist long after the edema is absorbed and define the site of swelling. Because the caput succedaneum develops in and under the scalp, it is movable over the skull surface. You can distinguish it from a cephalhematoma, an

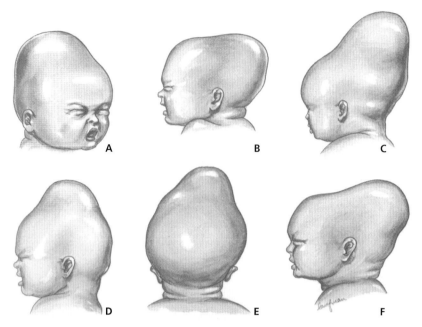

**Figure 4.14** Various types of caput succedaneum and molding of infants' heads.
**A**. Head shape after delivery from left occiput anterior position; **B**. breech presentation;
**C**. persistent occiput posterior with extended head; **D**. persistent occiput posterior
with flexed head; **E**. molding of head in flat pelvis; **F**. molding of head in generally
contracted pelvis.

accumulation of blood under the calvarial periosteum, because the hematoma is clearly delimited by the cranial sutures. The caput exaggerates the obliquity of the head produced by the depression of the parietal bone by the promontory of the sacrum or the pelvic floor. The caput is absorbed in 24–36 hours after delivery, and the asymmetry of the head disappears by the end of a week or so. Observation of the caput and the molding of the fetal head after delivery can provide important information about what the fetal position was during labor (Fig. 4.14).

## Method of clinical cephalopelvimetry

Clinical cephalopelvimetry is a requisite skill for everyone engaged in obstetric care because the architecture and the capacity of the pelvis may be critical in determining the course of events during labor. To achieve competence in this area, you should cultivate a thorough and systematic method of digital examination of the pelvis. To make each examination clinically meaningful, assess all of the pelvic characteristics listed in Table 4.1.

**Table 4.1** Observations for clinical pelvimetry

| Pelvic feature | Descriptors | | |
|---|---|---|---|
| Forepelvis (retropubic angle) | Wide | Moderate | Narrow |
| Subpubic arch | Wide | | Narrow |
| Pubic rami | Straight | Concave | |
| Pubic symphysis | Forward | Curved | Backward |
| Sidewalls | Divergent | Parallel | Convergent |
| Ischial spines | Blunt | Straight | Prominent |
| Sacrospinous ligaments | Thin, long | Average length, width | Thick, foreshortened |
| Sacral curve | Straight | Average | Hollow |
| Sacral inclination | Forward | Average | Backward |
| Terminal sacrum | Forward | Average | Backward |
| Coccyx | Backward/mobile | Average | Forward/fixed |

While Caldwell and Moloy identified four principal pelvic categories (gynecoid, android, anthropoid, and platypelloid), they recognized that pure examples of these archetypes are uncommon. The pelvis of most women shares characteristics of two or more types. You should reassess the architectural features of your patient's pelvis periodically during labor, especially with regard to their observed and predicted effects on the mechanism of labor and on the shape of the fetal head. Your ability to palpate changes in the presenting part will provide you with important insights into the adequacy of the pelvis in a particular situation.

Perform clinical pelvimetry for each of your patients during a prenatal visit. Doing so will give you the opportunity to obtain a general impression of the capacity of the pelvis and specific information about its bony architecture and capacity. You will, however, reap the most useful information during labor. At that time, the dynamic relationships between the pelvis and the fetal head can be assessed. In addition, the widening of the pelvic syndesmoses and head molding can be taken into account. You will obtain a great deal of information by vaginal examination if it is carried out in detail so that the essential features of the pelvis are studied carefully and methodically. The sequence in which the particulars are examined is not important so long as you establish a routine for yourself that will preclude omitting any significant landmarks.

Accurate quantitative measurement of pelvic diameters is important. It is far less critical, however, than determining the architectural features of the birth canal and relating them to what is happening in the labor and to how the shape of the head is changing. It should be obvious (but not always appreciated by those who dwell on pelvic mensuration rather than feto-pelvic relationships) that even a large pelvis may not safely accommodate

**Table 4.2** Interpretation of cephalopelvimetry

| Finding | Significance |
| --- | --- |
| Unengaged head | In nulliparas, risk factor for CPD.* Possible inlet disproportion or malposition |
| Large estimated fetal weight | Risk factor for CPD, dysfunctional labor pattern, shoulder dystocia |
| Malposition, malpresentation | May preclude further safe labor, or be risk factor for CPD, or signal nongynecoid architecture |
| Long, steeply inclined symphysis pubis | Suspect android pelvis |
| Sacrospinous ligaments short, thick | Possible narrow midpelvis posteriorly. Sacral curve may be shallow. Posterior space may be insufficient |
| Sacrospinous ligaments long | Suspect anthropoid pelvis with posteriorly recessed sacrum. Suspect flat pelvis with widely separated sidewalls |
| Diagonal conjugate short | Suspect flat or generally contracted pelvis. Consider inlet disproportion |
| AP of outlet short | May deliver occiput transverse |
| Narrow subpubic arch | Pelvis may have android or anthropoid features. High risk for perineal tears |
| Sidewalls convergent | Funnel pelvis. Suspect android or anthropoid pelvis |
| Ischial spines prominent | May prevent anterior or posterior rotation |
| Sacral curvature absent | May prevent posterior rotation of occiput |
| Occiput posterior | Suspect anthropoid or android characteristics. May be no room for internal rotation |
| Marked molding | Suspect disproportion |
| Anterior asynclitism | Suspect disproportion |
| Posterior asynclitism | Suspect disproportion; suspect flat contracted pelvis |

*CPD, cephalopelvic disproportion

a large fetus or one with a malposition, whereas a relatively small pelvis may readily accommodate an undersized fetus.

The sequential approach to clinical cephalopelvimetry that follows is an example of one you might consider for your practice (Tables 4.1 and 4.2).

**1.** Start at the abdomen. Determine the fetal lie and position and the degree of engagement of the presenting part. Estimate the fetal weight.

**2.** Determine the shape of the subpubic arch by external palpation of the inferior rami of the pubis (Fig. 4.15).

Align your thumbs along the rami so they meet near the inferior extremity of the symphysis pubis. Note the angle they subtend. Also note whether there is a concave curve in the contour of the inferior rami. This anatomic variation, a characteristic of an ample gynecoid pelvis, increases available space for the fetal head to pass beneath the subpubic arch. The angle of the subpubic arch is wide in the platypelloid pelvis; it is usually quite narrow in both android and anthropoid pelves.

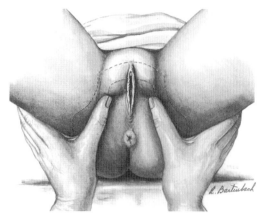

**Figure 4.15** The shape of the subpubic arch is determined by placing the examining thumbs along the inferior rami of the pubic bones.

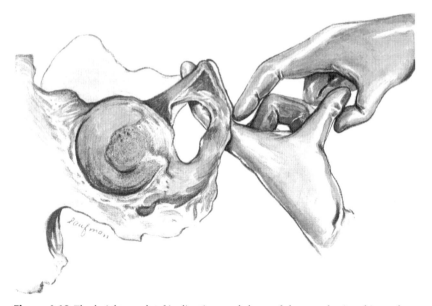

**Figure 4.16** The height, angle of inclination, and shape of the symphysis pubis can be determined digitally, as shown.

**3.** Estimate the height of the pubis and its inclination relative to the inlet (Fig. 4.16).

Insert two fingers of your examining hand into the vagina. Place the other hand gently on the mother's abdomen suprapubically and use the examining fingers of both hands to delineate the symphysis by palpation. The symphysis will be longest in the anthropoid pelvis (often more than 6 cm) and shortest in the flat pelvis. It may incline considerably posteriorly in the android pelvis.

**4.** Next examine the forepelvis at the inlet plane, located behind the symphysis pubis and radiating posterolaterally. Determine the angle that the walls of the forepelvis make with each other. A narrow angle is typical of the android pelvis. The forepelvis of the anthropoid pelvis is also narrow, but much deeper than that of the android type. The forepelvis of the gynecoid and the platypelloid pelvis is more rounded.

**5.** Move your fingers down from the forepelvis to evaluate the sidewalls and determine their inclination, i.e., whether they are parallel, convergent, or divergent.

To evaluate the slope of the sidewalls, move your intravaginal fingers to the base of the ischial spine as a referent landmark. Then palpate the ischial sidewall above the spine as far as you can reach and below this point down to the ischial tuberosities. This will allow you to sense the sidewall inclination. The sidewalls of an anthropoid pelvis may be convergent; a platypelloid pelvis may be divergent; those of the other types generally parallel.

**6.** Use your fingers to note the prominence of the ischial spines. Estimate the interspinous diameter digitally. Generally, a distance greater than 10 cm is considered normal.

Flat, indistinct spines are usually associated with wider interspinous diameters than are prominent, pointed spines. Overly prominent spines are found in the anthropoid and android pelvis. Flat spines are encountered in the platypelloid pelvis.

**7.** Then assess the length and thickness of the sacrospinous ligaments and the contours of the sacrosciatic notch.

Short, thick sacrosciatic ligaments (less than about 2.5 cm) are found in association with android pelves. The sacrosciatic notch will be narrow, and the sacral hollow will tend to be flattened in such cases. Elongated sacrospinous ligaments (more than 4 cm) occur in an anthropoid or platypelloid pelvis. The former has a deeply retrocessed sacrum, the latter a flat forward sacrum but widely separated sidewalls.

**8.** Ascertain the mobility of the coccyx by holding it between the examining fingers and attempting to move it backward and forward.

**9.** Note the inclination of the sacrum.

Move your examining fingers progressively up the sacrum in an attempt to reach the promontory. In so doing you will be able to determine how concave the sacral surface is. The sacrum tends to be broad and deeply curved in the gynecoid pelvis. The android pelvis, by contrast, has a narrower and flatter sacrum that is often angled forward.

**10.** If the promontory can be reached, measure from the lower border of the symphysis to the promontory, the diagonal conjugate.

**11.** Also measure the distance from the sacral tip to the underborder of the symphysis pubis, the anteroposterior diameter of the outlet, a useful indicator of outlet adequacy.

Extend the middle finger of your examining hand on the sacrococcygeal joint and mark off the point on the hand corresponding to the lower border of the symphysis. It is generally at least 12 cm, but will be shorter in android and platypelloid pelvic types.

**12.** Assess the fetal head. Determine its position, station, attitude, synclitism, presence and degree of molding, and caput succedaneum.

**13.** When appropriate in the late first stage or in the second stage of labor (see below) the Müller-Hillis maneuver may provide you with useful information about the dynamic fit of the head relative to the pelvis.

The best determination of the diagonal conjugate may be obtained by keeping your examining fingers and wrist straight in line with your forearm. With your fingers deep in the posterior vaginal fornix, depress your elbow toward the ground. The elbow may be rested on your knee while the fingers are advanced gently but firmly toward the sacral promontory. You may need to keep steady pressure on the perineum for some time before the patient relaxes her muscles sufficiently to allow any advancement. When the promontory is reached, keep your fingers there, but raise your elbow until your hand touches the lower border of the symphysis. Mark this point with a finger of the external hand and withdraw the internal hand. Use a ruler to make an accurate measurement of the diagonal conjugate. Subtracting 1.5 cm from this dimension will give a useful approximation of the true conjugate. If the pubis is unusually high, this may overestimate the true measurement, so you should then instead use a value of 2.0 cm or even 2.5 cm for subtraction.

Examining the fetal head for the presence of excessive degrees of molding and positional or attitudinal abnormalities provides you with valuable clinical clues to the suitability of the pelvis for safe vaginal delivery. The Müller-Hillis maneuver is a means for dynamically assessing the cephalopelvic relationship in terms of adequacy of fit and may be useful in this regard. With the cervix at least 5 cm dilated, have someone apply firm but gentle fundal pressure during a contraction while you do a bimanual abdomino-vaginal examination. Apply your suprapubic hand to the base of the fetal skull and your intravaginal fingers to the forward leading edge, thus holding the fetal skull between your hands. With the thrust of combined uterine contraction and downward fundal pressure, you should be able to assess descent, flexion, and rotation of the presenting part. You will garner the most useful information when you do this examination during the second stage. The maneuver is quite useful in late first stage to determine if the head is fixed in the pelvis or able to descend somewhat. It is much more predictive of safe vaginal delivery after the cervix is fully dilated. At that time, it helps to predict subsequent progress in descent and rotation, that is to say, how well the pelvis will accommodate the descending fetus.

## Significance of pelvimetric findings

Whether or not you consider evaluation of the pelvis to be useful depends on the information you expect from it. The term *cephalopelvic disproportion* is used frequently in conjunction with pelvimetry. In truth, pelvimetry is no more effective than any other technique in predicting safe vaginal delivery when applied in a clinical vacuum, i.e., without taking other relevant information into account. The mechanism of labor is influenced by many other factors, including fetal size, ability of the fetal skull to mold, the degree of flexion of the fetal head, distensibility of pelvic joints, uterine contractility, and the resistance of the pelvic soft tissues, among others.

Only by combining and interpreting information from these sources intelligently will you be able to make keen judgments. Knowledge of pelvic architecture and cephalopelvic relationships allows you to understand and explain the observed normal or abnormal mechanism of labor, to judge the effects of labor on the fetal skull, and thus to assess the prospects of a normal vaginal delivery. When you integrate such assessments with those obtained from serial evaluation of cervical dilatation and fetal descent, uterine activity, and fetal condition, you can make a decision about the advisability of conservative expectancy vs. more interventive uterine stimulation or operative delivery. This approach is preferable to administering oxytocin perfunctorily in every case of labor dysfunction and allowing the compressibility of the fetal head to dictate the route of delivery. The latter approach may increase the risk of harming the fetus.

For you to interpret the findings on examination properly, it is important to understand the typical characteristics of the various classic pelvic types and their relation to the probable mechanisms of labor. In the gynecoid pelvis, the most common position of the fetal head is obliquely anterior, i.e., right or left occiput anterior. In the android pelvis, posterior oblique positions are usually seen. The anthropoid pelvis is also commonly associated with posterior mechanisms because of its anteroposterior elongation and capacious posterior aspects. By contrast, occiput transverse is common in the transversely elongated flat pelvis.

*Failure of descent* (Chapter 5) is commonly the result of inlet disproportion. Absence of descent in the face of nearly complete cervical dilatation (or entry into the second stage), persistence of high fetal station, and poor response to oxytocin stimulation (which should rarely be used to treat this disorder) suggest mechanical obstruction. The likelihood of safe vaginal delivery is remote when this constellation is encountered. Early intervention under these circumstances is indicated if cephalopelvimetry supports a high probability of disproportion.

Consider some related scenarios. If you encounter a patient who has android midpelvic characteristics in association with a molded fetal head impinging on the crest of the symphysis pubis in the presence of a failure of descent, you can reasonably surmise that a safe vaginal delivery is highly improbable. Similarly, you can recognize the ominous prognosis for a fetus in occiput posterior position, even though engaged, in a patient whose midpelvis has prominent ischial spines (preventing anterior rotation) and a forward lower sacrum (not providing sufficient compensatory space for descent in the posterior position). However, when you find failure of descent (or other aberrations of descent) in the presence of a well-flexed unmolded head in a pelvis that seems ample, look for causes other than insurmountable cephalopelvic disproportion. Vaginal delivery is apt to occur in due course. Oxytocin infusion, if indicated, is safer and more likely to be efficacious under these more favorable circumstances.

If you determine that the ischial spines are very prominent and associated with foreshortened sacrospinous ligaments, both characteristic of an android pelvis, you can anticipate dysfunctional labor progress related to midpelvic contraction. Similarly, convergent sidewalls confirm funneling, which is often associated with midplane or outlet problems. Shortened sacrospinous ligaments result from forward inclination of the sacrum, or narrow transverse midplane dimensions, or both. Narrowing of the forepelvis of the inlet, which occurs in an android or anthropoid pelvis, constricts the transverse diameters. A narrow subpubic arch, which is similarly constrictive, but at the outlet, may also reflect a concurrent narrowing of the inlet forepelvis. A shortened anteroposterior diameter or true conjugate, such as seen in a platypelloid pelvis or one that has small overall dimensions, raises the specter of a serious inlet problem.

*Arrest of descent* and *protracted descent* (Chapter 5) are associated with several obstetric features, including malposition, excessive sedation or anesthesia, insufficient uterine contractility, chorioamnionitis, obesity, and cephalopelvic disproportion. You should undertake thorough evaluation of each of these factors when you are confronted with a patient who has these labor dysfunctions. When the likelihood of disproportion seems high based on your physical examination, you should avoid enhancing uterine contractility with oxytocin. Cephalopelvimetry will help to rule out positional abnormalities and disproportion.

Here are some more illustrative examples. Arrest of descent often occurs in the midpelvis with an occiput transverse position. This may be an entirely appropriate fetal position in a pelvis with quite ample transverse space throughout and straight or divergent sidewalls (typical of a flat pelvis). If the lower sacrum is straight or inclined backward or if the forepelvis is wide, you can usually demonstrate descent with the Müller-Hillis maneuver. Having reasonably ruled out disproportion at this level of the pelvis, you may safely administer oxytocin. As labor progresses, expect continued descent in the transverse position until internal rotation occurs when the fetal head reaches the levator ani muscular trough low in the pelvis. Similarly, you can successfully use uterotonic stimulation if the upper pelvis will accommodate anterior rotation and the lower pelvis will allow further descent in an anterior position. However, if you encounter arrest of descent with the occiput transverse in a pelvis with features that are unlikely to permit further descent easily, particularly if the head shows asynclitism or marked molding, you should be able to verify that a major degree of disproportion is present by clinical pelvimetry, including dynamic assessment with the Müller-Hillis maneuver. Then proceed expeditiously to cesarean delivery without a trial of oxytocin.

You can often gain valuable clues to the form and capacity of the pelvis and the evolving mechanism of labor by remembering two simple generalizations: (1) at any point in descent, the fetal occiput will usually rotate to the most ample available diameter of the pelvis; (2) the narrowest diameter of the fetal head tends to occupy the narrowest portion of the available pelvic plane. As demonstrative examples, consider the position of the fetal head in the midplane of a typical anthropoid pelvis as contrasted with the fetal position in a gynecoid pelvis.

In the anthropoid pelvis, you will commonly encounter an occiput posterior position. It occurs when the occiput occupies the ample posterior segment of the pelvis, and the biparietal diameter of the fetal head is accommodated in the narrower transverse axis of the pelvis. The situation is different under ordinary circumstances in a gynecoid pelvis, where the fetal head will pass the midplane at the level of the ischial spines with the biparietal diameter oriented between the spines, and the occiput directed anteriorly. If you find the head is in a transverse position, the pelvis may be relatively flattened in the anteroposterior diameter. Because there is not sufficient space anteriorly or posteriorly, the occiput cannot rotate in an occiput anterior or occiput posterior position. An alternative explanation is that the transverse diameter at the spines is exceptionally wide.

## Labor in the generally contracted pelvis

Marked pelvic contraction and deformities may result from vitamin D deficiency. They are uncommon in the industrialized world today. Nonetheless, various degrees of clinically significant pelvic contraction do occur. When you encounter a parturient with pelvic contraction, she can serve as a useful example to facilitate your understanding of the effects of

**Box 4.1 Characteristics of labor in the generally contracted pelvis**

- Malpositions and malpresentations common
- Marked caput succedaneum and molding occur
- Dysfunctional labor patterns, first and second stage
- Extreme flexion

pelvic anatomy on labor (Box 4.1). Abnormal fetal presentations (breech, face, brow, shoulder) are four times as frequent with a contracted pelvis as with a normal one. Prolapse of the arm, foot, and cord are also common, particularly in a woman with a flat pelvis. These complications occur because the fetal head is not firmly apposed to the lower uterine segment. It is displaced by the jutting promontory of the sacrum, thereby providing space for small parts to slip past.

Much depends on the size and moldability of the fetal head. If the bones are compliant and can overlap one another, they may adjust themselves to the shape of the pelvis and potential disproportion may thus be overcome. If the fetus is small, there may actually be no disproportion relative to the pelvic contraction. At the beginning of labor the fetal head is usually not engaged. It does not fit the lower uterine segment accurately. The membranes over the internal cervical os are exposed to the full force of the uterine contractions. This often results in membrane rupture, which in turn promotes prolapse of the cord or an extremity, or ascending uterine infection.

Differences are observed in the way the cervix dilates in obstructed labor. Typically, arrest of dilatation or descent is encountered in the presence of insurmountable obstruction. Prolonged deceleration phase and failure of descent are also common. In cases of labor allowed to continue for long periods in the presence of a severely contracted pelvis, the expanded and overstretched lower uterine segment may rupture. The risk of rupture becomes especially prominent in patients laboring with a uterine scar from a prior cesarean. Sometimes, the cervix is compressed between the bony plates of the head and the pelvis. The resulting edema is due to venous and lymphatic obstruction. The anterior lip is particularly likely to be caught between the head and the pubis and become quite swollen as labor continues. If neglected, it becomes markedly congested, or even necrotic. Later, it may form a cervicovesical fistula.

If the head is arrested at the inlet, you may find the uterine contractions becoming progressively stronger and the intervals between them shorter, but no advancement is perceptible. A large caput succedaneum forms. The scalp may even be visible at the vulva, although the head is actually not yet engaged, i.e., the biparietal diameter is still above the pelvic inlet.

This is particularly true in an occiput posterior position, which is commonly associated with deflexion of the head, advanced molding, and marked caput formation. The resulting elongation of the fetal head makes the forward leading edge seem to be descending. This leads in turn to sizeable and misleading overestimates of the degree of actual descent. In extreme cases, cerebral injury or hemorrhage may occur as the uterine forces compress the head through a passage that is too small.

The shape of the inlet determines the position of the fetal head at engagement and also the subsequent labor mechanism. In the gynecoid pelvis, the head enters the inlet and proceeds to descend normally unless the inlet is small or the fetus large. In the transversely contracted android or anthropoid pelvis, the area of the inlet might be sufficient to allow the head to pass, but the occiput rotates to the more ample posterior segment of the inlet; occiput posterior position results. When the contractions grow stronger, molding begins and the intrauterine pressures gradually force the head through the narrowed superior strait. Because the cranial bones are malleable and can overlap each other at the sutures, the head is capable of changing its form to accommodate itself to the shape of the inlet. The location of caput succedaneum and the nature of molding found in the newborn are characteristic of the fetal position during labor. You should, therefore, evaluate these neonatal features after delivery for their heuristic benefits.

Excess molding can occur in the contracted pelvis, sometimes with disturbing results. One of the parietal bones is first subjected to resistance from either the sacral promontory or the pubic bones. This parietal bone is thereby pressed under the opposite one. The plate of the occipital bone then comes to lie under the two parietal bones. This overlapping may be so pronounced that the dura mater begins to strip off and a row of minute hemorrhages forms on either side of the sagittal sinus. These effects can lead to fetal brain damage.

The very small gynecoid pelvis is generally narrow throughout. Progress of labor, therefore, is not rapid even if the presenting part successfully negotiates the inlet. The subsequent slow progress through the birth canal is often associated with protraction or arrest disorders. In general, you should not use oxytocin or instrumental delivery to treat protraction or arrest disorders in these cases, unless you are reasonably certain that disproportion is not present.

Three clinical signs can indicate the head is descending: the patient begins to bear down; she feels a desire to (or does) defecate; or cramps occur in the legs. The first two signs are due to pressure of the head on the rectum and the levator ani muscles; the last is due to irritation of the sacral plexus by contact with the advancing head. Because molding may be considerable in these cases, there is danger of mistaking elongation of the fetal head for true descent. You should assess fetal descent by both suprapubic palpation—to ensure the base of the fetal skull is descending as the leading edge does—and astute appraisal of the station of the head by vaginal examination. This combination will help you to differentiate descent from molding reliably. In true descent, the amount of the head palpable above the symphysis will diminish steadily over the course of serial examinations.

The fetal head usually fits well into the inlet of the small gynecoid pelvis. Abnormal attitudes, presentations, and positions are not as frequent as in flat pelves. Prolapse of the cord is rare because the head fits the inlet accurately. Early in labor, the head lies in flexion. As soon descent begins, this flexion can become extreme. You will be able to palpate the small posterior fontanel first. The sagittal suture most often lies in an oblique diameter. After labor has been in progress for some time, advanced head molding will displace the posterior fontanel toward the center of the pelvis, where it will usually be covered by substantial caput succedaneum. This extreme flexion is caused by an exaggeration of the same mechanism that produces flexion in normal labor. This occurs because the long sincipital pole of the leveraged head encounters greater resistance and, therefore, rises higher. The diagnosis is generally easy to make. Abdominally, the extreme flexion is indicated by the high forehead, which you can easily palpable over one pubic ramus, and by the deep occiput, usually not palpable. Vaginally, you will find the small fontanel, almost in the axis of the pelvis. The midline orientation of the sagittal suture confirms the extreme characteristic flexion.

### Labor in the flat pelvis

In the flat pelvis, resistance to fetal descent is encountered mostly at the inlet (unless the pelvic dimensions are small throughout). The first stage of labor is often completed without difficulty once the head engages. In multiparas, one or two powerful expulsive efforts in the second stage produce anterior rotation and delivery of the head. Overcoming the resistance of the soft tissues requires more time, and considerably more forceful effort in nulliparas. If the pelvis is generally contracted, the resistance continues all the way to the outlet and labor, if it progresses at all, is often prolonged and difficult.

Abnormalities of position and presentation are common in the platypelloid pelvis (Box 4.2). Because of the forward jutting of the sacral promontory, the head cannot enter the pelvis; therefore, it overrides the pubis. The biparietal diameter is often too large to engage in the true conjugate, which is the narrowest diameter. As a result, the head slides off to the side and the smaller bitemporal diameter comes to lie in the true conjugate while the biparietal diameter occupies the larger space in proximity to the sacroiliac joint.

---

**Box 4.2 Characteristics of labor in the flat pelvis**

- Abnormal presentations and position
- Persistent occiput transverse
- First stage labor dysfunctions
- Deflexion, sincipital presentation

---

**Box 4.3 Characteristics of labor in the funnel pelvis**

- Extreme flexion of head
- First and second stage labor dysfunction, especially failure or arrest of descent, prolonged deceleration phase
- Persistent occiput transverse common
- High risk of perineal damage

---

The forehead descends first because the resistance offered the occiput is greater. Thus, deflexion occurs instead of flexion, resulting in a sincipital presentation. Owing to the long transverse and short anteroposterior diameters of the inlet, the head seeks an occiput transverse position as the most accommodating position for its advance. You will find the sagittal diameter of the deflexed head in the transverse diameter of the pelvis. The space actually available for the fetal head is quite small. Active phase labor dysfunctions are common. The head may deliver in a transverse position if there is inadequate space in the mid- and lower pelvis to allow internal rotation.

### Labor in the funnel pelvis

In the funnel pelvis, the birth canal becomes progressively narrower from inlet to outlet (Box 4.3). Resistance to fetal descent increases steadily to a maximum at the pelvic outlet. Often descent of the head is arrested at or above this plane. Extreme flexion occurs, resembling that described for the generally contracted gynecoid pelvis.

The funnel pelvis is sometimes markedly contracted transversely at the outlet. This contraction lies between the inferior pubic rami and ischial tuberosities. The broad fetal occiput cannot utilize this space during the passage under the symphysis, but is forced instead backward onto the perineum and against the sacrum and coccyx. As a result, the perineum and levator ani muscles are often torn. Sometimes delivery is associated with fracture of the coccyx. If the sacrum curves too far forward, safe vaginal delivery may be impossible. In these cases instrumental delivery should be avoided because it may result in deep injury to the pelvic floor and vagina, and risks fetal trauma as well. In fact, the occiput posterior position may be an anatomic necessity for effecting vaginal delivery when-ever the midcavity and lower pelvis have android or anthropoid tenden-cies. If the sacrum is sufficiently posterior to accommodate the occiput and the forepelvis is narrow, you should not attempt to rotate the head to an anterior position manually or with forceps. Doing so will be coun-terproductive and potentially hazardous. Furthermore, you must beware of the risk of severe perineal damage if the subpubic arch is narrow, forc-ing the broad occiput to traverse the full length of the perineum. Indeed, the geometry of the outlet figures importantly in the risk of trauma to the vagina and the perineum. You should weigh it carefully as a factor in deciding whether or not an episiotomy is appropriate.

If the head does reach the pelvic floor in the funnel pelvis, descent often is arrested with the head impacted between the ischia. Descent does not continue here, even though the occiput rotates anteriorly, as it usually does, because of the limited space available for the large occiput. Strong maternal bearing-down efforts will produce no advance, beyond the spe-cious illusion of descent afforded by progressive molding of the head.

Your vaginal examination at this point will disclose the fetal head in exaggerated flexion, squeezed between the spines of the ischia and cov-ered with a large caput. As noted, you will usually find internal rotation is complete. Sometimes, however, you will encounter the sagittal suture lying in the transverse diameter. This occurs because the occiput cannot be accommodated by the equally constrained pelvic dimensions posteri-orly and anteriorly.

If the sacrum does not curve forward too much, there may still be ample room for the passage of the hyperflexed head. Nevertheless, deliv-ery is often difficult. In any patient with known or suspected pelvis con-traction, you must undertake thorough clinical pelvimetry. This applies especially in a patient who has a funnel pelvis or a transversely contracted pelvis. Your astute evaluation of the cephalopelvic relationship is vital to guide decision making about how to proceed with delivery. In the face of probable disproportion, you must consider whether the risk of undertak-ing a potentially traumatic operative vaginal delivery can be justified, as opposed to cesarean delivery.

## Labor in the transversely contracted pelvis

Mild degrees of contraction in the transverse diameter will not usually create serious problems. A circular pelvis has the largest area for a given diameter. A small round inlet, moreover, may have more available room than a large one that is rendered functionally inadequate by an anteriorly projecting sacral promontory, a narrow inlet forepelvis, or compressed sidewalls. In a pelvis with android or anthropoid characteristics (Box 4.4), the head fits better if it enters sagittally with its occiput posterior. When

> **Box 4.4 Characteristics of labor in the transversely contracted pelvis**
>
> - Occiput posterior common
> - Late or no rotation to occiput anterior
> - Attitude often deflexed
> - Descent disorders

the posterior segment of the inlet is larger, the occiput tends to rotate in that direction. If the sacrum projects more forward, as in an android type of pelvis, the whole head is moved anteriorly. Nevertheless, the occiput still favors the posterior or posterior oblique position after the fetal head becomes engaged.

The head will usually descend in the transversely contracted pelvis until it is arrested between the prominent ischial spines that are so often associated with transverse pelvic narrowing. Both characteristics commonly occur together in an android or an anthropoid pelvis and often result in arrest of dilatation or descent. If you encounter an arrest disorder in a patient with conspicuous transverse pelvic narrowing, this combination should suggest irremediable obstruction, especially if accompanied by marked molding of the fetal head. Abdominal delivery would be the most prudent alternative. However, if the head flexes well, it may be possible for additional descent to take place. If descent continues, the occiput will stay posterior if the sacrum is inclined posteriorly and has a good concavity. Alternatively, the fetal head may rotate in the midplane to an occiput anterior orientation. Sometimes, because of the considerable molding, this rotation may not occur until the leading edge of the head has descended to the point at which it is about to crown at the perineum.

## Anterior asynclitism

A most important abnormality of the descent mechanism is the lateral flexion of the head that is almost always encountered in the flat pelvis with anteroposterior narrowing. The parietal bone is inclined toward one or the other shoulder. The lateral flexion of the head relative to the pelvic plane is called parietal bone presentation or *asynclitism*. It is designated anterior or posterior asynclitism according to which parietal bone is lowermost in the pelvis (Figs. 4.17 to 4.19). You can diagnose posterior asynclitism if you find the sagittal suture positioned anterior to the midpoint of the pelvis. This results when the posterior parietal bone advances ahead of the anterior one, which is held up by the pubis. You can recognize anterior asynclitism when you encounter the sagittal suture posterior

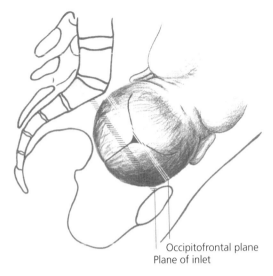

Occipitofrontal plane
Plane of inlet

**Figure 4.17** Lateral representation of normal synclitism showing parallelism of the fetal occipitofrontal plane and the pelvic superior strait.

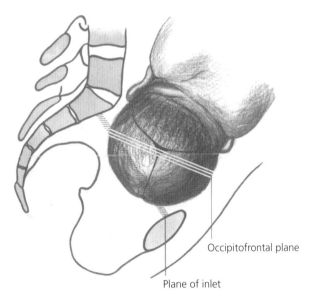

Occipitofrontal plane

Plane of inlet

**Figure 4.18** Posterior asynclitism (posterior parietal presentation), a common finding with the sagittal suture facing toward the symphysis pubis.

to the midpoint. Here the posterior parietal bone is held up on the sacral promontory as the fetal head descends.

In a normal pelvis, the head engages with the posterior parietal bone a little lower, i.e., in slight posterior asynclitism. However, in flat contracted pelves, anterior asynclitism is more common. It may even be exaggerated to the extreme in which the anterior ear is palpable behind the pubis. In the subsequent course of labor, the posterior parietal bone may roll over

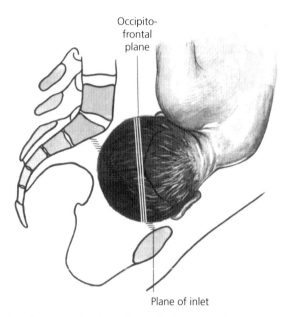

**Figure 4.19** Anterior asynclitism (anterior parietal presentation) is an uncommon event, with the sagittal suture facing toward the sacrum.

the promontory into the pelvis. If this happens, the anterior parietal bone acts like a sliding fulcrum on the posterior wall of the pubis, allowing the posterior parietal bone to descend still further.

As soon as the greatest dimension of the fetal head has passed the plane of the inlet, the head flexes. You can recognize this happening by palpation. You can feel the head descend and the occiput sink, while the large anterior fontanel ascends. If there is sufficient available space, anterior rotation can be expected to follow immediately. The subsequent mechanisms are as usual: flexion, descent, extension, restitution, and external rotation.

Abdominally, you may suspect deflexion of the head by observing the straightening of the fetal spine and lateral flexion at the neck. At vaginal examination, the sagittal suture lies in the transverse diameter, but very close to the sacrum, confirming that the head is in anterior asynclitism. The small posterior fontanel is on the same level as the large one, indicating deflexion, or sometimes it is even higher so that the brow comes down. The sutures are felt plainly at first because the cranial bones overlap. Later, the caput succedaneum obliterates the landmarks.

## Posterior asynclitism

In the posterior parietal bone presentation (posterior asynclitism), the head is inclined toward the anterior shoulder. The posterior parietal bone occupies the vault of the pelvis and, if lateral flexion is pronounced, the posterior ear may be palpable in front of the promontory. This mechanism is the reverse of what we have just considered. The anterior parietal bone stems on the symphysis pubis and the posterior one rolls down in front of the sacral promontory. In posterior asynclitism, the angle that the shoulder makes with the head can be felt just above the pubis. Often the rounded parietal bone can be felt also. Vaginally, the sagittal suture is just behind the pubis, usually in the transverse or slightly oblique diameter. The small and large fontanels are on a level with each other, or the small posterior fontanel is high and out of reach. Palpating the descended anterior fontanel permits you to diagnose head extension, which may indicate a brow presentation.

If the head can descend, the sagittal suture relocates from the pubis and approaches the sacrum. Later, descent and anterior rotation of the occiput bring this suture into an oblique diameter. The nape of the fetal neck stems from behind one ramus of the pubis and the head is delivered in the oblique.

When you encounter a marked degree of either form of asynclitism, you should suspect bony disproportion. Descent may be protracted, or even arrested if the narrowing of the lower pelvis is great enough to affect fetal descent or rotation adversely.

## Key points

- Clinical cephalopelvimetry is a requisite skill that must be developed by everyone engaged in obstetric care because the dimensional relationships of the pelvis may be critical in determining the course of events that transpire during labor.
- After every delivery, perform clinical pelvimetry and relate the findings to the previously observed mechanism of labor.
- The true pelvis can be considered to be a cylinder with a lower end that curves anteriorly. The entrance and the outlet of the true pelvis are smaller than the middle portion and have, therefore, been referred to as the *superior strait* and the *inferior strait*, respectively.
- The diagonal conjugate, the distance from the inferior margin of the pubis to the sacral promontory, measures about 12.5 cm or more in gynecoid pelves.
- Accurate quantitative measurements of pelvic diameters is far less important than determining the architectural features of the birth canal and relating them to extant circumstances in the labor and to changes in the fetal head.
- The fetal occiput will generally rotate to the most ample available diameter of the pelvis.

- When either form of asynclitism is marked, bony disproportion should be suspected.
- Descent may be protracted or even arrested if narrowing of the lower pelvis resists descent or rotation.
- In the funnel pelvis, the birth canal becomes progressively narrower from inlet to outlet. Resistance to fetal descent increases steadily to a maximum at the pelvic outlet. Descent of the head is often arrested at or above this plane.
- Abnormalities of position and presentation are common in the platy-pelloid pelvis.
- Abnormal presentations (breech, face, brow, shoulder) are four times as frequent with a contracted pelvis as with a normal one.
- The shape of the inlet determines the fetal position at the time of engagement and also the subsequent mechanism of labor.

## Further Reading

### Books and reviews

Abitbol MM. *Birth and Human Evolution. Anatomical and Obstetrical Mechanics in Primates.* Bergin & Garvey, Westport, CT, 1996.

Dietrichs E. Anatomy of the pelvic joints: a review. Scand J Rheum 1991;suppl 88:4–6.

Langnickel D. *Problems of the Pelvic Passageway.* Springer-Verlag, Berlin, 1985.

Rozenberg P. Quelle place pour la radiopelvimétrie au XXIe siècle? Gynécol Obstét Fertil 2007;35:6–12.

Thoms H. *Pelvimetry.* Paul B. Hoeber, Inc, New York, 1956.

Thurnau GR, Hales KA, Morgan MA. Evaluation of the fetal-pelvic relationship. Clin Obstet Gynecol 1992;35:570–581.

### Primary sources

Borell U, Fernstrom I. The movements at the sacro-iliac joints and their importance to changes in the pelvic dimensions during parturition. Acta Obstet Gynecol Scand 1957;36:42–57.

Caldwell WE, Moloy HC. Anatomical variations in the female pelvis and their effect in labor with a suggested classification. Am J Obstet Gynecol 1933;26:479–505.

Caldwell WE, Moloy HC, D'Esopo DA. Further studies on the pelvic architecture. Am J Obstet Gynecol 1934;28:482–500.

Danforth DN, Ellis AH. Midforceps delivery—a vanishing art? Am J Obstet Gynecol 1963;86:29–37.

Ince JGH, Young MD. The bony pelvis and its influence on labor. J Obstet Gynaecol Br Emp 1940;47:130–90.

March MR, Adair CD, Veille JC, Burrus DR. The modified Mueller-Hillis maneuver in predicting abnormalities in second stage labor. Int J Gynaecol Obstet. 1996;55:105–9.

Rustamova S, Predanic M, Cohen WR. Changes in symphysis pubis width during labor. J Perinat Med 2009;37:370–3.

Uonio S, Saarikoski S, Räty E, Vohlonen I. Clinical assessment of the pelvic capacity and outlet. Arch Gynecol 1986;239:11–16.

# CHAPTER 5

# Diagnosing and Treating Dysfunctional Labor

Most labors are normal, and would proceed to a safe and satisfactory outcome without any medical intervention. In some cases, however, events occur that place the fetus or the mother at risk. One of your primary roles during labor is to identify any potential adversity as early as possible and to intervene accordingly to minimize its impact.

Many factors influence whether labor will progress normally and terminate in a safe vaginal delivery. These include the maternal pelvic architecture and the mechanism of labor associated with it; the fetal presentation, position, and attitude; the fetal head size and its ability to be molded; the character of the uterine contractions; and the general health and condition of the parturient. Success in the conduct of labor depends on the proper evaluation of each of these factors and their interrelations.

Some conditions that can confound the expectation of an uncomplicated delivery are evident prior to or early in labor. For example, the presence of a malpresentation, a markedly contracted pelvis, a history of a uterine scar rupture during a prior pregnancy, or a serious maternal medical problem may sometimes make attempting labor imprudent. Much more commonly, events arise during labor that reduce the chance that an uncomplicated vaginal delivery will ensue. Recognizing and interpreting these events is the key to protecting mother and fetus from harm.

The process of labor assessment requires that you reappraise the situation every time you acquire new information regarding progress in cervical dilatation or fetal descent, the condition of the fetus or the mother, or the cephalopelvic relationships. At each interval assessment, you need to make a judgment about how the aggregate of available information affects the likelihood that a trouble-free spontaneous vaginal delivery will occur. Precise quantitation of such probabilities is not always possible, but with sufficient knowledge and experience you will be able to make good

*Labor and Delivery Care: A Practical Guide*, First Edition. Wayne R. Cohen and Emanuel A. Friedman. © 2011 John Wiley & Sons, Ltd. Published 2011 by John Wiley & Sons, Ltd.

decisions to minimize both the need for cesarean delivery and the risk of harm during vaginal birth.

## Cephalopelvic relationships

In Chapter 4 we stressed the importance of carrying out a systematic assessment of the pelvis during labor in all women, and explained in detail how you should do it. We also emphasized that information about pelvic architecture is of value only when you consider it in conjunction with its effects on the mechanism of labor, the molding of the fetal head, and the dynamic aspects of fetal descent and rotation. In determining whether it is likely that the fetus will go safely through the pelvis, you will need to perform and reevaluate the results of clinical cephalopelvimetry periodically during the labor.

The history of previous labors is of great value, but it must be weighed carefully. The notion that if a woman previously delivered a 4000 g baby without difficulty, she will be able to do the same in a subsequent pregnancy is not always correct. Fetal weight is but one of many factors to be considered. A fetus of the same size as one that delivered easily in a prior pregnancy may be encumbered by a malposition or an abnormal presentation. By contrast, abnormal labors do not always recur. A woman may have had a serious dysfunctional labor previously, and yet have a normal pelvis that will present no difficulty in the present labor. Nevertheless, if certain events occurred in a prior pregnancy (shoulder dystocia, maternal or fetal birth trauma, or the need for midcavity forceps or vacuum extraction), be especially wary about their potential recurrence, especially if a dysfunctional labor pattern develops.

### The importance of fetal station

You can use the station of the fetal presenting part in early labor as a prognostic indicator in nulliparas. The common belief, however, that the fetal head of nulliparas should be fully engaged by the onset of labor at term is incorrect; it is often not. If you find the vertex is indeed fully engaged in early labor, you can anticipate vaginal delivery in almost all such patients. By contrast, if the head is floating well above the inlet when labor begins, a higher likelihood exists that cesarean delivery will eventually be necessary. Most often, the fetal head is dipping into the pelvis at labor onset, but the biparietal diameter has not yet traversed the brim of the true pelvis. The degree of engagement depends in part on the fetal head size and position as well as the shape and dimensions of the pelvic inlet. Equally or more important is the degree to which the cervix has ripened and the lower uterine segment has expanded. Without thinning and stretching of the lower uterus, the head will not be able to descend sufficiently to engage.

Pay attention to your patient's rectosigmoid colon and bladder. If either is full, engagement of the head can be hindered. However, routine enemas are unnecessary and uncomfortable. Routine catheterization of the bladder should also be avoided, so as to obviate the associated risk of infection.

Later in labor, fetal station becomes more important in predicting the need for cesarean delivery, particularly in nulliparas. If the vault of the pelvis is empty and the head is found to be floating in late active labor, the pelvis is probably considerably contracted. In multiparas, however, you will commonly find that the head will remain well above the inlet until the deceleration phase, and then descend rapidly. You can obtain some information about the capacity of the pelvis to accommodate further descent by using the Müller-Hillis maneuver (Chapter 4).

## Trial of labor

The term *trial of labor* is usually applied to situations in which the prognosis for normal delivery is guarded. The most common example is that of labor in women with a uterine scar from a prior cesarean. In one sense, however, every labor is a trial, because it is rarely possible to predict at labor's onset what mode of delivery will be best. Each labor, therefore, requires your complete attention and thorough evaluation.

In most situations in which you suspect that disproportion may exist between the fetal head and the maternal pelvis, you can safely permit labor to evolve long enough to see if atraumatic vaginal delivery is feasible. The exceptions are those cases in which there is an exceptionally large fetus or an uncommonly contracted or distorted pelvis.

As described in Chapter 3, normal labors follow well-defined curves when cervical dilatation and station are plotted against time. Accordingly, a degree of predictability exists because the dilatation and the descent curves can be projected forward in time (Fig. 5.1). In the phase of maximum slope for example, in which dilatation proceeds essentially in a linear fashion, you can simply project the line upward to identify the expected progress in dilatation, assuming that no inhibitory or accelerative factors are imposed on the labor.

For a labor that has entered the active phase under observation and in which you have defined the maximum slope by two or more observations within this phase, you can project the graphed dilatation line as a straight line extension to about 9 cm dilatation. By adding to this line a representation of the maximum duration of the deceleration phase (3 hours in nulliparas, 1 hour in multiparas), you can determine the latest time when the second stage should be expected to begin. You can use the projected curve effectively to define expected normal active phase progress in an individual labor.

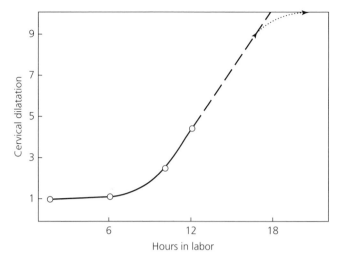

**Figure 5.1** Extrapolating the dilatation curve in the active phase by projecting the linear phase of maximum slope up to 9 cm. Deviations from this projection often signal problems in dilatation. By adding an appropriate duration for the deceleration phase, you can approximate when full cervical dilatation should occur.

## Identifying dysfunctional labor

The basis for defining normal labor in quantitative terms is the pictorial representation of the dilatation and descent patterns you create by graphing your observations of cervical dilatation and fetal station serially during the labor. Use the resulting curves to determine if the labor is progressing normally, or is characterized instead by some dysfunction.

To recognize abnormal patterns, you must have basic information about the nature of the patterns in the gravid population at large (Chapter 3). Normal ranges for the different component phases of the cervical dilatation and the fetal descent patterns were derived from measurements in large numbers of cases (Table 3.1). By convention, the 5% of the population that falls into the tail of the distribution curve for each aspect of labor is considered abnormal, analogous to how we define normal in most quantifiable medical evaluations. These cut-points logically define a subset of cases that warrant special clinical attention. These abnormal cases do not necessarily require active intervention for delivery, but rather astute evaluation and targeted management. In other words, using the labor curves provides you with an early warning system to identify labors at risk.

There are seven documentable dysfunctional labor patterns (Box 5.1; Fig. 5.2). These include those in which active cervical dilatation or fetal descent progresses linearly, but at a rate below the limit of normal (*protracted*

**Box 5.1 Classification of dysfunctional labor patterns**

- Disorders of dilatation
  - Prolonged latent phase
  - Protracted active phase
  - Arrest of dilatation
  - Prolonged deceleration phase
- Disorders of descent
  - Protracted descent
  - Arrest of descent
  - Failure of descent

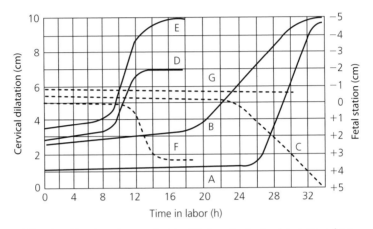

**Figure 5.2** Labor disorders that can be identified on the basis of deviations from the expected durations, slopes, and patterns of the dilatation and descent curves are illustrated graphically: **A**. prolonged latent phase; **B**. protracted active phase; **C**. protracted descent; **D**. arrest of dilatation; **E**. prolonged deceleration phase; **F**. arrest of descent; **G**. failure of descent. (Reproduced from Cohen WR and Friedman EA, in Kurjak A, Chervenak FA (eds) *Textbook of Perinatal Medicine,* 2nd edition. Informa UK, London, 2006, by permission.)

*active phase dilatation* and *protracted descent*); those in which progress in active phase dilatation or in descent begins, but then ceases (*arrest of dilatation, arrest of descent,* and *prolonged deceleration phase*), and those in which dilatation or descent does not accelerate normally into its active portion (*prolonged latent phase* and *failure of descent*). The diagnostic and therapeutic aspects of each kind of labor disorder are discussed below.

## Prolonged latent phase

When the latent phase lasts more than 20 hours in nulliparas or 14 hours in multiparas, it is considered prolonged. You will encounter a long latent phase most commonly when labor began with an unprepared cervix (i.e., one that was thick, uneffaced, and undilated). Sedation or anesthesia can also prolong the latent phase, which seems more sensitive to the inhibitory effects of drugs than does later labor. When labor begins with an unripe cervix, the long latent phase is necessary to allow maturation of the cervix, thus preparing it for subsequent active dilatation.

Determining the length of the latent phase can be imprecise, because you cannot always ascertain the exact time of labor onset. The simple recognition of the fact that the latent phase may normally be quite long is very important; knowing its precise length is less critical. Ignorance about the normal course of the latent phase sometimes leads to unnecessary cesarean delivery, under the erroneous assumption that continuous progress should be expected in all portions of labor, or that very long labors are always abnormal. About 10% of patients with what seemed to be an abnormally long latent phase are later found to have been in false labor. When the contractions finally stop, that diagnosis is apparent in retrospect.

Patients with prolonged latent phase (Fig. 5.3) are often quite exhausted and emotionally discouraged. Such women may benefit from a significant period of rest, induced by the use of a narcotic agent such as meperidine given in sufficient amounts (usually 100–150 mg intramuscularly) to suspend labor temporarily. Morphine (10–15 mg intramuscularly) can also be used, but may increase the risk of neonatal respiratory depression. The effectiveness of this treatment is equivalent to the alternative of oxytocin stimulation to manage this disorder, 85% of labors responding with active dilatation. Patients given therapeutic rest generally do not progress to delivery during the interval in which the opioid is most active, and neonatal depression is unusual. Make certain that a narcotic antagonist is available to treat the newborn should delivery occur sooner than expected, and always be sure the pediatrician is aware that a narcotic was used.

If there is a compelling reason not to lengthen the labor of your patient with a prolonged latent phase, such as the presence of preeclampsia, prolonged rupture of membranes or chorioamnionitis, oxytocin stimulation is appropriate. In fact, in such situations it is reasonable to begin oxytocin in the latent phase even before the limit of normal has been reached, in the hope of shortening the overall length of labor. When there are no such complications, therapeutic rest tends to be a better option because of the frequency of unrecognized false labor in these patients and in consideration of their emotional and physical needs. Your patient should have a voice in this decision. Many women prefer to have their labor augmented; others welcome the interposition of rest into an arduous and stressful experience.

As noted, following rest therapy about 10% of women awaken out of labor, and 85% are in the active phase. In the remaining 5%, the original condition recurs; contractions are ineffective in producing dilatation.

Only in this residual group is oxytocin therapy required. It is usually effective in terminating the latent phase and producing normal active phase progression.

Amniotomy is not consistently effective in stimulating advancement into active phase when the latent phase is prolonged. We therefore advise you not to perform amniotomy in these cases in an attempt to augment labor progress. Delivery may not occur for many hours, and having ruptured membranes raises the likelihood of infection.

Prolongation of the latent phase enhances fetal and maternal morbidity and mortality. This adversity can probably be minimized if the disorder is handled expeditiously when the diagnosis is made. Moreover, although the prognosis for vaginal delivery is worsened somewhat by prolongation of the latent phase, there is no reason to resort to cesarean section as a primary therapy for it. The cesarean delivery rate is, nevertheless, significantly higher among labors complicated by prolongation of the latent phase. This is in part because obstetricians sometimes mistake a long and slowly progressive latent phase for an abnormally redolent active phase. The distinction can be difficult.

As a general guideline to help you in this regard, remember that, although dilatation can progress during the latent phase, it is very unusual for it to advance at rates greater than about 0.6 cm/h. A slope of dilatation above that value is most likely active phase. Also, it is uncommon for labor to be still in the latent phase once the cervix has reached 6 cm dilatation, especially among nulliparas. Remember, however, that some gravidas, mostly multiparas, achieve this degree of dilatation before labor begins. Therefore, merely finding advanced dilatation does not necessarily guarantee that the active phase is in progress. A prior prelabor or early labor observation of dilatation gives you the information you need to make this important differentiation.

Although in most cases a long latent phase will eventually evolve into a normal active phase, sometimes the subsequent active phase dilatation pattern is also abnormally slow. In such cases, prolongation of the latent phase was probably a consequence of the same dysfunctional process that hindered active phase progress. There is no way to determine clinically when a prolonged latent phase is the consequence of a pathologic process, or simply a necessary physiologic component of a long labor. Pathology is more likely present if the latent phase is prolonged in the presence of a ripened cervix or a small pelvis.

## Protraction and arrest disorders

Once cervical dilatation begins to accelerate, the active phase has been reached (Fig. 5.4), and steady progressive dilatation will occur thereafter until the cervix begins to retract around the fetal head, usually at

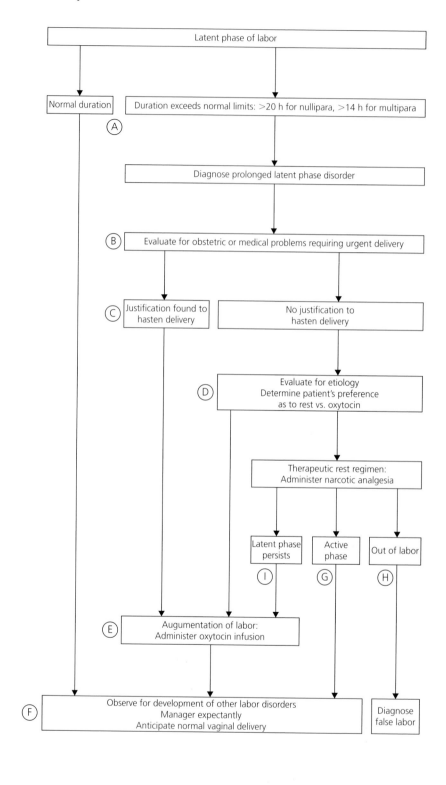

| Latent phase of labor |

Normal duration

Ⓐ   Duration exceeds normal limits: >20 h for nullipara, >14 h for multipara

Diagnose prolonged latent phase disorder

Ⓑ   Evaluate for obstetric or medical problems requiring urgent delivery

Ⓒ   Justification found to hasten delivery

No justification to hasten delivery

Ⓓ   Evaluate for etiology
Determine patient's preference
as to rest vs. oxytocin

Therapeutic rest regimen:
Administer narcotic analgesia

Latent phase persists

Active phase

Out of labor

Ⓘ   Ⓖ   Ⓗ

Ⓔ   Augumentation of labor:
Administer oxytocin infusion

Ⓕ   Observe for development of other labor disorders
Manager expectantly
Anticipate normal vaginal delivery

Diagnose false labor

8–9 cm of dilatation (Chapter 3). If dilatation advances linearly, but at a rate below the limit of normal (<1.2 cm/h in nulliparas; <1.5 cm/h in multiparas), you should diagnose a *protracted active phase*. If, once in the active phase, cervical dilatation ceases for two hours, diagnose an *arrest of dilatation*. A related abnormality is the *prolonged deceleration phase*, in which the deceleration phase exceeds 3 h in nulliparas or 1 h in multiparas. For practical purposes, you can use the time from 8 cm to complete dilatation to demarcate the deceleration phase.

There are analogous abnormalities of descent (Fig. 5.5). If fetal descent is progressive, but slower than the expected minimum (<1 station/h in nulliparas, each station representing a centimeter of progress; <2 stations/h

**Figure 5.3** Management of the latent phase of labor.

**A**. Time the latent phase from the onset of regular uterine contractions as perceived by the gravida until the upswing of the labor curve at the beginning of active phase dilatation. If the latent phase exceeds 20 h in a nullipara or 14 h in a multipara, diagnose prolonged latent phase.

**B**. Prolonged latent phase is not, by itself, an indication for active intervention. Evaluate to determine if there is any need for haste in effecting delivery, such as severe pregnancy-induced hypertension or chorioamnionitis.

**C**. If an indication exists for prompt delivery, augment labor with oxytocin, provided there are no contraindications to its use.

**D**. In the absence of any urgency to deliver, evaluate for any remediable cause of the prolonged latent phase, such as conduction anesthesia or heavy narcotic analgesia. These can inhibit the effectiveness of uterine contractions in the latent phase. Allow them to abate or counter their effect with oxytocin. If no cause is discernible, two options are available: augmentation with oxytocin or therapeutic rest with large doses of a narcotic analgesic. These latter agents will stop the contractions for a time and provide rest for the gravida. An important consideration in choosing between these options is the patient's preference.

**E**. Uterotonic stimulation is usually effective in propelling the labor into the active phase. It is less preferable than therapeutic rest because a proportion of cases (10%) are actually in false labor, even though they are not identifiable prospectively.

**F**. Although parturients with prolonged latent phase are not at increased risk of subsequent labor complications, they are not protected against them. Therefore, manage these patients expectantly with careful frequent reassessments for the development of other labor disorders. If none develops, anticipate a favorable outcome.

**G**. After gravidas awaken from the narcotic analgesic, most (85%) will be in the active phase of dilatation. Use of therapeutic rest helpfully serves to identify the gravida who is in false labor.

**H**. If her uterine contractions fail to resume after she awakens, it becomes clear by hindsight that the long period of contractions did not represent true labor at all. Without any overarching indication for intervention, no further care is required for her other than continued routine antepartum surveillance.

**I**. In a small fraction of women who have been managed with therapeutic rest (5%), ineffective uterine contractions resume when she awakens. She requires oxytocin augmentation at this point to effect transition to active phase. This is usually successful.

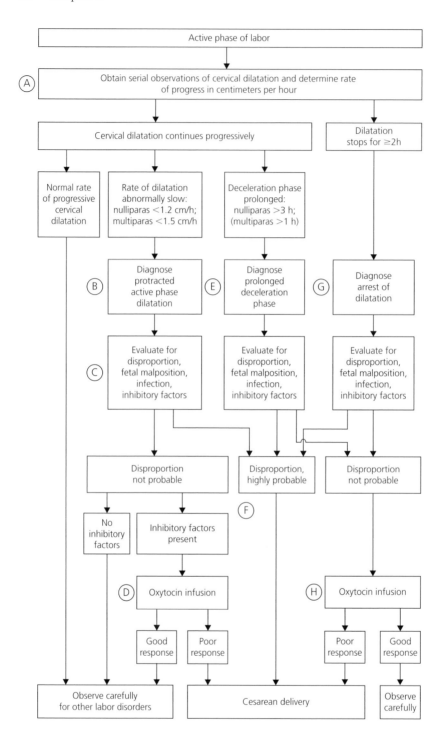

in multiparas), *protracted descent* is present. When descent has become linear, and then ceases for one hour, an *arrest of descent* has occurred. Another descent abnormality, *failure of descent*, is much less common, but very important because of its exceptionally strong association with disproportion. Diagnose failure of descent when you have observed no descent of the fetus from the latent phase through the deceleration phase or the beginning of the second stage. Table 5.1 lists the diagnostic criteria for dysfunctional labour patterns.

Although the underlying pathophysiology of arrest and protraction disorders is not known, they are all associated with one or more of several clinical

**Figure 5.4** Management of the active phase of labor.

**A**. Recognize when the labor has entered the active phase by noting the upswing of the cervical dilatation curve from the relatively flat line of the latent phase. With each subsequent evaluation of cervical dilatation, you can calculate the rate of dilatation in centimeters per hour.

**B**. If the rate of dilatation in a nullipara is less than 1.2 cm/h, or in a multipara less than 1.5 cm/h, diagnose the dysfunctional labor pattern of protracted active phase dilatation.

**C**. Evaluations for underlying predisposing factors are critical to management. The most important issue is to determine if disproportion is likely by undertaking detailed cephalopelvimetry. If findings show that disproportion is highly probable, proceed with cesarean delivery.

**D**. If disproportion is unlikely, the effects of inhibitory factors (such as excessive sedative-analgesic agents or high level of epidural anesthesia) can sometimes be overcome by the use of oxytocin. A good response in the form of more rapid dilatation indicates the likelihood of a successful vaginal delivery, whereas a poor response suggests that cesarean delivery is more appropriate.

**E**. Prolonged deceleration phase, in which the deceleration phase exceeds 3 h in nulliparas or 1 h in multiparas, is even more likely to be associated with cephalopelvic disproportion than protracted dilatation. Therefore, your first objective when you have diagnosed prolonged deceleration phase is to determine if there is likely to be disproportion present.

**F**. If the probability of cephalopelvic disproportion is high in the presence of a major labor disorder, such as a protraction of an arrest pattern, it is prudent to undertake cesarean delivery as the safest option for both mother and fetus.

**G**. Arrest of dilatation can be diagnosed in a labor that has entered the active phase by encountering cessation of dilatation for 2 h or more. This is one of the most serious of the labor dysfunctions because of its high frequency of association with cephalopelvic disproportion. As a consequence, do a thorough assessment of the cephalopelvic relation by cephalopelvimetry. If disproportion is highly probable, proceed without delay to cesarean delivery.

**H**. If you are able to show that disproportion is unlikely, oxytocin augmentation of uterine contractions should be done instead. After the dilatation process is reestablished, compare the postarrest slope of dilatation with the prearrest slope to help prognosticate: A postarrest slope slower than the antecedent pre-arrest rate is an ominous sign indicating that safe vaginal delivery will probably not be feasible. This finding warrants cesarean delivery. If the postarrest slope of dilatation is the same as (or faster than) the prearrest slope, the outlook is usually quite favorable.

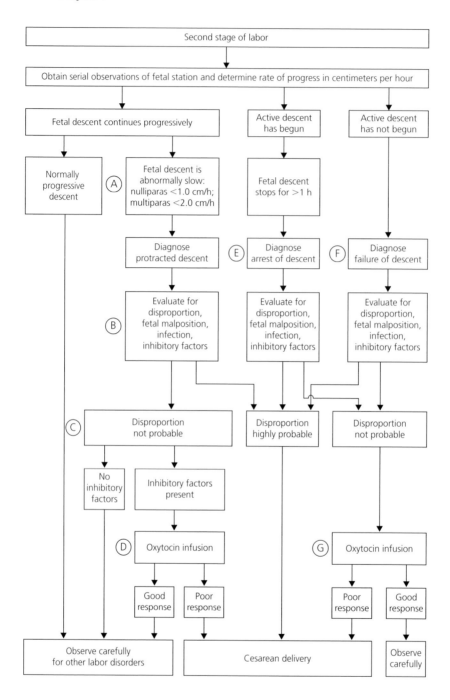

Second stage of labor

Obtain serial observations of fetal station and determine rate of progress in centimeters per hour

Fetal descent continues progressively

Active descent has begun

Active descent has not begun

Normally progressive descent

(A) Fetal descent is abnormally slow: nulliparas <1.0 cm/h; multiparas <2.0 cm/h

Fetal descent stops for >1 h

Diagnose protracted descent

(E) Diagnose arrest of descent

(F) Diagnose failure of descent

(B) Evaluate for disproportion, fetal malposition, infection, inhibitory factors

Evaluate for disproportion, fetal malposition, infection, inhibitory factors

Evaluate for disproportion, fetal malposition, infection, inhibitory factors

(C) Disproportion not probable

Disproportion highly probable

Disproportion not probable

No inhibitory factors

Inhibitory factors present

(D) Oxytocin infusion

(G) Oxytocin infusion

Good response

Poor response

Poor response

Good response

Observe carefully for other labor disorders

Cesarean delivery

Observe carefully

features (Box 5.2). Several of these factors probably exert their effects through impairment of uterine contractility (e.g., infection, excess analgesia, advanced maternal age, and obesity), and can therefore potentially be overcome with oxytocin therapy. In others (e.g., cephalopelvic disproportion) unwarranted uterotonic treatment might endanger the fetus.

The most common cause of protraction and arrest abnormalities is cephalopelvic disproportion. It is present in at least 25–30% of protraction and 40–50% of arrest disorders. The probability of associated disproportion varies according to circumstances. For example, when a failure of descent

**Figure 5.5** Management of the second stage of labor.

**A**. Evaluation of the rate of fetal descent is based on serial observations of fetal station, measured in centimeters above (minus values) or below (positive values) the plane of the ischial spines (station zero). For each pair of such observations, divide the change in station by the time it took for that change to take place. Once descent begins in late first stage (the deceleration phase) or in second stage, the rate of descent should normally be at least 1.0 cm/h in nulliparas or 2.0 cm/h in multiparas. If less, diagnose protracted descent, a disorder comparable to protracted dilatation because of its frequent association with disproportion.

**B**. Do detailed cephalopelvimetry to determine whether or not disproportion is likely to be present. If disproportion is highly probable based on the combination of protracted descent and the findings from this examination, cesarean delivery is justified.

**C**. In the absence of supportive clinical evidence of disproportion, investigate for inhibitory factors. If none is found, there is no benefit to administering an ecbolic agent because it is unlikely to change the rate of descent. Allowing the labor to continue is better. Given additional time in labor, there will usually be further progression in descent at the same languid rate. If allowed to continue long enough, the labor can be expected to result eventually in a safe vaginal delivery. In this regard, it is important to resist the temptation to intervene without a clear-cut indication. Some of these labors, however, may later become arrested. If that occurs, manage it in the same manner as an arrest of descent that arises de novo (see E, below).

**D**. Evaluation may reveal factors that inhibit labor progression, such as excessive analgesia or high conduction block. Allowing inhibitory conditions to abate may reestablish a more normal rate of descent. Alternatively, stimulate the uterus with oxytocin. While enhancing uterine contractility in the presence of a protracted descent pattern can seldom actually improve the rate of progress, it may sometimes do so. If there is no improvement, but it is urgent to effect delivery, consider cesarean delivery.

**E**. After active descent begins toward the end of the first stage or in the second stage of labor, you can expect uninterrupted descent to continue until the fetal head reaches the perineum. If descent stops for more than one hour, diagnose arrest of descent and evaluate for disproportion with cephalopelvimetry. If you find disproportion is likely to be present, undertake cesarean delivery.

**F**. If active descent fails to begin when it ordinarily does by the time the labor enters the second stage, diagnose failure of descent. Like arrest of descent, this pattern is commonly associated with disproportion. Carry out objective cephalopelvimetry.

**G**. If you find evidence of disproportion, proceed with cesarean delivery; if not, enhancing uterine contractions by oxytocin infusion may prove beneficial.

**Table 5.1** Diagnostic criteria for dysfunctional labor patterns

| Labor dysfunction | Nulliparas* | Multiparas |
|---|---|---|
| Prolonged latent phase | >20 h duration | >14 h duration |
| Protracted active phase | <1.2 cm/h active phase slope | <1.5 cm/h slope |
| Arrest of dilatation | 2 h without progress in active phase | 2 h without progress in active phase |
| Prolonged deceleration phase | >3 h duration | >1 h duration |
| Protracted descent | <1.0 cm/h slope | <2.0 cm/h slope |
| Arrest of descent | 1 h without progress after active descent has begun | 1 h without progress after active descent has begun |
| Failure of descent | No descent by deceleration phase or second stage onset | No descent by deceleration phase or second stage onset |

*Includes multiparous women who have never had a vaginal delivery

---

### Box 5.2 Factors associated with arrest and protraction disorders

- Cephalopelvic disproportion
- Fetal malposition
- Fetal malpresentation
- Infection (deciduitis or myometritis)
- Excess analgesia or anesthesia
- Maternal obesity
- Advanced maternal age
- Previous cesarean delivery
- Insufficient uterine contractility

---

occurs in the presence of oxytocin stimulation, the likelihood of a safe vaginal delivery is very low, probably less than 10%. An arrest of dilatation that develops in a morbidly obese woman with a capacious pelvis and average estimated fetal weight is much less likely to require cesarean delivery. When your clinical cephalopelvimetry (Chapter 4) identifies features consistent with a high probability of disproportion in the presence of any active phase or second stage abnormality, cesarean delivery is the safest approach.

### Diagnosing disproportion

*Cephalopelvic disproportion* is easier for the clinician to define than to identify. As a concept, it refers to a situation in which the potential for atraumatic vaginal delivery is negligible, owing to a mismatch between the size of the presenting part and the capacity of the pelvis. Unfortunately, there is no single clinical assessment or laboratory test that is highly specific for the diagnosis. Rather, the probability of disproportion is determined from the aggregate of clinical findings. Accurate diagnosis requires experience, keen observation, and good judgment.

Skillful cephalopelvimetry (Chapter 4) is the key to identifying labors in which disproportion is unlikely. If that is the case, then oxytocin stimulation, or simply allowing more time in labor, is appropriate. For example, an arrest of dilatation in which the engaged fetal head is in an occiput anterior position and well flexed, there is minimal cranial molding and caput formation, the estimated fetal weight is not excessive, and the pelvic architecture is favorable collectively suggests disproportion is unlikely. Another cause for the arrest should be sought. By contrast, if examination reveals an unengaged head with marked cranial molding and a small pelvis, disproportion is likely. The association of probable bony disproportion and arrest of dilatation or descent constitutes a significant warning. Patients with this combination warrant cesarean delivery as the safest and most conservative approach.

Patients frequently present with an arrest of dilatation pattern as the first sign of disproportion. Under these circumstances, you can use the pattern of dilatation as a prognostic index. If the arrest was preceded by a protraction abnormality, disproportion is more likely than if the preceding active phase was normal. Remember, however, that most labors with arrest or protraction disorders can end with a safe vaginal delivery, and you need to develop the ability to recognize those cases.

It is easy to understand why descent disorders can signal the presence of disproportion. If descent of the fetus is mechanically impeded by the pelvis, a protracted descent or an arrest of descent would result during the second stage of labor. Why dilatational abnormalities are so closely associated with disproportion is less obvious, because these labor dysfunctions are diagnosed prior to the time when the fetus is actively descending through the birth canal. While it is tempting to assume that dilatational disorders are purely the result of inadequate uterine contractility, that is probably not often so. Some arrest or protraction abnormalities occur despite strong uterine contractions, and empiric observations strongly suggest that arrest and protraction disorders of dilatation are associated with disproportion. Whether the uterus somehow "recognizes" disproportion and responds with diminished contractility to protect itself and the fetus is a tantalizing hypothesis that so far lacks confirmation. What is important for you to remember is that any protraction or descent disorder may be a manifestation of disproportion that is not safely surmountable, and requires your careful evaluation.

## Treatment

You should not institute any therapy for arrest or protraction disorders before you adequately investigate the fetopelvic relationships. If you find that disproportion is not likely present in a patient with arrest of dilatation or descent, treatment can then be chosen according to the existing circumstances.

If an arrest of dilatation has resulted from excessive sedation or anesthesia, expectancy alone may suffice while the effects of the drugs are allowed to dissipate; alternatively, the inhibitory effects of drugs can usually be counteracted by oxytocin. In the occasional patient who is thoroughly exhausted, providing parenteral analgesia or, preferably, epidural anesthesia, may allow her some rest and respite from pain. In the remaining patients, as well as in those who have had adequate rest but who have failed to reinstitute labor spontaneously, stimulation with oxytocin infusion should be undertaken, barring contraindications. Most patients respond well to such stimulation as primary therapy if it is administered cautiously and in sufficient doses to stimulate normal active phase labor.

Most arrest disorders will respond to oxytocin with additional progress in dilatation or descent within four hours, and it is rarely necessary to administer the drug for longer than this. Exceptionally, you might continue the oxytocin if you are convinced that disproportion is quite unlikely, and some inhibitory factor (say, excessively high level of neuraxial anesthesia) requires more time to abate. In other situations, you can make a decision to perform a cesarean delivery before four hours have elapsed if new evidence of disproportion develops.

If you graph the labor progress carefully, you can determine the prognosis by comparing the rate of progression in dilatation or descent that existed prior to the arrest with the rate that occurs after you begin oxytocin therapy. Delivery prognosis improves with the increment in slope. The more rapid the postarrest slope, the more likely that delivery can be vaginal.

If, after 2–4 hours of oxytocin stimulation with a good contractile pattern, there has been no further dlatation, the chance of vaginal delivery is very small. If progress in dilatation has occurred, but with a slope lower than that prior to the arrest, the likelihood of safe vaginal delivery is also minimal. In both circumstances, cesarean delivery is appropriate. If, however, the postarrest slope is the same or better than the prearrest rate of progress, the prospect for a vaginal delivery is much better, and you should allow the labor to continue while you observe for the development of other labor disorders.

Many obstetricians perform artificial rupture of the membranes when faced with an arrest disorder, although there is no objective proof that it is a useful treatment. You may want to rupture the membranes for other reasons, such as to facilitate internal fetal monitoring or to evaluate the amniotic fluid; but while amniotomy seems occasionally to be effective in treating an arrest disorder, it is not reliably so. If patients do respond with further dilatation, they do so promptly. Thus, there is no reason to wait more than one hour to determine if amniotomy has affected labor progress. We do not generally recommend amniotomy purely for the purpose of treating an arrest disorder.

Although, as noted, protraction and arrest disorders are associated with the same pathogenetic factors (Box 5.2), the treatment of protracted active phase or protracted descent differs somewhat from that of the corresponding arrest disorders. Contrary to common expectation, the treatment of protraction disorders with oxytocin when they arise de novo is uniformly ineffectual. That is to say, protraction disorders do not respond with more rapid dilatation or descent to uterotonic stimulation or artificial rupture of membranes. The exception is when an inhibitory factor is present. Labor progress in protraction disorders is quite sensitive to the inhibitory effects of sedation or regional block anesthesia, and when a protraction abnormality seems to have developed in response to their use, oxytocin is appropriate if you and the patient would rather not allow the anesthesia to abate. The same may be true in cases of intrauterine infection, maternal obesity, or a malposition if you are reasonably certain that disproportion is not present.

If you find evidence of bony disproportion in a patient with a protraction abnormality, you can justifiably elect cesarean section. Doing so avoids subjecting mother and fetus to a long tedious labor with the risk of ascending infection and potential injury.

If a protracted labor is allowed to proceed, support is essential to provide for the parturient's emotional and physical needs, because these labors are grueling and strenuous. Expect continued progress if patients with a protraction disorder are properly managed conservatively, and disproportion is absent. The prognosis remains good as long as progress continues. The risks to mother or fetus from these conditions appear to be only slightly increased, provided that no ill-advised measures for uterotonic stimulation or, even more important, for potentially traumatic instrumental delivery are undertaken.

If your patient with a protraction disorder develops a further complication in the form of arrest of dilatation, prolonged deceleration phase, or arrest of descent, the outlook becomes considerably worse. Here fetal risks increase substantially, making cesarean delivery advisable. The risk to the fetus in protraction disorders is primarily related to the type of delivery utilized. Midforceps procedures are especially hazardous. Conservative management must be employed to optimum advantage in these cases. If spontaneous delivery is not feasible, limit vaginal delivery techniques to gentle outlet vacuum or forceps procedures, although even these can sometimes cause harm after a protracted descent. Patience and watchfulness are preferable.

Protracted descent is often accompanied by considerable cranial molding and overlying caput succedaneum formation. Sometimes the fetal scalp can be seen parting the labia during a contraction, while the biparietal diameter of the elongated head remains above the inlet. Do not succumb to the temptation to do an operative vaginal delivery without demonstrating that the head is completely engaged and that the skull has reached the pelvic floor. Conversely, do not be deluded into thinking that progress in descent is occurring just because the scalp steadily approaches the introitus. Allowing labor to continue when descent is obstructed can result in fetal harm.

## Prolonged deceleration phase

The terminal portion of dilatation, when the cervix makes its journey around the edges of the fetal head and retracts beyond its widest diameter, is a period of great importance. Unfortunately, its significance is often overlooked on the assumption that, if the cervix has reached near-complete dilatation, it will surely finish that task. Worse, impatient practitioners sometimes push a lingering rim or anterior lip of cervix over the fetal head to force full cervical dilatation artificially. You must avoid doing this. Rather, ask yourself why the cervix is lingering, and address the root of the problem. By this we mean that you must recognize that cephalopelvic disproportion is a common cause of the problem, evaluate for it, and if you find it, proceed with cesarean delivery. If the cephalopelvic relations are satisfactory, allow labor to continue to evolve with additional time or, if urgency dictates, carefully supplement uterine contractility with oxytocin.

The deceleration phase is important because the terminal events of dilatation will usually not occur unless some fetal descent is also taking place. Thus, attainment of complete dilatation is an important milestone in descent. Any delay in the initiation of descent at this point in labor is frequently associated with cephalopelvic disproportion, abnormalities of the second stage, and difficult shoulder delivery.

A prolonged deceleration phase has the same associations and etiologies as arrest and protraction disorders, and is treated in much the same manner. It is of particular importance because of its strong association with disproportion, as well as with shoulder dystocia if vaginal delivery occurs. It is a harbinger of second stage labor dysfunction, and is frequently accompanied by failure of descent. The combination of prolonged deceleration phase with any disorder of fetal descent makes safe vaginal delivery very unlikely.

## Combined labor dysfunctions

Some patients will manifest more than one labor dysfunction. With each successive active phase or second stage abnormality, the likelihood of an uncomplicated vaginal birth diminishes. If serial labor dysfunctions arise in the presence of oxytocin stimulation, atraumatic vaginal delivery is even less likely than when they occur de novo.

## Precipitate labor

An abnormally fast, tumultuous labor in which cervical dilatation occurs quickly and descent of the presenting part is rapid is called *precipitate labor*. It has been variously defined according to length as a labor of two to four hours. A better approach is to consider the rate of cervical dilatation in the active phase or of fetal descent during the second stage. This perspective disregards the latent phase, which may or may not be short, and concentrates on unusually rapid dilatation and descent. Using this approach, when cervical dilatation or fetal descent is greater than 5 cm/h in nulliparas or 10 cm/h in multiparas, you can diagnose *precipitate dilatation* or *precipitate descent*. This is an objective clinical entity and can be identified graphically. Etiologic factors are not clearly defined, but precipitate labor may occur even in the presence of heavy sedation, relative bony disproportion, and minor malpositions. It can sometimes be a factor in the development of shoulder dystocia.

Precipitate labor presumably results from uterine contractions that occur too frequently and too intensely in conjunction with negligible resistance of maternal soft parts. When precipitate labor occurs spontaneously, it is generally unpredictable and unpreventable. Excessive oxytocin administration is an iatrogenic cause.

Precipitate labor may be injurious to both mother and baby. It is often associated with fetal bradycardia, presumably from head compression during rapid descent, meconium passage, and birth canal trauma. Fetal injury, in the form of brachial plexus palsy or, in rare cases, intracranial bleeding, can occur.

Under no circumstances should you forcibly attempt to hold the head back during a precipitate delivery, because you may cause serious injury to mother or fetus. The most you can do is try to control the expulsion of the fetus, making sure the head extends as it crosses the perineum. Thoroughly examine the birth canal after delivery to detect and then repair injuries to uterus, cervix, vagina or perineum that commonly result.

## Effects on the fetus

All the labor dysfunctions we have described are associated with increased perinatal morbidity in comparison to normal labors. Much of this adversity is related to the type of delivery that is undertaken. The near disappearance of complex forceps operations has done much to improve outcome. Nevertheless, even when such delivery hazards are taken into consideration, excess morbidity persists. On this basis, dysfunctional labor must be considered inherently deleterious to the fetus.

Your response to this concern is not to avoid abnormal labor by undertaking cesarean delivery on everyone prior to labor. That would simply exchange one set of risks for another, arguably more serious, set of dangers.

Prompt diagnosis followed by timely and prudent evaluation and treatment are the keys to minimizing risk. For example, if an arrest of dilatation is identified promptly, disproportion is ruled out, and then oxytocin is given, the vast majority of fetuses will suffer no adverse effects, even if there is a poor response to the drug after a few hours and a cesarean delivery is required. If, however, an arrest disorder is not diagnosed until it has persisted for many hours, or if oxytocin is administered for too long, the fetus will be at risk of serious harm.

Unfortunately, we do not know the answers to some pertinent questions. What makes some fetuses vulnerable to the adverse effects of abnormal labor? Will intrapartum cesarean delivery negate those effects? How closely are the hazards of a labor disorder related to the timeliness of diagnosis and treatment?

These issues need to be addressed in a contemporary population. In the absence of definitive studies, we must practice with the best information available. With that perspective in mind, we can draw several conclusions:

- It is important to follow labor progress using a graphic approach, because this is the best way to identify deviations from normal as early as possible. Delay in diagnosis is probably detrimental to the fetus.
- Once a dysfunction is discovered, do a thorough analysis to determine the likely etiology and assess the probability that cephalopelvic disproportion is present.
- If you find strong evidence of disproportion, consider prompt cesarean delivery. Continuing labor in this situation may expose the fetus to further hazard.
- If disproportion is unlikely, give oxytocin if the disorder is one that can respond to it, such as one of the arrest disorders (but not a protraction disorder).
- Monitor oxytocin use to avoid producing excess contractility. Simultaneously follow progress in dilatation or descent. Once it is clear that oxytocin is not effective, usually requiring a trial of about four hours, discontinue it and proceed to cesarean delivery.
- Avoid operative vaginal delivery whenever possible in the presence of dysfunctional labor patterns.

## Oxytocin and uterine activity

Uterine contractions are obviously a prerequisite for labor and vaginal delivery to occur. While we know a great deal about the physiology and biochemistry of myometrial smooth muscle contraction, the precise manner in which the uterus generates the optimally timed and coordinated bursts of contractile energy that first dilate the cervix and then propel the fetus through the birth canal is little understood.

There is an impressively large range of contractility patterns (based on the frequency, duration, and amplitude of contractions) in normal labor. Not surprisingly then, using contraction pattern characteristics to distinguish normal from abnormal labor is, for the most part, a futile exercise. This may be in part because none of the techniques we use to measure contractions during labor (manual palpation, surface tocodynamometry, and intrauterine pressure transducer) provide a means to judge the overall efficiency of contractility in effecting change in dilatation or descent.

Some classifications of abnormal labor are based on the presence of "inadequate" uterine activity. In clinical practice, this approach is difficult to apply and the distinctions between adequate and inadequate contractility are not always clear. Unless normal labor and its limits can be defined objectively, as described in Chapter 3, the diagnosis of an abnormality is at best nebulous. It is a rather difficult matter to study labor in detail and to analyze it critically because of the dynamic nature of the several changes that take place simultaneously. The simple, clinically applicable, and objective method of graphic evaluation is most useful in this regard.

The goal of oxytocin therapy for dysfunctional labor is to produce regular, strong uterine contractions that recur at intervals of 2–3 minutes, with a maximum of five contractions in a 10-minute interval. If the patient is having spontaneous strong contractions at this frequency, further uterotonic stimulation is generally unacceptable.

Several models for oxytocin infusion are in common use (Chapter 10). We recommend starting most cases with a low-dose approach. Begin the infusion at 1 mU/min, and increase the dose by 1–2 mU/min every 20–30 minutes until the uterus is contracting at the desired intensity and spacing. Occasionally, a patient will need higher doses at more frequent intervals to achieve an increase in contraction frequency.

Some obstetricians prefer to use a device to monitor intrauterine pressure continuously during oxytocin administration. This approach has some virtues. It is useful when tocodynamometry does not provide a clear contraction profile, as is often the case in obese women. Also, it can detect increases in baseline tone, which frequently precede development of excess contraction amplitude or frequency. There is no compelling evidence, however, to suggest that this is a better approach than external monitoring of contractions. In fact, transabdominal palpation of the uterus is usually sufficient to determine if the contractions are strong, and if there is relaxation of the uterus between them.

Intrauterine pressure measurements make it possible to quantitate uterine activity using Montevideo units or similar measures. While it may seem appealing to use this kind of objective approach to define the adequacy of spontaneous or oxytocin-stimulated contractions, its value is not established, and dubious. Moreover, use of the intrauterine transducer is not without risk, particularly with regard to increased infections.

## Second stage problems

The second stage encompasses most of the process of fetal descent and culminates in the thrilling and dramatic events of delivery. The rate at which the fetus descends through the birth canal is influenced by several factors, including uterine contractile force, voluntary maternal expulsive efforts, fetal size, position and attitude, pelvic architecture, and, terminally, by the configuration and tone of the pelvic floor.

You must pay scrupulous attention to the progress of descent if you are to make the most appropriate judgments about the need for intervention during the second stage. Integrate the observations of the progress of fetal descent that you record on the labor graph with your assessment of other clinical events. Development of progressive molding of the cranial bones, inadequate rotation, malposition, and other abnormalities distinguishable by examination are equally important and must be considered in the assessment of each labor.

## Duration

An issue of critical importance concerns the appropriate duration of the second stage. In fact, most controversies regarding this aspect of labor relate directly or indirectly to notions regarding acceptable time limits for the second stage. Decisions to use oxytocin, instrumental delivery, and episiotomy, and to accept alternative maternal postures or bearing-down techniques depend on the perceived (often erroneously) need to shorten the second stage.

Opinions about the propriety of a long second stage vary considerably, and derive from considerations of both maternal and fetal safety. In fact duration, per se, of the second stage has little influence on neonatal outcome. This applies to second stages of at least three hours, and probably of longer duration, provided that the slope of descent is normal and that there is no evidence of fetal oxygen deprivation.

Using the rate of descent to judge the normality of the second stage is a more rational tactic than is relying on somewhat arbitrary time limits. The assessment of descent is, however, difficult and requires you to employ good physical examination skills. A long second stage may be of no consequence to the fetus or mother if the rate of descent is normal, cranial molding is not excessive, and fetal position is appropriate to the pelvic shape. By contrast, a second stage of even one hour might confer risk in a situation where there is a failure of descent and clinical suspicion of disproportion, because dysfunctional descent patterns are associated with increased neonatal morbidity. There is no virtue, and some risk, in allowing a labor to continue once you have established that the chance of a safe vaginal delivery is small.

Although, as noted, most studies have not found a strong relation between neonatal morbidity and length of the second stage, that observation has been misinterpreted by some to imply that it never matters how long the second stage lasts. This unfortunate inference has resulted in justification of extraordinarily long second stages, sometimes to the detriment of mother and baby.

A decision to terminate labor during the second stage should be based on a careful evaluation of maternal and fetal condition and of progress in descent, not on the passage of an absolute amount of time. Some fetuses may descend at a normal rate and take several hours to deliver, and to subject such patients to potentially traumatic operative procedures merely because they have not delivered within two hours after the second stage has begun should be decried. A long second stage, however, should not be ignored. On the contrary, it may signify an important labor disorder that must be evaluated. Your neglecting to diagnose and treat abnormal descent can have serious consequences.

### Bearing-down styles

The second stage is often managed in "cheerleader" style. The mother is encouraged to bear down with contractions as soon as the cervix becomes fully dilated. She is urged to push with sustained Valsalva maneuvers, during which she is exhorted to progressively greater feats of strength and endurance by a cacophony of cheers and approbations from everyone in the room.

Adverse effects of prolonged pushing on fetal acid–base balance have been reported. Nevertheless, most women deliver normally oxygenated fetuses even if they have been pushing in the traditional manner for prolonged periods. Occasionally, animated and heroic bearing-down efforts do seem necessary to effect spontaneous vaginal delivery.

A more restrained approach to the second stage involves the mother pushing only when she feels an overwhelming urge to do so. This may coincide with full cervical dilatation, but in some labors the need to push is delayed until some descent has occurred without maternal efforts. This is logical, given that the bearing-down reflex is stimulated when the descending fetal head stretches the vagina and perineum. Bearing-down activity need not occupy the entire contraction, and can even be exerted with a partially open glottis. Moreover, it is not always necessary to bear down with every contraction, and some women may benefit from an occasional respite from the energy-consuming efforts to expel the fetus.

Either pushing style is reasonable and safe for most women. Exceptions are those situations in which there is a maternal medical indication to avoid the dramatic fluctuations in blood pressure that accompany the Valsalva maneuver, or cases in which fetal oxygenation is compromised. Whether pushing technique influences the risk of pelvic floor injury is not known. It seems logical that an unhurried gradual descent would be kinder to the pelvic floor tissues than would an unrestrained sprint to delivery. In this regard, the widespread use of epidural anesthesia may have some benefits, in that it tends to make descent more gradual.

Intermittent, delayed, or energy-conserving pushing efforts may result in a longer second stage, but this should not generally be a concern. The choice of pushing methods in a normal pregnancy should depend on the preference of the patient and, to a lesser extent, her caretakers.

## Maternal posture

Disagreement exists about whether maternal position influences the efficiency and comfort of the second stage. Women in many cultures have used some variation of upright posture (standing, sitting, or squatting) during childbirth, but upright postures have been generally eschewed by Western obstetrics. Most deliveries today are done with the mother sitting semi-upright on a specially designed labor and delivery bed. Her back is buttressed, and her feet pressed against supports that allow her to have her hips and knees partially flexed. This is comfortable for most women, and is much preferred to the dorsal lithotomy position that was popular for many years. In fact, dorsal lithotomy position is best avoided entirely because it is recognized to be potentially hazardous to mother and fetus as the consequence of supine hypotension.

Some patients and practitioners prefer delivery in the lateral recumbent position, which works nicely. So does almost any other posture, including squatting, sitting, or the hands and knees position. As long as the mother is content and the labor is progressing normally, it makes little difference what her position is, and she should be encouraged to assume the position in which she feels most composed and comfortable in coping with her contractions. The presence of an epidural anesthetic will, of necessity, limit the parturient's options if she has some motor blockade.

Under most circumstances, maternal position probably has little influence on labor. There are, however, data to support the notion that variants of upright posture, including sitting and squatting, may optimize descent in the second stage by enlarging some pelvic diameters and maximizing the efficiency of voluntary bearing-down efforts. We know of no adverse implications of upright positions and they should probably be encouraged during the pelvic division of labor (deceleration phase and second stage), particularly if abnormal descent is present or anticipated. Upright or lateral positions may also be valuable in the prevention or resolution of shoulder dystocia (Chapter 13).

## Pain management during labor

Labor is a painful process, and all women can benefit from pain-reduction techniques to help them manage the experience. The amount of pain your patient perceives depends on many factors, including her parity, the speed of dilatation and descent, psychological factors, fatigue, and her personal pain threshold. Pain relief can be obtained from nonpharmacologic techniques or from the use of various medications.

Regardless of what your patient desires in this regard, two things will ease her way through labor: knowledge and emotional support. Each patient should have some form of childbirth education, especially during her first pregnancy. Knowledge about what to expect during labor serves to reduce anxiety and fear, both of which can increase the need for analgesia or sedation. The presence of a supportive partner during labor is quite advantageous for the same reason. Most important is your expressed support of her choice of pain relief, and your encouraging and sympathetic presence during her labor.

Nonpharmacologic approaches to labor pain, termed psychoprophylactic techniques, work remarkably well for many women. These use various relaxation, focusing, and breathing techniques to help the parturient cope with the pain. They have the obvious advantage of not exposing mother or fetus to the potentially adverse effects of medications. Psychoprophylactic techniques do not, however, always suffice. If so, patients may benefit from parenteral medication or conduction anesthesia.

Narcotic and sedative drugs can be used to assist in coping with pain. Meperidine is used commonly, although opioid agonist-antagonist drugs like nalbuphine or butorphanol cause less nausea and respiratory depression. Fentanyl has become popular recently. It has a relatively short duration of action and relatively little sedation and respiratory depression compared to meperidine. Neonatal respiratory depression is possible after use of any opioid, and naloxone should always be available for treatment of a depressed neonate.

The opioids in general provide only moderate pain relief during labor but, used properly, can work well for patients who need an adjunct to their psychoprophylactic techniques, or for those who do not want (or, for medical reasons, cannot have) epidural block.

Epidural anesthesia provides the most complete relief of labor pain, and is the best option for women who desire medical analgesia during labor. Pain signals during the first stage are carried in sensory fibers of the paracervical and inferior hypogastric plexuses. These fibers join the lumbar sympathetic chain at L2–3, and enter the spinal cord via the lower thoracic nerve roots (T10–12). Cutaneous nerves from these roots innervate the skin of the lower back. That is why some patients feel the pain from contractions referred to their lumbosacral region.

The most commonly used epidural anesthetic agents are bupivacaine and ropivacaine. This combination, properly administered, gives a strong sensory block with relatively little motor inhibition. Sometimes one of these drugs is combined with an opioid such as fentanyl or sufentanyl. This approach further diminishes motor blockade and reduces the amount of anesthetic required. The combination of drugs gives good pain relief and causes less hypotension and less shivering than when anesthetic drugs are used alone for an epidural block.

Various other approaches to conduction anesthesia have been used, including combined spinal and epidural block, and patient-controlled epidural infusions, each of which works well in experienced hands. Epidural anesthesia is, of course, not risk-free. The anesthesia can sometimes be inadequate or spotty; hypotension (generally manageable with ephedrine and volume expansion) occurs in some patients, and pruritis (if an opioid is used) is not uncommon. Headaches from dural puncture in combined spinal/epidural techniques, or from accidental dural entry during epidural placement, and low-grade fever also occur. Fortunately, severe side effects are quite rare. These include high spinal block if the epidural catheter is actually in the subarachnoid space, epidural hematoma or abscess, and nerve toxicity.

The most germane question to pose about epidural block anesthesia in its various forms is whether it affects the course of labor. The summary answer is that a properly administered block (one that achieves no higher than a T10 level of analgesia using dilute solutions of anesthetic drugs) will have little or no perceptible effect on the course of normal active phase labor. The second stage and deceleration phase, however, will tend to be lengthened.

If anesthesia extends above the tenth thoracic dermatome level, inhibition of labor is more likely. Many obstetric services have reported enhanced instrumental delivery and cesarean section rates among parturients with epidural anesthesia, but this has not been a universal finding. Moreover, operative delivery under these circumstances is often done without clear-cut justification, i.e., with no obstetric indication other than the desire to hasten delivery. If the anesthetic is properly administered and the labor intelligently managed, epidural block anesthesia need not increase the incidence of operative delivery.

Neuraxial blocks have the potential to retard progress in the latent phase. For that reason, you should ideally institute epidural anesthesia early in the active phase. You can, however, certainly use it in the latent phase if your patient is having difficulty coping with her labor. Be aware that you might thereby prolong the latent phase, and need to consider oxytocin administration to overcome the inhibitory effects of the analgesia.

Similarly, excessively high epidural blocks can probably cause protraction and arrest disorders. Even appropriate anesthetic levels have a propensity to inhibit progress in abnormal labors, further slowing a protracted active phase or converting it to an arrest of dilatation. These inhibitory effects may be more pronounced in the second stage, when motor block reduces the mother's bearing-down power in addition to affecting contractility. These consequences can usually be overcome with oxytocin.

Some practitioners allow epidural anesthesia to abate during the second stage, arguing that descent and rotation may be delayed by inhibition of uterine contraction, reduced maternal bearing-down force, and relaxation of the pelvic floor. While this can happen, modest lengthening of the second stage, as long as the fetus manifests no evidence of oxygen deprivation, seems to cause no harm and, as noted, more leisurely descent may even be salutary for the pelvic floor. In addition, having to cope with the sudden return of pain after hours of anesthesia can be difficult. Under most circumstances, it is preferable to continue epidural anesthesia during the second stage. If you are patient, this approach will not increase the need for operative vaginal delivery or neonatal depression. Women with an epidural block may need more coaching to help them push effectively, because the sensations from stretching of the vagina and perineum that create an irresistible urge to push will be blunted.

It is likely that much of the controversy over the influence of anesthesia relates more to obstetric attitudes than to documentable adverse affects of anesthetics on labor progress. Epidural block does slow descent in some patients; but these inhibitory effects can generally be overcome with oxytocin if necessary. Sometimes it is best simply to allow the labor to continue to evolve, even if it means the second stage will be somewhat lengthened. More important, if the conservative approach to management of the second stage described here is used, excessive rates of operative delivery are avoidable.

## Key points
- Labor assessment requires you reappraise the situation each time you acquire new information regarding cervical dilatation, fetal descent, the condition of the fetus or mother, and the cephalopelvic relationships. At each assessment judge how available information affects the likelihood of a trouble-free vaginal delivery.

- Use the station of the fetal presenting part in early labor as a prognostic indicator in nulliparas.
- Use the graph of dilatation and descent patterns you create to determine if the labor is progressing normally, or is characterized by some dysfunction.
- There are seven documentable dysfunctional labor patterns: those in which cervical dilatation or fetal descent progresses linearly, but at a rate below the limit of normal (*protracted active phase dilatation* and *protracted descent*); those in which progress in active phase dilatation or in descent begins, but then ceases (*arrest of dilatation, arrest of descent,* and *prolonged deceleration phase),* and those in which dilatation or descent does not accelerate normally into its active portion (*prolonged latent phase* and *failure of descent*).
- A prolonged deceleration phase is of particular importance because of its strong association with disproportion, as well as with shoulder dystocia if vaginal delivery occurs.
- The combination of prolonged deceleration phase with any disorder of fetal descent makes safe vaginal delivery very unlikely.
- With each successive active phase or second stage abnormality in a parturient, the likelihood of an uncomplicated vaginal birth diminishes.
- Delay in diagnosis of dysfunctional labor is probably detrimental to the fetus.
- There is a large range of contractility patterns in normal labor. Using contraction pattern characteristics to distinguish normal from abnormal labor is not helpful.
- The goal of oxytocin therapy for dysfunctional labor, when its use is indicated, is to produce regular, strong uterine contractions that recur at intervals of 2–3 minutes, with a maximum of five contractions in a 10-minute interval. If the patient is having spontaneous strong contractions at this frequency, further uterotonic stimulation is generally not warranted.
- Begin an oxytocin infusion at 1 mU/min, and increase the dose by 1–2 mU/min every 30 minutes until the uterus is contracting at the desired intensity and spacing. Sometimes, higher doses will be required.
- All women can benefit from pain-reduction techniques to help them manage labor.
- Once a dysfunction is discovered, do a thorough analysis to determine the likely etiology and assess the probability that cephalopelvic disproportion is present.
- If you find strong evidence of disproportion, consider prompt cesarean delivery. Continuing labor in this situation may expose the fetus to further hazard.
- If disproportion is unlikely, give oxytocin if the disorder is one that can respond to it, such as one of the arrest disorders (but not necessarily a protraction disorder).

- Monitor oxytocin use to avoid producing excess contractility.
- Avoid operative vaginal delivery whenever possible in the presence of dysfunctional labor patterns.
- The opioids in general provide only moderate pain relief during labor but work well as an adjunct to psychoprophylactic techniques, or for those who do not want or cannot have an epidural block.
- Each of your patients should have some form of childbirth education, especially during her first pregnancy. Knowledge about what to expect during labor serves to reduce anxiety and fear, both of which can increase the need for analgesia or sedation.
- Epidural block can slow dilatation and descent in some patients; these inhibitory effects can generally be overcome with oxytocin.

## Further Reading

### Books and reviews

Cardozo LD, Gibb DMF, Studd JWW, Vasant RV, Cooper DJ. Predictive value of cervimetric labour patterns in primigravidae. Br J Obstet Gynaecol 1982;89:33–8.

Cohen WR. Controversies in the assessment of labor. In: Studd J, Tan SL, Chervenak FA (eds) *Progress in Obstetrics and Gynaecology* 2006; 17:231–44.

Cohen WR, Friedman EA. The assessment of labor. In: Kurjak A, Chervenak FA (eds) *Textbook of Perinatal Medicine*, 2nd edition. Informa UK, London, 2006: 1821–30.

Cohen WR. Normal and abnormal labor. In: Reece EA, Hobbins J (eds) *Clinical Obstetrics: The Fetus and Mother*, 3rd edition. Blackwell Publishing, London, 2007: 1065–76.

Friedman EA. Effects of labor and delivery on the fetus. In: Kurjak A, Chervenak FA (eds) *Textbook of Perinatal Medicine, 2nd edition*. Informa UK, London, 2006: 1989–97.

Friedman EA. Dystocia and "failure to progress" in labor. In: Flamm BL, Quilligan EJ (eds) *Cesarean Section: Guidelines for Appropriate Utilization*. Springer-Verlag, New York, 1995: 23–42.

Friedman EA. The functional divisions of labor Am J Obstet Gynecol 1971;109:274–80.

Friedman EA. *Labor: Clinical Evaluation and Management*, 2nd edition. Appleton-Century-Crofts, New York, 1978.

Leighton BL, Halpern SH. The effects of epidural analgesia on labor, maternal, and neonatal outcomes: a systematic review. Am J Obstet Gynecol 2002;186:S69–77.

Schifrin BS, Cohen WR: Labor's dysfunctional lexicon. Obstet Gynecol 1989;74:121–4.

### Primary sources

Chazotte C, Madden R, Cohen WR. Labor patterns in women with previous cesareans. Obstet Gynecol 1990;75:350–5.

Clark S, Belfort M, Saade G, Hankins G, Miller D, Frye D, et al. Implementation of a conservative checklist-based protocol for oxytocin administration: maternal and newborn outcomes. Am J Obstet Gynecol 2007;197:480.e1–e5.

Cohen WR. Influence of the duration of second stage labor on perinatal outcome and puerperal morbidity. Obstet Gynecol 1977;49:266–9.

Cohen WR, Newman L, Friedman EA. Frequency of labor disorders with advancing maternal age. Obstet Gynecol 1980;55:414–16.

Cohen WR, Mahon T, Chazotte C. *The Very Long Second Stage of Labor. Proceedings of the Third World Congress on Labor and Delivery.* Parthenon Publishing, New York, 1998: 348–51.

Friedman EA, Sachtleben MR. Dysfunctional labor III: secondary arrest of dilatation. Obstet Gynecol 1962;19:576–91.

Friedman EA, Niswander KR, Sachtleben MR, Nemore J. Dysfunctional labor VIII: relative accuracy of clinical and graphic diagnostic methods. Obstet Gynecol 1969;33:145–52.

Friedman EA, Sachtleben MR. Station of the fetal presenting part VI: arrest of descent in nulliparas. Obstet Gynecol 1976;47:129–36.

Garrett K, Butler A, Cohen WR. Cesarean delivery during second stage labor: characteristics and diagnostic accuracy. J Mat Fetal Neonat Med 2005;17:49–53.

Henry DEM, Cheng YW, Shaffer BL, Kaimal AJ, Bianco K, Caughey AB. Perinatal outcomes in the setting of active phase arrest of labor. Obstet Gynecol 2008;112:1109–15.

Kjaergaard H, Olsen J, Ottesen B, Dykes A. Incidence and outcome of dystocia in the active phase of labor in term nulliparous women with spontaneous labor onset. Acta Obstet Gynecol Scand 2009;88:402–7.

Mahon T, Chazotte C, Cohen WR. Short labor: characteristics and outcome. Obstet Gynecol 1994;84:47–51.

March MR, Adair CD, Veille J, Burrus DR. The modified Mueller-Hillis maneuver in predicting abnormalities in second stage labor. Int J Gynecol Obstet 1996;55:105–9.

Murphy K, Shah L, Cohen WR. Labor and delivery in nulliparas who present with an unengaged fetal head. J Perinatol 1998;18:122–5.

Seitchik J, Castillo M. Oxytocin augmentation of dysfunctional labor III: multiparous patients. Am J Obstet Gynecol 1983:145:777–80.

Towner D, Castro MA, Eby-Wilkens E, Gilbert WM. Effect of mode of delivery in nulliparous women on intracranial injury. N Engl J Med 1999;341:1709–14.

Verdiales M, Pacheco C, Cohen WR. Effect of maternal obesity on the course of labor. J Perinat Med 2009;37:651–5.

# CHAPTER 6

# Managing the Third Stage

The third stage of labor may seem banal in some respects when compared to the arduous and exhilarating events of the first and second stages, but it requires vigilance. Any obstetrician or midwife who has dealt with severe postpartum uterine bleeding approaches the third stage and immediate puerperium with respect and attentiveness. Remember, more women die from complications of the third stage (primarily hemorrhage) than from any other portion of labor. Properly managing this stage will reduce the risk of postpartum hemorrhage, ensure the expulsion of the complete secundines, enhance the likelihood of smooth convalescence during the puerperium, and avoid potential threats to the patient's subsequent health.

Two mechanisms are involved in placental delivery: its *separation* from the uterine wall and its *expulsion*. Placental separation occurs in most women very promptly after delivery of the fetus. It is generally said to result from mechanical shearing forces that occur when the uterine wall contracts beneath the broad placental surface. This is a reasonable, but perhaps overly simplistic, explanation. Undoubtedly, placental separation is a complex process, and the precise mechanisms remain uncertain.

Expulsion of the placenta begins when its separation is complete. Uterine contractions force the placenta into the lower uterine segment, and finally through the cervix into the vagina. The patient bears down; if this fails to deliver the placenta, you can usually expel it with gentle pressure on the uterus. A full description of normal placental delivery is found in Chapter 3.

Once the placenta has separated, large vascular sinuses in the placental bed are exposed, and can bleed. Excess hemorrhage from this area is controlled primarily by powerful contractions of the uterine muscular fibers. The shifting and shortening of the muscle fibers compress, twist, and bend the thin-walled vessels so that they become physically occluded, reducing the bleeding considerably, if not entirely. This reduced blood

---

*Labor and Delivery Care: A Practical Guide*, First Edition. Wayne R. Cohen and
Emanuel A. Friedman. © 2011 John Wiley & Sons, Ltd.
Published 2011 by John Wiley & Sons, Ltd

flow allows for the formation of platelet aggregates and, eventually, firm clots. You can feel the uterus become a small round organ lying low in the abdomen during this time.

## Normal limits

Because of our penchant for intervening in third stage events, and because of the difficulty in clinically distinguishing the processes of placental separation and expulsion, it is difficult to assign precise normal limits for the third stage. Some useful generalizations can, nevertheless, be made. After the fetus is delivered, the placenta will usually separate from its attachment promptly. Once separated, it will emerge from the uterus with minimal manipulation. Having entered the vagina, the placenta can be expressed by fundal pressure within about 5 minutes. By 15 minutes after fetal delivery, about 90% of placentas have delivered; by 30 minutes, only 2–3% are still retained. It is, therefore, reasonable to refrain from active attempts at placental delivery before 30 minutes of third stage have elapsed, unless there is excessive bleeding or other factors that militate against waiting. Some authorities advocate a 60-minute wait.

## Clinical signs of separation

Separation of the placenta in most normal deliveries begins as the fetus leaves the uterus. Clinical signs of separation and inauguration of descent of the placenta include a change in uterine shape from discoid to globular, the appearance of more exposed umbilical cord at the introitus, and vaginal bleeding, often appearing as a surprising gush. These signs frequently lag behind actual separation. Also, the signs may appear even though a small part of the placenta is still attached in the upper uterine segment. The generally accepted clinical signs are not, therefore, entirely reliable.

Delivery of the placenta will usually require some assistance from you. This may be an artifact of our general use of recumbent postures for delivery. If birth occurred in an erect position, gravity (and perhaps minimal gentle assistance from mother or attendant) would probably create more spontaneous expulsions.

## Management of the third stage

After you have delivered a healthy baby, hold it at or below the level of the placenta for about 1–2 minutes before clamping the cord. This allows some placental blood volume to enter the newborn's circulation—a so-called placental transfusion. The benefits of these extra red blood cells are expressed in both term and premature newborns by better iron stores and reduced frequency of anemia. Mild polycythemia and hyperbilirubinemia may sometimes occur from these extra red cells, but no serious adverse effects have been reported.

Apply a clamp to the cord 2–4 cm from the baby's abdominal wall. Divide the cord distal to the clamp, and place the newborn in the mother's arms. A nurse or the patient's partner should ensure the baby's safety there. Palpate the abdomen to assess the condition of the uterus. To avoid contaminating your gloved hands, do this through a sterile towel or drape. With one hand resting on the uterus, note its firmness. Its consistency may vary, owing to contraction and relaxation. If time permits, place a fresh sterile sheet under your patient's buttocks. Hold a sterile basin against the perineum to catch the emerging placenta (Fig. 3.7). Use a gauze sponge to compress an episiotomy wound or perineal laceration temporarily. If bleeding is heavy, take the time to clamp and ligate bleeding vessels. A surprising amount of blood can be lost from such wounds, even in the few minutes you await placental delivery. Wound repair can be done before placental delivery, but this risks disruption of the sutures by the emerging placenta or, even more so, by your hand should a manual removal of the placenta prove necessary. Thus, the episiotomy or laceration wound may prudently be left open until after the placenta has delivered, but active bleeding should be quelled early.

Now, sit or stand facing the perineum and wait. By palpating the uterus through the abdominal wall, you will be able to determine the frequency and strength of contractions and observe signs of placental descent. Observe the amount of blood accumulating in the basin. Nothing need be done if the uterus remains firm and does not balloon with blood, and there is no external bleeding. Be patient. Under no circumstance should you pull hard on the cord. Vigorous traction may tear the cord from its placental moorings. In addition to embarrassing you, this event usually results in the requirement for manual removal of the placenta, which exposes the patient to discomfort and the potential morbidity of retained secundines or uterine inversion (see below).

If the uterus softens and there is associated external bleeding, you can often stimulate myometrial contraction with massage. Gently grasp the uterus through the abdominal wall with one hand. With your thumb on the anterior uterine wall and the other four fingers on the posterior wall, make gentle but firm circular compressions of the posterior wall of the corpus. As soon as the uterus becomes firm, the oozing will cease and you can discontinue the massage, always prepared to reinstitute it. Meanwhile, inspect the vulva, vagina, and cervix to ensure that excessive

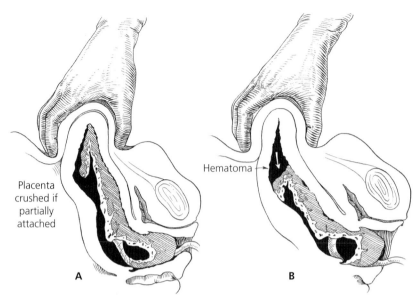

Placenta
crushed if
partially
attached

Hematoma

A

B

**Figure 6.1** Expression of the placenta (**A**) incorrectly by the Credé method of squeezing the fundus before separation, an inadvisable procedure, and (**B**) correctly, by using the corpus as a piston after the placenta has separated and entered the vagina.

bleeding is not coming from a tear in these areas. If there are no lacerations, blood coming from the cervical canal indicates bleeding from higher in the birth canal. If the uterus remains atonic—that is, does not contract firmly—and bleeding is heavy, prompt manual removal of the placenta and treatment with ecbolic agents is appropriate.

Wait for the signs that indicate the placenta has been expelled from the upper to the lower uterine segment. Three indicators of this event are strong uterine contractions, advancement of the cord segment protruding from the introitus, and the uterus assuming a globular shape. When the placenta is out of the uterine cavity and has moved into the vagina there is no need to wait any longer for its delivery; in fact, it is best to express it at this time so as to minimize blood loss. Ask the mother to bear down while you hold the cord in place (without pulling on it) in one hand, with the placental basin in the other. She will probably expel the placenta herself. If she cannot, grasp the uterus in the whole hand with the thumb in front (Fig. 6.1) and gently, without squeezing, push down on the uterus in the axis of the inlet. The uterus is thus used simply as a piston to exert pressure on the placenta lying in the vagina.

An alternative is the Brandt maneuver (Fig. 6.2). After the placenta has separated from the uterus, hold the cord at the introitus in one hand. Place your other hand suprapubically and press backward (dorsally) and slightly cephalad on the corpus. If separation has occurred, it will usually

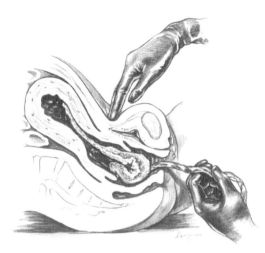

**Figure 6.2** The Brandt method of expressing the placenta. After the placenta has separated from the uterus, the cord is held in one hand. The other hand is placed suprapubically. By gently pressing backward and slightly cephalad on the corpus one can easily determine if separation has occurred. Once this is verified, the placenta and membranes are easily expelled.

be evident because the cord will not be pulled cephalad as the uterus is elevated. You can then easily extract the placenta and membranes.

As the vulva is distended by the placenta, women usually bear down reflexively and expel it. It should be allowed to fall under its own weight the short distance into the basin by gravity and to drag the attached chorioamniotic membranes after it. If the membranes do not come out by this means, exert gentle steady traction on them with your fingers or a Kelly clamp. Twisting the emerging membranes around the clamp seems to assist their removal and reduces the risk of tearing them. Grasp the membranes near the vulva from above to avoid contaminating your gloves by contact with the perineal and anal areas. If the membranes begin to tear, grasp their proximal end with two clamps. Place these progressively higher and higher, using gentle traction as the membranes emerge.

Some obstetricians perform the Credé maneuver for placental delivery (Fig. 6.1). It differs from simple expression in that when you force the uterus down into the pelvis, you squeeze it as well from all sides so that its contents are expelled. This maneuver can injure the uterus or bladder and provoke retained secundines and bleeding. We do not recommend it. As a general rule, the less intervention used in the third stage, the lower the risk of complications. This advice does not apply, of course, if there is too much bleeding or other third stage pathology evident that requires prompt placental delivery and reestablishment of uterine tone.

After delivery, examine the placenta to be sure it is complete, and note in the medical record any observed abnormalities (Table 6.1). In particular, be alert for missing cotyledons, vessels that end at the margin alerting to an accessory or succenturiate lobe, large adherent clots, and avascular areas of infarction. Histologic examination of every placenta is impractical, but can be especially valuable in certain circumstances (Box 6.1).

**Table 6.1** Features to note on gross placental examination

| Tissue | Normal feature | Significance |
|---|---|---|
| **Fetal membranes** | | |
| Meconium staining | None | Staining of chorion and umbilical cord surface suggests meconium present for at least several hours |
| Clarity, luster | Translucent, shiny | Cloudiness suggests infection |
| Odor | Odorless or clean metallic character | Foul odor suggests infection |
| Exudate | None | Exudate suggests infection |
| Amnion nodosum | None | Associated with chronic oligohydramnios, e.g., from renal agenesis |
| Venous thrombi | None | Associated with thrombophilia, severe chorioamnionitis |
| **Umbilical cord** | | |
| Number of arteries | Two | One artery sometimes associated with fetal anomalies |
| Diameter | 2.0–2.5 cm | Thin cord with deficient Wharton jelly associated with IUGR, postmaturity, torsion. Edematous cord (focal) associated with trisomy 18, omphalocele |
| Firmness | Firm, rubbery | Soft compressible cord associated with IUGR, vulnerability to occlusion |
| Knots, strictures, hematomas | None | True knots may rarely cause fetal compromise or death. Hematomas and strictures associated with mortality |
| Thrombosis | None | Associated with hematomas, knots, stricture, funisitis |
| Coiling | 1 coil/5 cm | Lean cord with diminished coiling associated with IUGR; excess coiling with reduced fetal maturation and fetal death |
| Length | 40–90 cm (median about 60 cm) | Long cord associated with knotting, prolapse, wrapping around neck or body. Short cord associated with trisomy 21, perhaps delayed descent |
| Attachment | Central or eccentric on chorionic plate | Marginal (battledore) or velamentous may accompany IUGR and make cord vulnerable to intrapartum compression |
| **Parenchyma** | | |
| Completeness | Complete | Consider retained cotyledon or succenturiate lobe if incomplete |
| Shape | Round to oval, average diameter 22 cm | Extra lobes may be retained or associated with vasa previa |
| Vessels | Arborized throughout | Vessels that end abruptly at placental margin indicate missing succenturiate lobe |
| Calcifications | Present at term | No known relevance |
| Thickness | 2.0–2.5 cm | Thinner associated with IUGR; thicker with diabetes mellitus, fetal hydrops, fetal infections |
| Color | Maternal surface maroon | Pallor suggests fetal anemia |

**Table 6.1** Continued

| Tissue | Normal feature | Significance |
|---|---|---|
| Edema | None | Immune or nonimmune fetal hydrops, diabetes mellitus, preeclampsia, syphilis |
| Infarction (firm pale areas) | None or scattered small | Associated with thrombophilias, systemic lupus erythematosus, IUGR |
| Adherent clot | None | Clots on maternal surface suggest abruptio placentae, especially if central and compress parenchyma |
| Tumor | None | Chorioangioma usually of no clinical significance; if large, may be associated with IUGR and fetal hydrops |

IUGR, intrauterine growth restriction

Every obstetric service should have a set of criteria for mandated pathologic examination.

## Active third stage management

There is a spectrum of opinion and practice regarding management of the third stage of labor. It is common practice to expedite placental delivery with uterotonic adjuvants, such as oxytocin or methergine. These drugs cause powerful contractions that might encourage separation, and certainly help force the placenta into the lower uterine segment and upper vagina. Use of such agents probably shortens the third stage by several minutes and may reduce the risk of postpartum hemorrhage. Often this approach is combined with moderate cord traction to further encourage delivery, a practice that cannot be condoned because of its known risks of uterine inversion, retained placental tissue or umbilical cord avulsion. None of these is a common consequence of active third stage management, but when they occur they may cause considerable morbidity.

It is obvious that the vast majority of women fare perfectly well in the third stage without any active intervention. That notwithstanding, the potential benefits of reducing postpartum blood loss and modifying the risk of hemorrhage justify the routine use of oxytocin or another ecbolic in the third stage, and this has become recommended standard practice in many countries. While some advocate administering oxytocin when the baby's anterior shoulder emerges, it probably makes no difference if you wait until the baby has delivered, especially if the drug is given intravenously. If the intramuscular route is used, somewhat earlier intervention makes sense. Use caution for gravidas who have had no prenatal care (and therefore no imaging studies) or in regions where sonography

## Box 6.1 Indications to perform placental histopathologic examination

- Fetal and neonatal indications
  - ○ Hydrops fetalis
  - ○ Intrauterine growth restriction
  - ○ Fetal/neonatal anemia
  - ○ Hydrops fetalis
  - ○ Major congenital anomalies (structural, chromosomal or functional)
  - ○ Multiple gestation
  - ○ Neonatal macrosomia (>4500 g birth weight)
  - ○ Neonatal fever, infection, sepsis, seizures
  - ○ Oligohydramnios
  - ○ Polyhydramnios
  - ○ Preterm birth (<37 weeks' gestational age)
  - ○ Stillbirth or perinatal death
- Maternal indications
  - ○ Diabetes mellitus
  - ○ Preeclampsia/eclampsia
  - ○ Chronic hypertension
  - ○ Rheumatic disease
  - ○ Drug abuse
  - ○ History of abdominal trauma in pregnancy
  - ○ Fever or infection during labor
  - ○ Malaria, toxoplasmosis, syphilis, herpes simplex
- Placental indications
  - ○ Abruptio placentae
  - ○ Velamentous cord insertion
  - ○ Single umbilical artery
  - ○ Unusual placental size or shape
  - ○ Unusually long (>100 cm) or short (<30 cm) umbilical cord
  - ○ Cord with increased or decreased vascular spiraling (normal 1 coil/5 cm)
  - ○ Venous thrombi seen on chorionic plate
  - ○ Edematous or pale placenta
  - ○ Succenturiate lobes
  - ○ Placenta previa
  - ○ Vasa previa
  - ○ Maternal floor infarcts
  - ○ Prenatal ultrasound, MRI or CT imaging abnormalities (e.g., cysts, chorioangiomas, suspected accreta, accessory lobes, etc.)

is unavailable because of the risk of entrapping an undiagnosed second twin and exposing that fetus to hypoxia from uterine hypercontractility.

A reasonable approach, based on available literature and experience, is to allow delivery of the fetus, administer oxytocin (10 U IM or 50–150 mU/min IV) and then assess the condition of the uterus and placenta. If bleeding is not excessive, and no other factors require prompt placental delivery, periodically perform the Brandt maneuver, with minimal tension on the umbilical cord. If you do it gently, this maneuver will result in placental delivery in most instances. In the absence of hemorrhage or other serious complication, there is no reason to hurry.

Nipple stimulation (which causes release of endogenous oxytocin) has been suggested as a replacement for drug therapy in the management of the third stage, but there is no objective evidence of its effectiveness. Consider its use only when drug resources are limited.

## Retained placenta

Diagnose failure of placental delivery (*retained placenta*) if 30 minutes have passed without spontaneous placental separation or delivery. There may be several causes for this situation: (1) the placenta has separated, but a contracted lower uterine segment impedes its expulsion; (2) a normally implanted placenta has failed to separate from the uterine wall or has only partially separated; or (3) the placenta is abnormally implanted (*placenta accreta*).

Of these possibilities, you will find the first most commonly. Sometimes the placenta per se has separated, but adherence of membranes to the surrounding decidua may prevent expulsion. Also, unusually broad, flat placentas or those with accessory lobes may not separate completely or in a timely manner. Always be aware of the possibility of a Müllerian duct anomaly (especially an arcuate, subseptate or bicornuate uterus) when a retained placenta is encountered.

The problem of a separated but retained placenta is generally easily remedied by manual removal (Fig. 6.3). Some analgesia or anesthesia is usually required because this process can be painful. Occasionally, you will find it difficult to insert your hand into the endometrial cavity because of persistent contraction of the lower segment. In that case, a short-acting tocolytic drug (e.g., nitroglycerin) or uterine relaxant anesthesia (a halogenated inhalational agent) may be necessary to relax the myometrium and allow entry of the examining hand. Be extremely careful in such circumstances, because the pharmacologically relaxed uterine wall is highly vulnerable to perforation, especially at the placental site, where the wall is thin. Moreover, the induced atony may produce uterine bleeding, thereby causing the very problem you are trying to prevent. Be prepared to use an ecbolic drug, if necessary, after you remove the placenta, and immediately turn off the inhalational agent if it was used.

Dislodging a still-implanted placenta is more difficult and imposes greater risks. Sometimes expulsion may be delayed by inadequate contractions and, to the extent that this mechanism is operative, oxytocin or

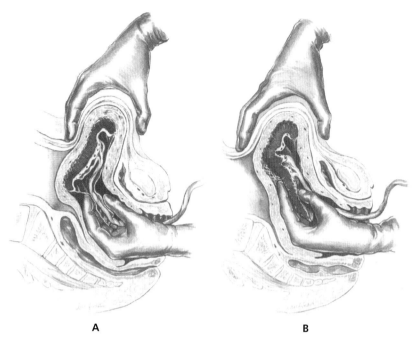

A                                         B

**Figure 6.3** Method for manual removal of the placenta showing (**A**) the hand being introduced in a cone shape into the uterus and (**B**) separating the placenta from its attachment to the uterus by gently dissecting the cleavage plane with lateral movements of the fingers.

ergot derivatives may be salutary. Their advantages in promoting separation must be weighed against the fact that manual uterine exploration and placental extraction may be more difficult with a firmly contracted lower uterine segment.

In most cases it is not known what causes the placenta to remain adherent to the uterus even after 30 minutes of the third stage. Most often you can readily remove these placentas manually. To do so, insert one hand in a cone shape (i.e., with fingertips together) into the uterine cavity and steady the uterus through the abdominal wall with the other hand. Usually, you can easily develop a cleavage plane between the placenta and the decidua by the hand exploring the uterus. Gently separate the entire placenta using lateral sweeping movements of the hand, taking care to keep your fingers in the same plane. Once the entire placenta is separated from its attachment to the uterine wall, grasp and remove it. Manual extraction of the placenta must always be done with great care to ensure the placenta is completely removed and to minimize patient discomfort and the risk of genital tract trauma. Uterine wall perforation, although rare, can result from careless attempts at placental removal. If there is any doubt that the whole placenta has been removed, you should reinsert a hand wrapped in a laparotomy pad and firmly wipe the surfaces of the uterine cavity. The friction provided by the pad is helpful in dislodging any remaining placental fragments and membranes.

There are a few procedures you can try prior to attempts at manual removal if a placenta is retained. The placenta can be drained of its blood content via the umbilical vessels. This is a harmless maneuver touted by some to ease placental separation or expulsion, although without objective support. The infusion of 10–20 units of oxytocin diluted in 20 mL of saline into the umbilical vein may also have some value in expediting placental delivery, and is worth trying.

### Placenta accreta

Rarely, the placenta implants without an intervening layer of decidua spongiosum, and is attached directly to, or invades, the myometrium. Abnormal attachment is called *placenta accreta*. When the placenta accreta invades the underlying myometrium it is referred to as *placenta increta*; when it grows through the full thickness of the uterine wall, it is a *placenta percreta*. Such cases can even invade the bladder or other adjacent structures. In any of its forms, abnormal placentation of this nature is a serious complication. These various degrees of abnormal placentation are being seen with increasing frequency owing to the rise in the cesarean delivery rate over the past several decades. The number of previous cesarean deliveries seems to be directly related to the likelihood of placenta accreta. There is also an association of placenta accreta with placenta previa, especially when the latter occurs over a previous uterine incision.

Placenta accreta can cause torrential bleeding during attempts to remove the retained placenta. When the entire placental bed is involved, no plane of separation can be found. It is important to recognize the condition so you do not make forceful efforts to create a plane and thereby damage the myometrium and cause heavy bleeding. Sometimes only focal areas are involved, and these situations are often associated with the most severe hemorrhage because persistent inappropriate attempts are made to remove the adherent placenta.

Hysterectomy is usually necessary for a gravida with placenta accreta. Occasionally, hysterectomy can be avoided if the adherent portion of the placenta accreta is focal, blood loss is not excessive, and bleeding is controllable by other measures. Case reports of placenta accreta treated by leaving the placenta in situ and treating with methotrexate have appeared. The safety of this approach has not been established.

The definitive diagnosis of placenta accreta can only be made histologically, but you should presume the problem exists whenever a distinct cleavage plane cannot be developed between the placenta and the uterine wall or, during the process of developing the plane, you encounter a firmly adherent area. Ideally, in high-risk cases, prenatal placental imaging by ultrasonography, and sometimes magnetic resonance imaging, can provide strong suspicion of the diagnosis and allow delivery plans to be made to optimize outcome. When the diagnosis is firm, no attempts should be made to remove the placenta. Perform hysterectomy after cesarean delivery instead, leaving the placenta undisturbed in place.

## Uterine inversion

Acute puerperal inversion of the uterus is an uncommon cause of severe postpartum hemorrhage, and sometimes of shock. The patient usually complains of pain. The bleeding that occurs in these cases may be sudden and profuse. The inverted fundus often presents as a mass visible at the introitus (Fig. 6.4). Less commonly, you may discover the mass in the vagina when you attempt routine examination of the cervix after delivery.

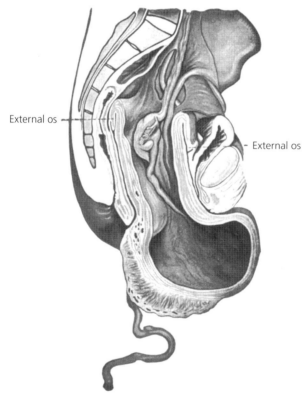

External os

External os

**Figure 6.4** Illustration of a case of total uterine inversion with the placenta still attached to the posterior endometrial surface. Note the tube and ovary pulled down into the intraabdominal inversion funnel.

Inversion is sometimes iatrogenic, the result of overzealous traction on the umbilical cord prior to placental separation during the third stage, especially if such traction is applied to the cord when the uterus is atonic. Many cases, however, occur spontaneously in the presence of uterine atony or without apparent cause or provocation. Prompt replacement of the fundus is important to minimize bleeding and to prevent or reduce hypotension. The latter is said to occur out of proportion to the blood loss, perhaps the result of a vasovagal response to peritoneal stretching. We are not sure whether that occurs, but it is certain that inversion of the uterus can be associated with rapid and severe blood loss. When inversion occurs, summon help promptly. An anesthesiologist is usually required, and the help of another experienced obstetrician and a nurse is invaluable.

The traditional approach to this disorder was to attempt replacement of the fundus under general anesthesia, but today this is rarely necessary. Modern obstetric drugs have led to new management methods that are quite effective. If anesthesia is required, the regional anesthetic block used for delivery will usually suffice.

When the inversion is identified, give a tocolytic drug to relax the uterus. Terbutaline, magnesium sulfate, or nitroglycerin are options. Use caution, however, if there is considerable bleeding because all of these agents have the potential to reduce maternal blood pressure. If your patient has no existing regional anesthesia and is too uncomfortable to tolerate the procedure without pain relief, consider deep halothane, isoflurane or sevoflurane anesthesia. These inhalational agents will effectively and profoundly relax the myometrium, and can be stopped as soon as the fundus is replaced. They also have hypotensive properties and potential cardiotoxicity, so discuss the situation with the anesthesiologist and decide together the safest approach for the situation. Once the uterus is relaxed the fundus can usually be replaced with relative ease.

To replace the inverted fundus, place as much of the palm of your hand and extended fingers as you can over the dome of the inverted fundus. This will distribute the applied force over the greatest possible area, thereby minimizing the risk of damaging the exposed myometrium. Above all, never push on the fundus with your fingertips. Such concentrated force can result in uterine perforation, making a bad situation much worse. Elevate the uterus into the abdominal cavity. Push cephalad, spreading the constricting cervical ring with the fingers and thumb, and steadily forcing the fundus upward with the palm, so as to create firm and persistent pressure at the junction of the uterine corpus and cervix with your examining hand (Fig. 6.5). In 3–5 minutes, the fundus usually begins to recede, perhaps aided by the tension you create on the uterine ligaments. Be patient. Correction can take time. While awaiting resolution, be sure to attend to your patient's fluid replacement needs.

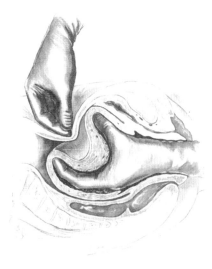

**Figure 6.5** Mechanism for replacing the inverted uterus, showing the intravaginal hand grasping the inverted corpus, spreading the constricting cervical ring with the fingers and thumb and steadily forcing the fundus upward with the palm.

After you have successfully replaced the fundus, give uterotonic agents. High dose oxytocin infusion (50–200 mU/min in an electrolyte solution to help prevent water intoxication) or intramuscular 15-methyl prostaglandin $F_2\alpha$ (250 μg) is usually effective. Grasp the uterus through the abdominal wall and massage it to promote contractions. Do not release it until it has contracted firmly! Sometimes inversion will recur, and you will need to repeat the treatment. In obdurate cases, in which nothing you do seems to prevent recurrent inversions, consider placing an intra-uterine tamponade balloon for several hours. Deflate it very gradually as you maintain uterine contractility with prostaglandins.

When none of the above resolves the situation, a laparotomy will be necessary. A small transverse abdominal incision will suffice. Under uterine relaxant anesthesia, first place a traction suture into the inverted dome of the uterus. This can be difficult, because the inverted fundus is very far down in the pelvis. Pull upward on the traction suture while an assistant applies intravaginal upward pressure on the inverted fundus, as described above. If this does not work, identify the contraction ring that surrounds the inverted dome and incise it vertically at its posterior rim. The fundus can now be readily replaced by a combination of pressure from below by your assistant and traction on the suture previously placed on the fundus, or by placing two fingers into the incision to reach the lowest point on the inverted fundus and then pulling the fundus back into place. Discontinue the halogenated anesthetic as soon as the uterus has been successfully reposited. This will minimize the time it takes for good uterine contractility to resume, and thereby reduce the risk of bleeding. Repair the posterior incision and give oxytocin or prostaglandins to maintain uterine tone, as described above. A recommended sequential approach to uterine inversion is provided in Fig. 6.6.

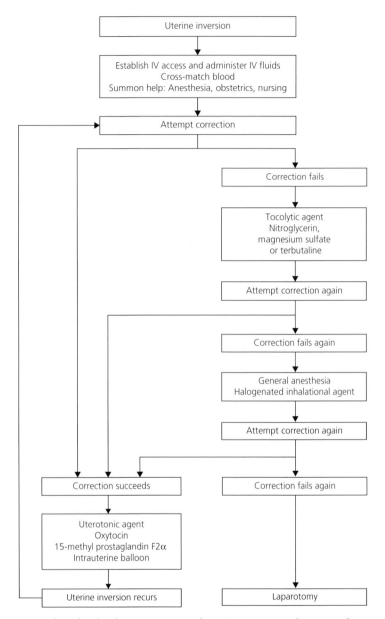

**Figure 6.6** Algorithm for the management of uterine inversion. The sooner the diagnosis is made, the easier will be replacement of the fundus. Anesthesia is usually necessary, and measures to deal with uterine atony and hemorrhage must be prepared. Place the inverted fundus in your palm and push upward, holding steady pressure. A uterine relaxant drug may be necessary. Once the inversion is corrected, give an ecbolic agent to help prevent reinversion. In rare cases, laparotomy may be necessary.

## Key points

- Placental delivery involves two discrete mechanisms: *separation* from the uterine wall and *expulsion*.
- Most placentas emerge within about 5 minutes; after 30 minutes, diagnose retained placenta.
- Clinical signs of placental separation are a change in uterine shape from discoid to globular, appearance of more exposed cord at the introitus, and a short burst of bleeding.
- After delivering a healthy baby, hold it at or below the level of the placenta for about 1–2 minutes before clamping the cord to permit placental transfusion.
- After delivery, examine the placenta to be sure it is complete and send it for histopathologic examination in selected cases.
- The potential benefits of reducing postpartum blood loss justify the routine use of oxytocin in the third stage.
- When the placenta does not deliver promptly, consider that it may have separated, but contraction of the lower uterine segment may be obstructing placental descent. Abnormal adherence of the placenta to the myometrium (placenta accreta) may also explain it.
- Unusually broad flat placentas or those with accessory lobes may not separate in a timely manner.
- Be aware of the possibility of a uterine anomaly when the placenta is retained.
- Be extremely careful when performing manual placental removal, especially if a tocolytic agent or a uterine-relaxing anesthetic has been used, because the relaxed uterine wall is highly vulnerable to perforation.
- The number of prior cesarean deliveries is directly related to the likelihood of placenta accreta, especially in association with placenta previa when the placenta has implanted in the uterine scar.
- Acute puerperal inversion of the uterus can cause severe postpartum hemorrhage. Prompt diagnosis and treatment are necessary.
- When the inversion is identified, administer a tocolytic drug to relax the uterus. Once the fundus is replaced, give a uterotonic agent.

## Further Reading

### Books and reviews

California Society of Pathologists. Guidelines for placental examination for the general practicing surgical pathologist. (www.calpath.org/docs/placental.pdf)

Gülmezoglu AM, Souza JP. The evolving management of the third stage of labour. BJOG 2009;116 (suppl1):26–8.

Hutton EK, Hassan ES. Late vs early clamping of the umbilical cord in full-term neonates: systematic review and meta-analysis of controlled trials. JAMA 2007;297:1241–52.

Leduc D, Senikas V, Lalonde AB, Ballerman C, Biringer A, Delaney M, et al. Active management of the third stage of labour: prevention and treatment of postpartum hemorrhage. J Obstet Gynaecol Can 2009;31:980–93.

Rajan PV, Wing DA. Postpartum hemorrhage: evidence-based medical interventions for prevention and treatment. Clin Obstet Gynecol 2010;53:165–81.

Su LL, Chong YS, Samuel M. Oxytocin agonists for preventing postpartum haemorrhage (Review). Cochrane Database Syst Rev 2007:CD005457.

Weeks AD. The retained placenta. Best Pract Res Clin Obstet Gynaecol 2008;22:1103–17.

Yetter JF III. Examination of the placenta. Am Family Physician 1998;57:1045–54.

## Primary sources

Achanna S, Mohamed Z, Krishman M. Puerperal uterine inversion: a report of four cases. J Obstet Gynaecol 2006;32: 341–5.

Brandt ML. The mechanism and management of the third stage of labor. Am J Obstet Gynecol 1933;25:662–7.

Catanzarite VA, Moffitt KD, Baker ML, Awadalla SG, Argubright KF, Perkins RP. New approaches to the management of acute puerperal uterine inversion. Obstet Gynecol 1986;68:75–105.

Chestnut DH, Wilcox LL. Influence of umbilical vein administration of oxytocin on the third stage of labor: a randomized, double-blind, placebo-controlled study. Am J Obstet Gynecol 1987;157:160–2.

Fliegner JR, Hibbard BM. Active management of the third stage of labour. Br Med J 1966;2:622–3.

Fliegner JR. Third stage management: how important is it? Med J Aust 1978;2:190–3.

Golan A, Lidor AL, Wexler S, David MP. A new method for the management of the retained placenta. AmJ Obstet Gynecol 1983;146:708–9.

Hibbard BH. The third stage of labor. Br Med J 1964;1:1485–8.

Ibrahim HM, Krouskop RW, Lewis DF, Dhanireddy R. Placental transfusion: umbilical cord clamping and preterm infants. J Perinatol 2000;20:351–4.

Jahazi A, Kordi M, Mirbehbahani NB, Mazloom SR. The effect of early and late umbilical cord clamping on neonatal hematocrit. J Perinatol 2008;28:523–5.

Mercer JS, Vohr BR, McGrath MM, Padbury JF, Wallach M, Oh W. Delayed cord clamping in very preterm infants reduces the incidence of intraventricular hemorrhage and late-onset sepsis: a randomized, controlled trial. Pediatrics 2006;117:1434–5.

Robson S, Adair S, Bland P. A new surgical technique for dealing with uterine inversion. Aust NZ J Obstet Gynaecol 2005;45:250–1.

Sorbe B. Active pharmacologic management of the third stage of labor. Obstet Gynecol 1978;52:694–7.

Thiery M, Delveke L. Acute puerperal inversion: two-step management with a β-mimetic and a prostaglandin. Am J Obstet Gynecol 1985;153:891–2.

# CHAPTER 7

# Dealing with Malpositions and Deflexed Attitudes

## Occiput posterior

### Diagnosis

Ordinarily, the fetal head undergoes internal rotation during its descent through the midpelvis so that the occiput comes to lie beneath the symphysis pubis in an occiput anterior position (OA). In some cases, such rotation will not occur, or will take place so that the occiput will turn toward the sacrum. In that event, you will diagnose an occiput posterior (OP) position.

It is not easy to identify an OP position by abdominal examination. In thin women, you may suspect it if you are unable to feel the prominent posterior part of the fetal head by suprapubic palpation, using the fourth Leopold maneuver (Chapter 2). The fetal shoulder is located far laterally in the uterus, and can be difficult to feel.

On vaginal examination early in labor you will generally find the head high in the pelvis. Usually, the head is partly deflexed. This will be apparent to you when you encounter the small posterior fontanel higher than (i.e., more cephalad) or on the same level as the large anterior fontanel. You will also be able to recognize that the anterior fontanel is nearer to the center of the pelvis. These findings reflect the relative deflexion of the head usually present in the fetus in OP position. As you follow labor in an OP case, you will be able to determine whether the head is flexing, or becoming more extended over time. The head is usually synclitic, i.e., you feel the same portion of each parietal bone presenting on either side of the sagittal suture.

During descent, the head destined to deliver in the direct OP position (with the occiput in the midline directed toward the sacrum) will often rotate there progressively from an oblique posterior position (ROP or

*Labor and Delivery Care: A Practical Guide*, First Edition. Wayne R. Cohen and Emanuel A. Friedman. © 2011 John Wiley & Sons, Ltd. Published 2011 by John Wiley & Sons, Ltd.

LOP), from an occiput transverse position (ROT or LOT), or even occasionally from an anterior position (ROA, OA or LOA), depending on the bony structure of the pelvis. If the posterior orientation is to persist, the head descends in moderate extension. You can sometimes detect whether the head that is in a transverse position (ROT or LOT) or an oblique posterior position (ROP, or LOP) is not going to rotate anteriorly by vaginal examination. Your examining fingers will often sense the tendency of the small fontanel to turn posteriorly during a contraction, especially if you use the Müller-Hillis maneuver. If anterior rotation is going to occur spontaneously, flexion will take place with descent.

As the occiput descends into the pelvis and turns into the hollow of the sacrum, you can find the posterior fontanel deep in the pelvis, the head firmly pressing on the rectovaginal tissues. The sagittal suture occupies the midline. You can readily palpate the large anterior fontanel behind the pubis if the head is flexed. If extension has persisted during descent, you will feel the anterior fontanel in the center of the pelvis and the glabella (root of the nose) behind the pubis.

Most fetal heads that descend in the OP position tend to have considerable molding of the cranial plates and much caput succedaneum formation, especially if descent has been protracted. Because of these changes, you may find it difficult or impossible to outline the sutures, particularly in late labor. In such cases, you can usually verify position by passing a finger alongside the head and identifying the fetal ear; the direction of the tragus will reveal the diagnosis. Be careful: because the ear is soft, discerning its orientation requires you to concentrate on its anatomic features.

The importance of following the position of the head from early in labor, when molding and caput do not generally obscure anatomic landmarks, cannot be overemphasized. Knowing the fetal position from the outset and how it changes over the course of time will serve you well as important guides to the events that occur later in labor. Sometimes, fetal position is erroneously diagnosed as OA when in fact the head delivers as an OP. When this occurs, it tends to be written off as a trivial oversight. It may, however, have considerable consequences. If you fail to identify an OP position, you may overlook the cause of dysfunctional labor (Chapter 5), and treat it inappropriately. Moreover, you will be more likely to abet pelvic floor and perineal injury, misapply a vacuum extractor or forceps, or force restitution of the head at delivery in the wrong direction.

## Clinical course

Fetal position early in labor is often OP. Engagement may occur in this position when the pelvis is quite large relative to the fetus, and rotation to accommodate the inlet shape is, therefore, not necessary for engagement to occur. Alternatively, when the fetal head is large enough to occupy most of the available space, engagement in the OP position will occur when the forepelvis is narrow relative to the posterior segment of the inlet. This occurs mostly in anthropoid and android pelvic types (Chapter 4).

Most of the time, a head that is OP early in labor will rotate to an OA position as descent progresses. Sometimes, however, it will remain OP well into the second stage, and even deliver in that position if the pelvic structure favors that mechanism. Sometimes, you will observe the head rapidly rotate to OA very late in the second stage once the head encounters the pelvic floor or immediately prior to the delivery. Remember also that the reverse situation is possible in some fetuses, with the head engaging in a transverse or anterior orientation and then later in labor rotating into a posterior position.

While OP position is generally categorized as a *malposition*, it is in fact sometimes an appropriate accommodation to the pelvic architecture that the fetus is encountering. Thus, for example, finding a fetus in an OP position in a spacious anthropoid pelvis suggests good adaptation to the available space. Persistence of the occiput in this position throughout descent would be expected, and labor progress would probably be normal. Were the head in OA position, it might not fit as well in such a pelvis. By contrast, a persistent OP position in a gynecoid pelvis would not be adaptive, thus representing a true malposition in which the position might hinder fetal descent.

Sometimes, inadequate uterine contractility will result in a persistent OP position during labor. More commonly, the position is mandated by the architecture and restraining capacity of the encircling bony pelvis. Sometimes, for example, very prominent ischial spines may resist internal rotation. In that situation, if the posterior pelvis is ample with a deep sacral hollow and there is a relatively narrow anterior pelvis, descent may continue unimpeded with the fetal head remaining as an OP. If, however, the sacrum is forward or the sidewalls of the lower pelvis are convergent, descent may become arrested.

When you find an OP position any time in labor, be concerned about the possibility of dysfunctional labor progress and structural pelvic pathology. As noted, most OP positions found in early labor are innocuous. At least 85% self-correct during the course of labor, most often late in the active phase of dilatation when descent begins. This occurs by internal rotation through a long arc to an OA orientation. Expect the subsequent mechanism of labor to be entirely normal after rotation has occurred. The remaining 15% of cases persist in the OP position. A small number of other fetuses who deliver in OP position began labor in an OA or OT position and then rotated posteriorly during the descent process.

The mechanism of labor associated with a persistent OP position is depicted in Fig. 7.1. Engagement may take place with the fetal head

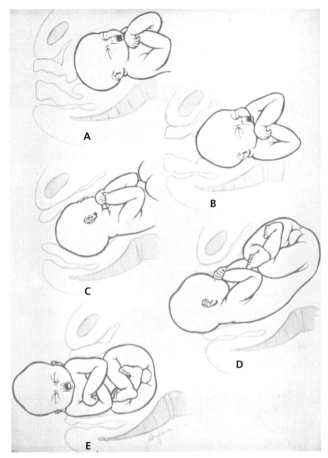

**Figure 7.1** Mechanism of labor in right occiput posterior position as it evolves into a direct occiput posterior position. **A**. Engagement of the deflexed head in right oblique diameter with occiput posterior. **B**. Descent with partial internal rotation of the occiput to the posterior, but with little flexion. **C**. Internal rotation completed to the direct occiput posterior position. **D**. Flexion of the head in the pelvic outlet under the symphysis and delivery. **E**. Restitution and external rotation.

assuming any variant of posterior oblique or transverse occiput positions, usually with some degree of deflexion. During subsequent descent, internal rotation takes place through a short arc, bringing the occiput to the sacrum. The head is later brought under the symphysis by flexion along the curvature of the lower pelvis and is delivered over the distended perineum, face up. After the head delivers, restitution occurs as the head aligns with the shoulders once again. External rotation follows as the shoulders internally rotate. The mechanisms of delivery of the shoulders and the rest of the body are the same as for the OA position.

Although labor patterns in most cases of OP presentation are normal, protraction and arrest disorders of dilatation and descent are more likely to occur than in anterior positions of the occiput. The presence of an OP position itself causes dysfunctional labor in some cases. More commonly, the malposition is probably a consequence of other factors that have perturbed the labor (such as abnormal pelvic capacity, inadequate contractility, excess anesthesia, etc.) rather than the direct cause of the dysfunction.

The latent phase in unaffected by an OP position, but the active phase tends to be longer and often protracted. In persistent OP positions, the progress of labor is especially likely to be slowed toward the end of the first stage and during the second stage. Cervical dilatation may proceed well to the deceleration phase, but may then be prolonged or even arrested. Descent may also be impeded because the head does not fit well into the pelvis. Spontaneous delivery requires more uterine and abdominal effort than for a comparable OA mechanism. To aid in this regard, vacuum extraction or a forceps procedure is often used to shorten the second stage, although allowing the gravida to labor longer will usually accomplish the same objective with greater safety.

Perineal lacerations are common when the fetus delivers as an OP, particularly in nulliparas, unless the fetal head is small. Injuries occur because the head presents larger planes than usual to the outlet, and also because the perineum is forcibly stretched and displaced posteriorly by the head during the terminal portion of descent. The presenting fetal diameter (the occipitofrontal) is 2.5–3.0 cm larger than that of a flexed head in OA position, which presents its much smaller suboccipitobregmatic dimension to the pelvis. Also, as noted above, instrumental delivery, which predisposes to lacerations, is done more commonly in OP positions.

## Prognosis

Since most fetal heads in OP position rotate spontaneously to an OA position and deliver uneventfully, the overall risks are small. The troublesome cases are those in which the occiput remains persistently posterior in spite of a long labor. In such cases, delivery may be difficult and accompanied by extensive maternal lacerations and even damage to the fetus. This is particularly true if the correct diagnosis of fetal malposition is not made before instruments are applied for the delivery.

There is controversy about the long-term effects of labor and delivery for fetuses in an OP orientation. Some data suggest that babies who delivered OP are predisposed to neurologic problems. It is uncertain whether that is a consequence of their malposition in utero or of the dysfunctional labor and instrumental delivery that follows.

## Management

When you identify an OP position, carry out meticulous and thorough manual pelvimetry. Determine whether the pelvis is contracted overall, and be sure to evaluate for pelvic characteristics that might require specific treatment or consideration. Focus especially on identifying an anthropoid pelvis, which is commonly encountered in these cases. Establish whether the pelvis is more likely to accommodate a fetus to aid its anterior rotation or to maintain its posterior orientation when descent occurs.

If protraction or arrest disorders occur, they should be treated in the standard manner (Chapter 5). Be particularly attentive to the deceleration phase. In OP cases, the anterior lip of the cervix tends to linger, sometimes prolonging this phase. Resist the temptation to force the first stage to end by pushing the remaining rim or lip of cervix over the head. The failure to achieve full retraction of the cervix may signal that disproportion is present. If you force entry into the second stage, you will lose an important clinical marker of whether or not safe vaginal delivery will ensue. Furthermore, pushing the cervical lip over the fetal head may damage the cervix and cause bleeding.

To make matters worse, the cervix can occasionally become strongly compressed between the fetal head and the pubic symphysis. It may thus not be possible for the cervix to achieve full dilatation because it is prevented from being retracted around the fetal presenting part in the course of late labor. That problem is compounded by the ensuing cervical congestion and edema. This tends to happen when the head is large relative to the pelvis, or when the sacral curve is flat, displacing the head anteriorly. In such cases, it is best to assume the worst (i.e., that adverse bony pelvic factors are preventing further dilatation) rather than that the edema per se is the problem and that it can safely be overcome by forcing the cervix around the head.

It can be difficult to determine by vaginal examination if the fetal head is actually engaged in the pelvis when the head is in an OP position. The general rule is that one can assume engagement (that is, the widest diameter of the fetal head has advanced to or below the plane of the pelvic inlet) when the leading edge of the skull reaches the plane of the ischial spines. This clinical guide, however, applies only to well-flexed OA positions without extensive molding of the cranial bones. For the fetus in an OP position, the head is usually extended and there is often considerable molding and caput formation. In some cases in which these changes are extreme, the fetal skull can even begin to distend the perineum and be visible at the introitus before the head has engaged. Ignorance of this fact can lead to inappropriate attempts at instrumental delivery, exposing both mother and fetus to possible trauma. What you presume to be an outlet forceps (or vacuum extractor) operation based on the station of the forward leading edge of a molded head can actually be a dangerous midforceps or even high forceps (or midcavity or high vacuum extraction) procedure with an unacceptably high associated risk of fetal injury. In labors with the fetus in an OP position, therefore, you should always confirm engagement by suprapubic palpation of the fetal head. By this clinical means, you can readily distinguish true descent from simple elongation of the fetal head by molding (Chapter 4).

After the head has engaged, you will find that most will undergo internal rotation to an anterior or obliquely anterior position, followed in due course by spontaneous delivery. If the posterior head is descending in an OP position with good flexion, the perineum is not endangered as much as when the head is deflexed. In either case, a deep episiotomy is indicated, unless the patient is a multipara with elastic perineal tissues. While we generally advocate a median episiotomy, the chance of sphincter or rectal laceration is considerable when the head emerges in an OP orientation, so a mediolateral incision is justified instead.

If you choose to use forceps or vacuum extraction for delivering a fetus in OP position, be sure the skull is on the perineum and that the head is actually deeply engaged. Be certain of the precise fetal position before you attempt any instrumental application. Forceps rotation through 180° used to be common practice for delivering a fetus from the OP position. Today, this approach can no longer be justified because it is known to be associated with trauma to mother or fetus. It is difficult to rationalize this risk if the rotation is being done ostensibly to avert trauma due to the aberrant position. It is better to deliver the fetus in the direct OP position, taking as much care as possible to protect the perineum. Manual rotation from OP to OA, a somewhat safer alternative to forceps rotation, was once commonly attempted for arrest of descent in which the lower pelvis was deemed adequate to accommodate the fetus for anterior rotation. However, it has fallen out of favor because it is not as safe as spontaneous rotation. If the lower pelvis is truly adequate for rotation, then rotation is likely to occur spontaneously if further labor is allowed. Once the fetal head has rotated, descent and delivery can be expected to follow in due course. Thus, manual rotation of an OP presentation is almost never advisable in modern obstetric practice. It might be an option when cesarean delivery is not available, and there is no time to await spontaneous rotation.

If you feel you must do manual rotation because facilities for abdominal delivery are not immediately at hand, it can be accomplished with the head low in the pelvis by grasping the occiput in one hand, distributing the applied force over as great an area as possible. For example, if the head is ROP, insert your left hand into the vagina, grasp the posterior portion of the head, flex it if necessary (it usually is necessary), and rotate your hand so as to bring the occiput to a direct OA position. This is easier described than accomplished because there is very little room in which to maneuver your hand, especially if the head is large. Applying a large amount of surgical lubricant into the vagina can help. Anesthesia will usually be necessary. Once you have rotated the head, hold it in its new position for a few minutes, because there is a tendency for it to return to its original OP position. If the head does return to OP, it is prudent not to persist and use multiple attempts at rotation. Do not dislodge the head upward during manual rotation. This undoubtedly makes the rotation easier, but risks having to deal with a prolapsed cord or arm, and can injure the head.

If it is not possible to grasp the head, you can try exerting gentle rotational pressure with the lateral part of your index finger along the lambdoidal suture edge, which is usually raised and prominent because of molding. If you use this approach, called digital rotation, abandon efforts if more than minimal force is required, and never exert pressure downward toward the cranial cavity. Whenever manual rotation is attempted with the head low in the pelvis, have an assistant help by rotating the shoulders in the appropriate direction with transabdominal pressure.

## Deflexion attitudes

As noted, it is not uncommon during an examination early in labor to find the fetal head deflexed. After labor becomes established, the head will usually flex and a normal mechanism will ensue. If the malposition fails to correct itself spontaneously, the prognosis is poor that flexion will be possible. A pathologic mechanism will result.

Three deflexion attitudes are recognized as distinct presentations. In order of their degree of deflexion they are *sincipital, brow,* and *face* presentations (Fig. 7.2). Each has a clearly defined course and mechanism. The fetal spine becomes extended so it is straight in sincipital presentations and S-shaped in brow and face presentations instead of its normal flexed condition or C-configuration. An approach to the diagnosis of fetal presentation is presented in Fig. 7.3.

### Sincipital presentation

#### Diagnosis
On abdominal examination, you will find that the trunk of the fetus is straight. You will usually feel the shoulder in the midline, just above the pubis. If the head is floating, you can easily recognize the occiput and the chin on about the same level. If the head is engaged, determining deflexion

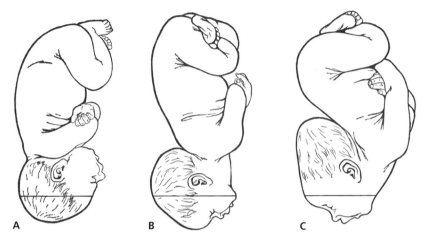

**Figure 7.2** Gamut of deflexion attitudes from (**A**) sincipital and (**B**) brow presentations to (**C**) face presentation, showing altered presenting fetal diameter from occipitobregmatic to mentobregmatic to trachelobregmatic.

is a bit more difficult, but insinuating your fingers suprapubically into the pelvis will help demonstrate it. Internally, you can feel the two fontanels in the same plane with the sagittal suture often transverse in the pelvis. Usually, the head is synclitic; but be aware that asynclitism is not uncommonly encountered with sincipital malpresentations after a long time in labor as a hallmark of associated cephalopelvic disproportion. The occiput is still considered the point of reference.

### Clinical course

With the fetal head in only slight deflexion, you can anticipate a labor similar to that in OP positions. Keep careful track of the head's attitude over time. Because a sincipital presentation is unstable, it will usually change in the course of labor so that it converts to a vertex presentation as the head flexes. Sometimes, however, you will notice the deflexion becoming more marked, even to the point at which the forehead presents. It has thereby become a brow presentation and is potentially much more hazardous. Treatment of labor with sincipital presentation is the same as described above for OP positions.

### Prognosis and management

Labor may be long in association with sincipital presentations, and protraction and arrest disorders can occur. Often you will find that, after the head reaches the pelvic floor, the contractions improve, flexion takes place, and the head is expelled without further difficulty.

## Brow presentation

### Diagnosis

With somewhat more deflexion of the fetal head than in the sincipital presentation, the brow (also called the bregma or forehead) of the fetus becomes the leading portion of the presenting part. Abdominally, the diagnostic findings are similar to those seen in a face presentation. The uterine ovoid is elongated and the cephalic prominence can be felt on the same side as the fetal back. Vaginally, the bregma is the lowest point and occupies the center of the pelvis (Fig. 7.4). The large anterior fontanel is palpable on one side and the root of the nose and orbital ridges are palpable on the other. The nose, mouth and chin are high up and out of reach most of the time. The orbital ridges are on a level with the posterior border of the large fontanel. The small posterior fontanel cannot be reached because it, too, is so high.

The kind of molding of the fetal head that takes place in association with a brow presentation is characteristic. The head acquires a three-cornered outline. The face is flattened; the distance from the chin to the top of the forehead is great; and this is exaggerated temporarily by the large caput that forms over the dependent brow. These features are shown in Fig. 7.5.

Transitory presentation of the brow in the beginning of labor is occasionally observed. Descent of the occiput usually occurs as the head engages in the pelvis. This converts the brow presentation into a vertex presentation. You can expect a more normal mechanism to follow. Sometimes, but less often, the fetal head will extend further instead. If this additional deflexion continues, it can produce a face presentation.

### Clinical course

Engagement in brow presentation occurs transversely with the fetal head deflexed so that the plane of the mentoparietal diameter presents. As many as 75% of brow presentations that are diagnosed early in labor later convert, the vast majority through further flexion to vertex presentations or, infrequently, by extension to face presentations. If the brow presentation persists, safe vaginal delivery will prove unlikely unless the fetus is very small. The associated labor will be dysfunctional. If conversion to a face presentation is to take place, it will usually occur late in descent, most often during the second stage. By contrast, conversion to a vertex, in our experience, tends to occur as the head engages, although it can also sometimes occur later in labor. Extensive molding and caput formation may make flexion during descent impossible in some cases.

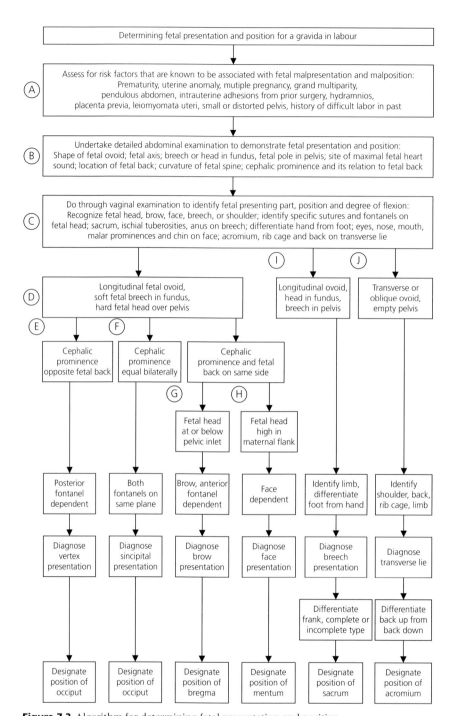

**Figure 7.3** Algorithm for determining fetal presentation and position.
**A**. Flag gravidas likely to develop a fetal malpresentation or malposition by identifying predisposing factors.
**B**. Abdominal examination reveals clues to fetal presentation and position, although you may be limited by maternal obesity, tense abdominal muscles or a hypertonic uterus. The uterine ovoid will be longitudinal in cephalic and breech presentations but will be transverse or oblique in transverse lie. Leopold maneuvers provide

additional information. Determine if the hard round fetal head is located in the pelvis or the uterine fundus, and where the soft breech is. Finding the back is important in conjunction with the location of the cephalic prominence to help recognize extension of the head in brow and face presentations. You can use auscultation (with a fetoscope, not Doppler ultrasound) to inform your palpatory findings. The heart is generally best heard through the back of the fetal thorax. Heart sounds tend to be found in the lower maternal abdomen in cephalic presentation, and the upper abdomen in a breech.

**C**. Provide additional details to document presentation and position and flexion or extension by vaginal examination. Confirming what the presenting part is, find the referent point (e.g., occiput for vertex, bregma for brow, chin for face, etc.), and determine its orientation in the pelvis. For cephalic presentations feel for the sutures and fontanels to help evaluate flexion and fetal position.

**D**. Verify a cephalic presentation if the fetal ovoid is longitudinal and the head is in the pelvis. To differentiate a well-flexed head (vertex presentation) from one that is somewhat deflexed (sincipital presentation) or more extended (brow or face presentation) learn where the cephalic prominence is in relation to the back. Recognize vertex presentation when the prominence is opposite the back; a sincipital presentation when both front and back of the head are equally prominent; and a brow or face presentation when the prominence is on the same side as the back. Brow can often be differentiated from face presentation by the brow dipping or engaged in the pelvis, while the face presents with the head located laterally in the lower abdomen.

**E**. The cephalic prominence found opposite the back signifies a well-flexed vertex presentation. Confirm by vaginal palpation of the posterior fontanel at or near the lowermost edge of the head. The sagittal suture adjacent to the fontanel tells you fetal position.

**F**. Suspect sincipital presentation when both sides of the fetal head are equally prominent on abdominal palpation. Verify by palpating both anterior and posterior fontanels in the same plane on vaginal examination. Diagnose position based on the orientation of the sagittal suture.

**G**. Both brow and face presentations show the cephalic prominence on same side as the back. The head in brow presentation is usually in the pelvis, while it remains high and off to the side in face presentation. Confirm brow presentation by identifying the brow vaginally. The brow is flanked on one side by the large diamond-shaped anterior fontanel and by the orbits and bridge of the nose on the other. Describe fetal position relative to the bregma. If the brow is on the left side of the pelvis and the sagittal suture runs transversely fetal position is left bregma transverse.

**H**. Suspect face presentation when the cephalic prominence is on the same side as the fetal back, but the head is unengaged and in the maternal flank. The fetal spine will be S-shaped from extreme extension of the head, in contrast to the usual C-shaped vertebral column of other cephalic presentations. Vaginally it can be difficult to identify the face because its features may be distorted by edema. If facial landmarks cannot be identified, reach for an ear. Another aid is the relations among the three bony prominences of the face, the malar protuberances of the zygoma and the nasal bone, all in a row. By contrast, the ischial tuberosities and sacrum in breech presentation form a triangle.

**I**. In breech presentation the head is found in the uterine fundus and the sacrum, natal cleft, and anus are recognized vaginally. The type of breech is not always apparent from the abdominal findings, but you should be able to distinguish among frank, complete, and incomplete breech vaginally. The location of the sacrum and the orientation of the natal cleft tell you fetal position. If a limb presents, distinguish hand (compound presentation) from foot (single or double footling presentation). The distal ends of the fingers align in spade fashion, whereas the ends of the toes are straight across.

**J**. Consider a transverse lie if the fetal ovoid is transverse or oblique and the pelvis is empty of a palpable presenting part. Confirm vaginally by finding the presenting part high out of the pelvis. Try to determine whether the fetal back is up or down in location. This can usually be done by abdominal palpation in which you will encounter either the fetal small parts or the back occupying the ventral aspect of the uterus.

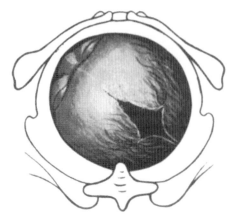

**Figure 7.4** Palpatory findings in brow presentation, right bregma anterior position, showing large centrally located anterior fontanel and root of nose within reach.

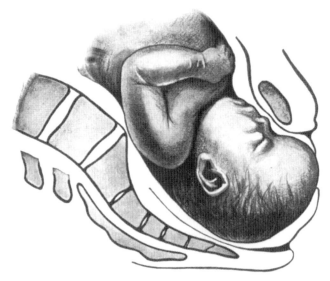

**Figure 7.5** Brow presentation, bregma anterior, demonstrating deflexion of the head and considerable caput succedaneum formation.

## Prognosis and management

Persistent brow presentation is potentially hazardous because of its frequent association with prolonged and difficult labor. The treatment of brow presentation is intelligent expectancy, with neither uterotonic stimulation nor operative intervention. This practice is warranted because spontaneous flexion to vertex presentation or, less often, extension to face presentation will usually take place in the course of a normal progressive labor. You should not manage these cases expectantly, however, when the pelvis is contracted or the fetus is unusually large. In these circumstances, perform cesarean delivery early in labor instead. As long as labor is progressing normally in dilatation and descent, there is no reason for you to interfere. If arrest of dilatation in the active phase or of descent in the second stage should occur, cesarean delivery is prudent. Manual or forceps conversion of a brow to a vertex presentation may be possible, but these potentially unsafe manipulations are rarely, if ever, done today because of their difficulty and the risks they pose of attendant fetal and maternal injury. To the point, their risks outweigh their ostensible benefits.

## Face presentation

With maximal deflexion (hyperextension) of the fetal head, the entire face comes to lie in the presenting plane (Figs 7.2 and 7.4) and is readily felt on vaginal examination. Major anomalies, especially anencephaly, account for about 5% of face presentations. Prematurity is common. At term, cephalopelvic disproportion is often present. The chin or mentum is the point of reference. Mentum positions are analogous to the occipital positions from which they develop. For example, marked deflexion of an LOT position will bring the face down in a right mentum transverse (RMT) position.

Face presentations may exist prior to labor, presumably because of congenital shortening or spasm of the extensor muscles of the head and neck. More commonly, a face presentation develops fully only after labor has been in progress for some time. What began as a sincipital presentation gradually extends to create a brow presentation and, finally, a face presentation. While labor progress is most often normal at first, the presenting trachelobregmatic (also called submentobregmatic) diameter predisposes to disproportion, manifested in both first and second stage labor dysfunction. This diameter is actually only a little larger than the suboccipitobregmatic that would negotiate the pelvis in a vertex presentation, but the face does not lend itself to the degree of molding that generally occurs in the head.

### Diagnosis

Early in labor the longitudinal ovoid of the uterus will seem decidedly elongated, and the maternal flanks are flat. You can feel the head easily over the inlet; engagement in early labor is unusual. The hard, rounded prominence of the occiput is felt to one side and above the inlet on the same side as the back. This is an important feature differentiating a face presentation from a vertex presentation in which the occipital prominence is on the side opposite the back. The occiput is separated from the back by the deep furrow of the fetal neck. On the other side, the inlet feels empty.

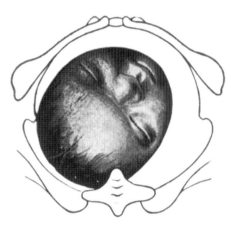

**Figure 7.6** Face presentation in left mentum anterior position. The brow, nose, orbits, mouth and chin can be recognized on examination.

However, if the abdominal wall is relaxed and the patient is thin, deep pressure with your examining fingers will detect the horseshoe-shaped jaw. Because the vertebral column is S-shaped (in contrast to the C-shape associated with vertex presentation) with marked extension of the back, the fetal chest protrudes anteriorly. The chest is often mistaken for the back, making the diagnosis quite challenging. In fact, the diagnosis is most often made by vaginal examination done late in labor when the presenting part has descended down far enough for detailed examination.

Vaginally, you will usually find the pelvis empty early in labor. Reach high into the pelvis and you will often recognize the brow. If the lower uterine segment has become very thin you might be able to identify the orbital ridges, if not the root of the nose. Once the membranes rupture, you will have less difficulty recognizing the eyes, mouth, nose, and jaw (Fig. 7.6). Careful palpation is very important to be sure that what you feel is a face and not the buttocks of a fetus in breech presentation. That mistake is often made, especially late in labor when the face has become quite edematous and landmarks are more difficult to identify. The distinction is obviously important because the management of face and breech presentations is very different. Sometimes, an accurate diagnosis cannot be made until the cervix is quite dilated. If it is a face presentation, even if the face is so swollen that the landmarks are obliterated, you should still be able to identify the saddle of the nose and the gums.

Remember to correlate your vaginal findings with those from your abdominal examination. Confusion between a face and breech presentation can usually be resolved by identifying the head and the breech abdominally.

An important point in the diagnosis is the determination of station. Engagement in face presentations usually occurs in the mentum transverse position. By definition, the fetal head is engaged only when the biparietal

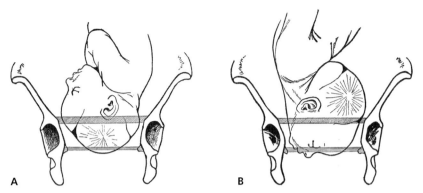

**Figure 7.7** Diagrams showing the relative degrees of engagement of vertex (**A**) and face (**B**) presentations when the forward leading edge of the head has advanced to the plane of the ischial spines. The parietal bosses are at or below the inlet with the vertex presentation, but well above the inlet in the face presentation. Any degree of extension of the head negates the general principle that the head is likely engaged once its leading part had descended to station 0.

diameter has passed the inlet. In occipital presentations with the fetal head well flexed, the parietal bosses are just below the plane of the inlet when the lowest part of the head, the vertex, is at or below the plane of the ischial spines. In face presentation, however, when the brow or the root of the nose (the lowest portion of the presenting part) lies in this plane, the parietal bosses are still at least 2–3 cm above the plane of the inlet (Fig. 7.7). With molding, moreover, the distance will be even greater. Only when the face is deep down in the pelvis, sometimes even on the pelvic floor and distending it, may the head be considered to have engaged.

When internal examinations are made in face presentations, try to avoid the introduction of mucus, meconium, or antiseptic solutions into the eyes of the fetus. Applying a fetal monitoring electrode should be avoided, if possible; if it is required, take special care to attach it to the forehead, avoiding the eyes or other areas of the face where it may do harm.

### Clinical course

Contrary to widely-held opinion, labor is usually uncomplicated in face presentations, and vaginal delivery is likely. That said, we must acknowledge that the cesarean rate in these cases is justifiably high because dysfunctional labor and disproportion do often exist. Disproportion is perhaps more the cause of the malpresentation, however, than its consequence.

The molding of the fetal head in face presentations causes the parietal bones to be depressed, unlike in vertex presentations, in which they are elevated. Molding generally starts when the fetal head is in the upper part

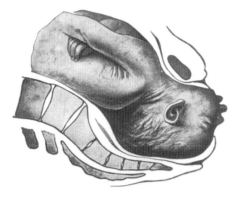

**Figure 7.8** Face presentation with mentum anterior position, showing extreme extension of the fetal head under the symphysis pubis and beginning flexion as the face is delivered over the perineum. Compare with Fig. 7.9.

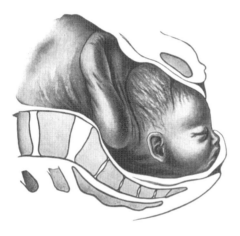

**Figure 7.9** Face presentation with the particularly hazardous mentum posterior position. The fetal chin has rotated into the hollow of the sacrum and the head is fully extended. Vaginal delivery would require further extension, and is therefore impossible unless rotation to mentum anterior position can be safely accomplished.

of the birth canal. Internal rotation from the mentum transverse to the mentum anterior position (Fig. 7.8) takes place in the lower midpelvis, somewhat below the level of comparable rotation in vertex presentation. If the mentum rotates to an anterior position, delivery will generally follow without complication. This rotation may not occur until the face is on the pelvic floor. Waiting for this to occur takes great patience on your part. If the face presents to the outlet as a mentum posterior, safe delivery is impossible unless the fetus is very small (Fig. 7.9).

Management of cases in which the mentum is anterior through most of descent need not differ from that of vertex presentations. If the face is transverse as it nears the pelvic floor, expect that it will almost always rotate to a favorable mentum anterior orientation. Use the Müller-Hillis maneuver (Chapter 4) to help evaluate whether or not disproportion is likely to exist. In addition, if the face tends to rotate toward a mentum anterior position during the maneuver, it will most likely rotate anteriorly as descent progresses. Be prepared to perform a cesarean if the head is fixed or if it prefers to rotate to mentum posterior. For cases in which the fetal head descends as a mentum posterior, anterior rotation might occur, although rarely. Nonetheless, cesarean delivery is probably the best approach.

Be aware, however, that cesarean delivery for a face presentation with the presenting part deeply wedged into the pelvis can be difficult. Take great care not to damage the fetus or the uterus during extraction of the fetus. Manually dislodging the fetal head gently upward is preferable to attempting to do so through the uterine incision. The dislodgement process should be done by someone who is experienced in and knowledgeable about it. It is important to spread the palm and fingers widely to distribute the pressure and thus avoid damaging any of the facial structures. After the delivery, whether by cesarean or vaginal approach, allow the head to remain in hyperextension. Do not try to straighten it forcibly.

The face of the newborn is often disfigured, especially if labor has been prolonged after the membranes have ruptured. Caput forms over the whole face. The eyes bulge, the lids are swollen, and a mucoserous discharge escapes from the eyes. The baby's mouth is open because the lips are tumid, and the tongue sometimes protrudes. Minute hemorrhages under the conjunctiva and in the skin, intense venous congestion, and cracks in the skin of the neck give the child a most alarming appearance. The shape of the head is extremely dolichocephalic. After delivery, the baby lies on its side with its head and neck extended and its back straight. It may sometimes retain this attitude for more than a week. The mother should be reassured that the child's features and its odd habitus will soon gain their proper appearance. Contrary to expectation, they do.

### Prognosis

Maternal morbidity is increased with face presentation because of the higher rates of long labor and of cesarean delivery. Infant mortality is also increased due to the same factors as in brow presentation. Edema of the glottis and fracture of the larynx have been reported rarely, and should be carefully watched for in the neonate.

Factors that affect the course of labor with vertex presentation act similarly in these cases. Progress is influenced not so much by the face presentation as by associated phenomena, particularly disproportion. Delivery will be spontaneous and uneventful most times. There is a higher rate of operative intervention, especially among women with very large babies.

### Management

Not all face presentations require special treatment (Fig. 7.10). Although there has been a recent tendency to undertake cesarean delivery for any

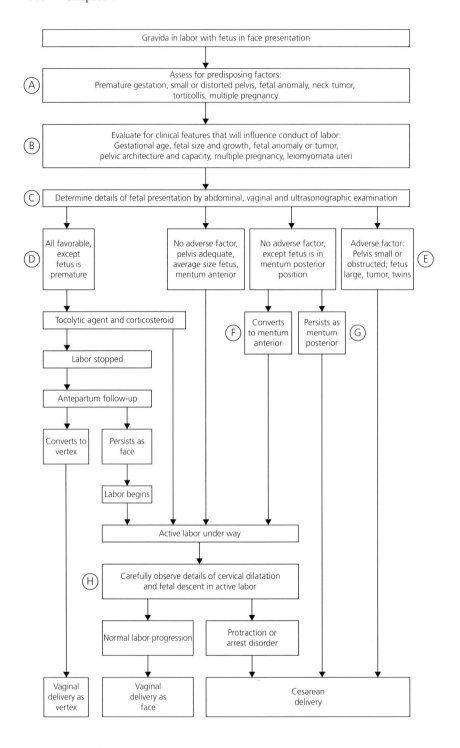

Gravida in labor with fetus in face presentation

(A) Assess for predisposing factors:
Premature gestation, small or distorted pelvis, fetal anomaly, neck tumor,
torticollis, multiple pregnancy

(B) Evaluate for clinical features that will influence conduct of labor:
Gestational age, fetal size and growth, fetal anomaly or tumor,
pelvic architecture and capacity, multiple pregnancy, leiomyomata uteri

(C) Determine details of fetal presentation by abdominal, vaginal and ultrasonographic examination

(D) All favorable, except fetus is premature

No adverse factor, pelvis adequate, average size fetus, mentum anterior

No adverse factor, except fetus is in mentum posterior position

Adverse factor: Pelvis small or obstructed; fetus large, tumor, twins (E)

Tocolytic agent and corticosteroid

(F) Converts to mentum anterior

Persists as mentum posterior (G)

Labor stopped

Antepartum follow-up

Converts to vertex

Persists as face

Labor begins

Active labor under way

(H) Carefully observe details of cervical dilatation and fetal descent in active labor

Normal labor progression

Protraction or arrest disorder

Vaginal delivery as vertex

Vaginal delivery as face

Cesarean delivery

**Figure 7.10** Management algorithm for face presentation.

**A**. Some predisposing factors for face presentation require special consideration in the care of the fetus. Preterm labor, an especially common concurrent condition, may warrant treatment. Recognizing that the maternal pelvis is inadequate in size or shape to accommodate the fetus may lead you to undertake cesarean delivery. Fetal anomalies (e.g., anencephaly) may be so severe as to preclude heroic measures, whereas tumors (e.g., large goiter) or neuromuscular disorders (e.g., torticollis) deserve labor management aimed at ensuring fetal well-being. The same applies to multiple pregnancy.

**B**. Carry out detailed evaluation for conditions that may limit your options in regard to how you handle the labor. Careful assessment of gestational duration and fetal weight estimation is important because prematurity, growth restriction or macrosomia will influence management, as would the presence of fetal anomalies.

**C**. Obtain essential details of the face presentation by a combination of abdominal, vaginal and ultrasonographic examinations. Aside from verifying the presentation itself, ascertain the orientation of the referent point on the face, namely the chin (mentum). The optimal fetal position for safe vaginal delivery is mentum anterior, although most fetuses with face presentation are in mentum transverse position during early labor and only rotate toward mentum anterior later in the course of the active phase and second stage. Critical to labor management is identification of the mentum posterior position, which requires special attention if it fails to convert spontaneously to mentum anterior.

**D**. Face presentation is much more common among premature fetuses. Apart from the maturational advantages to the newborn if delivery can be postponed, the longer the labor can be delayed, the greater the possibility of spontaneous conversion to vertex presentation.

**E**. In the presence of conditions that make vaginal delivery unsafe, it is prudent to proceed directly to cesarean delivery. A maternal pelvis that is clearly inadequate to accommodate the fetus by virtue of its small capacity or architectural distortion is one example. Another is fetal macrosomia. Additionally, if the fetus has a large tumor that cannot be delivered vaginally without trauma, if at all, attempting such a delivery is unwise.

**F.** The mentum posterior position is quite unfavorable for vaginal delivery. However, about half the cases in which mentum posterior is recognized in early labor will spontaneously convert to mentum anterior in advanced labor. If this occurs, allowing labor to proceed to vaginal delivery is appropriate.

**G.** Attempts to effect rotation of a fetal head in persistent mentum posterior position by digital or instrumental means are sometimes possible, but they require special skill and may be traumatic even in the best of hands. They are, therefore, not generally recommended. Prudence makes cesarean delivery preferable.

**H.** The pattern of progression of cervical dilatation and fetal descent is an important objective indicator of whether or not safe vaginal delivery is likely to occur. Normal progress presages safe vaginal delivery. Protraction and arrest disorders signal the probability of cephalopelvic disproportion. While the labor abnormalities are not actually diagnostic of obstructed labor in the individual case, it is far safer to assume disproportion is present under these circumstances than to expose mother and fetus to its risks. Cesarean delivery is, therefore, indicated.

fetus in face presentation, the majority can in fact deliver spontaneously without complications. The parents must be prepared in advance, because the facial edema and the extended neck noted above can be disturbing to the uninitiated.

Once a diagnosis is made, determine, if possible, the cause of the face presentation. Anencephaly, hydrocephaly, and other major anomalies can usually be ruled out by ultrasonographic imaging. If an anomaly exists, plan the delivery route accordingly, i.e., avoid operative intervention for fetal indications alone if the malformations are not compatible with survival. Rarely, the extension of the head is caused by a large neoplasm in the fetal neck and, if diagnosed by imaging, prompt cesarean is indicated. If you find the pelvis is contracted, deliver by cesarean. Without these special indications, intelligent expectancy should be pursued. You and your patient will usually be rewarded by a spontaneous delivery. If a labor abnormality occurs, you should not administer oxytocin unless you have first ruled out disproportion. While forceps can be used to aid delivery, and even to effect rotation, these procedures are potentially quite traumatic and we recommend against them. Obviously, never apply a vacuum extractor to a face!

When the mentum is anterior, normal descent and spontaneous delivery are the rule. Mentum posterior presentations are of concern, although, as noted, in about half the cases the chin rotates spontaneously to the anterior late in the second stage. If it does not, cesarean delivery, even with the face deep in the pelvis, is the best option.

If cesarean delivery is not an available option, you can attempt to rotate the face from MP to MA when it has reached the perineum. To do so, place one hand in the vagina and obtain purchase on the malar and frontal bones using the extended fingers and, if room permits, the palm. During a contraction, exert gentle traction, rotating the face toward the anterior quadrant while pulling forward (caudad) with the fingers in an attempt to bring the chin under the pubis. This maneuver is aided by simultaneous external abdominal pressure on the fetal shoulder by an assistant. If rotation is successful and the new position is retained with a few contractions, the prognosis for vaginal delivery is good. If manual rotation cannot be accomplished, or the fetus returns to a mentum posterior position, cesarean delivery is necessary.

In all vaginal deliveries of fetuses in face presentation, the diameters and circumferences presented to the pelvic outlet are not as favorable as in vertex deliveries. The pelvic floor is stretched markedly and pushed farther downward, putting it at risk of damage. Use a deep mediolateral episiotomy to help avert both maternal and fetal injuries. Always be especially careful not to injure the fetal face when making an episiotomy or performing any other manipulation.

## Key points

- Early in labor, the OP head is often high in the pelvis and partly deflexed. The small posterior fontanel, located posteriorly in the pelvis, is felt higher or on the same level as the large anterior fontanel.
- Most heads that descend in OP position have considerable molding and caput succedaneum formation, especially if descent has been protracted.
- Most of the time, a head that is OP early in labor will rotate to an OA position as descent progresses. Sometimes, it will remain OP and deliver in that position.
- While OP is generally categorized as a *malposition*, it is in fact sometimes an appropriate accommodation to the extant pelvic architecture.
- When you find an OP position any time in labor, be concerned about the possibility of dysfunctional labor progress and structural pelvic pathology.
- Although most labor patterns in OP positions are normal, there is a higher associated frequency of protraction and arrest disorders of dilatation and descent.
- Perineal lacerations are common when the head delivers in an OP position.
- Most brow presentations diagnosed early in labor later convert through flexion to vertex or by extension to face presentations. If the brow persists, it is unlikely to be safely deliverable vaginally.
- With the slight deflexion of a sincipital presentation, anticipate a labor similar to that in OP positions.
- Face presentations may exist prior to labor, but most develop fully after labor has been in progress for some time.
- Once a face presentation is diagnosed, try to determine the cause.
- When the face is mentum anterior, anticipate normal descent and spontaneous delivery. Most mentum transverse and mentum posterior presentations will rotate to mentum anterior late in the second stage.
- Oxytocin should not be used in deflexion attitudes unless disproportion is judged very unlikely.

## Further Reading

### Books and reviews

Cruikshank DP, Cruikshank JE. Face and brow presentation: a review. Clin Obstet Gynecol 1981;24:333–51.

Novak-Antolic Z. Transverse lie, brow and face presentations. In: Kurjak A, Chervenak FA (eds) *Textbook of Perinatal Medicine*, 2nd edition. Informa Healthcare, London, 2006: 1912–17.

## Primary sources

Borell V, Fernstrom I. The mechanism of labor in face and brow presentation: a radiologic study. Acta Obstet Gynecol Scand 1960;39:626–44.

Cheng YW, Shaffer BL, Caughey AB. The association between persistent occiput posterior position and neonatal outcomes. Obstet Gynecol 2006;107:837–44.

Fitzpatrick M, McQuillan K, O'Herlihy C. Influence of persistent occiput posterior position on delivery outcome. Obstet Gynecol 2001;98:1027–31.

Meltzer RM, Sachtleben MR, Friedman EA. Brow presentation. Am J Obstet Gynecol 1968;100:63.

Gardberg M, Laakkonen E, Sälevaara M. Intrapartum sonography and persistent occiput posterior position: a study of 408 deliveries. Obstet Gynecol 1998;91:746–9.

Kutcipal RA. The persistent occiput posterior position: a review of 498 cases. Obstet Gynecol 1959;14:296–304.

Le Ray C, Serres P, Schmitz T, Cabrol D, Goffinet F. Manual rotation in occiput posterior or transverse positions: risk factors and consequences on the cesarean delivery rate. Obstet Gynecol 2007; 110: 873–9.

Lowenstein A, Zevin R. Digital rotation of the vertex. Obstet Gynecol 1970;37:790–1.

Pearl ML, Roberts JM, Laros RK, Hurd WW. Vaginal delivery from the persistent occiput posterior positon. J Reprod Med 1993;38:955–61.

Shaffer BL, Cheng YW, Vargas JE, Laros RK, Caughey AB. Manual rotation of the fetal occiput: predictors of success and delivery. Med Image Analysis 2006;194:e7–e9.

Sizer AR, Nirmal DM. Occipitoposterior position: associated factors and obstetric outcome in nulliparas. Obstet Gynecol 2000;96:749–52.

Yancey MK, Zhang J, Schweitzer DL, Schwarz J, Klebanoff MA. Epidural anesthesia and fetal head malposition at vaginal delivery. Obstet Gynecol 2001;97:608–12.

## CHAPTER 8

# Managing Breech Presentation and Transverse Lie

## Breech presentation

### Etiology

About 3–5% of all deliveries occur with the fetus presenting as a breech. In most cases, the precise cause of this malpresentation is unknown. It is recognized to be associated with prematurity, placenta previa, multiple pregnancy, and fetal or uterine malformations (Box 8.1). Higher fetal and neonatal morbidity and mortality occur among fetuses with breech presentation than corresponding fetuses with vertex presentation. As a consequence, the question of how to manage the breech presentation has generated a vast literature and no shortage of polemic.

Not all of the excess morbidity and mortality that accrues to fetuses in breech presentation is related to their delivery mode. In fact, most of the adversity derives from the factors that predispose to breech presentation, especially prematurity (Boxes 8.1 and 8.2). You should identify these sundry conditions whenever possible because they might affect decisions that you make about management of the labor and the mode of delivery.

During the course of labor and vaginal delivery, a number of serious, even lethal, complications can befall the fetus (Box 8.3). These can usually be avoided if properly selected cases are managed expertly. One of the prerequisites for such expert management is the presence of attendant personnel with the necessary knowledge, skills, and experience to perform vaginal breech delivery safely. Those same skills are equally important for the cesarean delivery of a fetus in breech presentation.

The notion that cesarean delivery is safer for breech presentation than vaginal birth is not new. Abdominal section was used increasingly, beginning in the 1970s and 1980s. Many studies supported the virtues of cesarean delivery, and by the early 2000s vaginal breech delivery was no longer considered appropriate by most authorities. That stance has softened

*Labor and Delivery Care: A Practical Guide*, First Edition. Wayne R. Cohen and Emanuel A. Friedman. © 2011 John Wiley & Sons, Ltd. Published 2011 by John Wiley & Sons, Ltd

**Box 8.1 Obstetric factors associated with breech presentation**

- Placenta previa
- Müllerian anomalies (maternal)
- Prematurity
- Multiple gestation

**Box 8.2 Congenital abnormalities associated with breech presentation**

- Central nervous system
  - Hydrocephaly
  - Anencephaly
  - Meningomyelocele
  - Familial dysautonomia
- Urinary system
  - Renal agenesis
- Musculoskeletal system
  - Congenital hip dislocation
  - Myotonic dystrophy
- Chromosome abnormalities
  - Trisomy-13
  - Trisomy-18
  - Trisomy-21
- Other disorders
  - Prader-Willi syndrome
  - Werdnig-Hoffman syndrome
  - Smith-Lemle-Opitz syndrome
  - deLange syndrome
  - Fetal alcohol syndrome

**Box 8.3 Fetal injuries that can occur during vaginal breech delivery**

- Brachial plexus injury
- Long bone fractures
- Cervical spinal cord injury
- Asphyxia
- Traumatic hip dislocation
- Adrenal hemorrhage

recently. There is now considerable evidence that, in properly selected candidates, long-term outcome for babies born vaginally in breech presentation is not different from results in comparable vertex presentations.

There is a perverse irony in these shifting views. Managing a breech delivery safely requires considerable skill and experience. Because concerns about the safety of vaginal breech birth led to its near-eradication from residency training for many years, there are now few obstetricians who feel sufficiently comfortable with the procedure to do it safely. With few willing and able teachers, breech delivery has, for better or worse, become increasingly rare.

In this chapter we describe in detail the basic maneuvers necessary to perform vaginal breech delivery and to manage its common complications. We urge you to master them because they will prove useful to you if you wish to perform planned breech delivery. Even if you do not, they will serve for those inevitable situations in which a patient presents in advanced labor and there is no time to resort to cesarean. Also, you will find that delivery of a fetus in breech presentation through a cesarean incision is not always easy; the difficulties you encounter will require you to understand the same basic principles and apply the same skills as in vaginal delivery.

## Diagnosis

The types of breech presentations are named according to the posture of the fetus. Most common is the *frank breech* presentation, in which the legs are extended against the trunk so that the feet lie against the face (Fig. 8.1). In the *complete breech*, the fetus is in the same attitude as in a vertex presentation, but with reversed polarity. The thighs are flexed against the body, and the lower legs flexed on the thighs so that the buttocks, with the feet alongside them, present at the internal cervical os (Fig. 8.2). *Incomplete breech* presentations are of two types. One or both feet may prolapse into the vagina, producing a single or double *footling presentation* or, more rarely, one or both knees are prolapsed, called a *knee presentation*.

In describing the orientation of the breech presentation in the pelvis, use the fetal sacrum as the point of reference. The most common presentations are left sacrum anterior (LSA) and right sacrum posterior (RSP). The natal cleft (the groove between the buttocks) is used for orientation in the same way that the sagittal suture is used for vertex presentations.

Abdominal examination will show the ovoid to be longitudinal. Instead of the hard, round head you are accustomed to feeling in cephalic presentations, you will feel a softer, more yielding, irregular mass over the inlet. As you press your hands alongside the presenting part toward the inlet, the unengaged breech will often tend to slip upward between them. You will generally feel the head lateral to the midline in the fundus. If the head is in the midline, it is more consistent with a frank breech, in which the fetal back has been straightened and splinted by the extended legs. In a thin patient, the feet may sometimes be felt in the upper uterus alongside the head.

Carry out a vaginal examination to confirm your impressions from the Leopold maneuvers. Because the breech often remains high in the pelvis

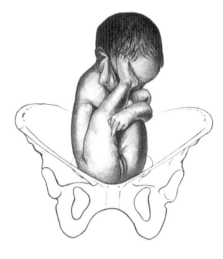

**Figure 8.1** Fetus in frank breech presentation, right sacrum posterior position, with lower extremities extended fully across abdomen, chest and face.

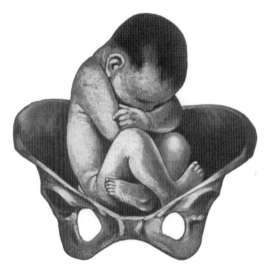

**Figure 8.2** Fetus in complete breech presentation with buttocks and both feet presenting at the pelvic inlet, right sacrum posterior position.

during most of the first stage of labor, reaching the presenting part may be difficult. You will not feel a hard, convex skull; instead, you will palpate a roundish, soft mass of prominences and depressions. These are the buttocks with the natal cleft between them. At one end of the crease, you can distinguish the hard sacrum (Fig. 8.3), which you will use to describe the fetal position. To confirm position, follow the crease until the scrotum or the vulva can be distinguished. Higher up and to one side, you may feel one or both feet, although usually in a complete breech only the heels are within your reach.

Mistakes are common in the diagnosis of breech presentation by vaginal examination. This is in part because it can be difficult to feel the high

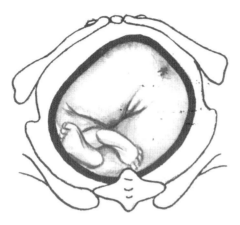

**Figure 8.3** Findings on vaginal examination in a complete breech presentation, left sacrum anterior position, with natal cleft in the oblique diameter, sacrum and anus in the left anterior quadrant, and the feet palpable in the right posterior quadrant.

presenting part, or to distinguish its features until the cervix is at least 3–4 cm dilated. Also, once dilatation and descent are sufficiently advanced for identification, considerable edema may obscure landmarks. While the presence of soft irregularities in the presenting part may make it obvious that you are not dealing with a vertex presentation, the breech is often mistaken for a face, a shoulder, or an anencephalic head. Careful examination and correlation of vaginal with abdominal findings are necessary to confirm your diagnosis.

## Mechanism

Safe management of vaginal breech delivery, particularly if manipulations of the fetus are involved, requires a good understanding of the normal mechanism of labor. Application of that understanding minimizes risk, even when you are delivering the breech through a hysterotomy incision.

The mechanism of labor (Fig. 8.4) is essentially the same whether the breech is frank, complete, or incomplete. The breech often remains high in the pelvis until labor is well advanced and dilatation of the cervix is nearly complete. Descent occurs at about the same rate as in vertex presentations. We will consider the mechanism of a left sacrum anterior position (LSA).

*Lateral flexion* of the lower trunk occurs as soon as the breech reaches the perineum. The posterior buttock is held back and the anterior buttock stems under the pubis. This movement is always associated with *internal anterior rotation*. In the LSA position, the breech descends in the left oblique. That is, the fetal sacrum is in the left anterior part of the maternal pelvis; the bisiliac diameter lies in the oblique diameter of the pelvis; the natal cleft lies in the opposite oblique; and the anterior hip points to the right pubic tubercle and is a little deeper in the pelvis than the posterior hip. Anterior rotation occurs as the anterior hip rotates to the midline

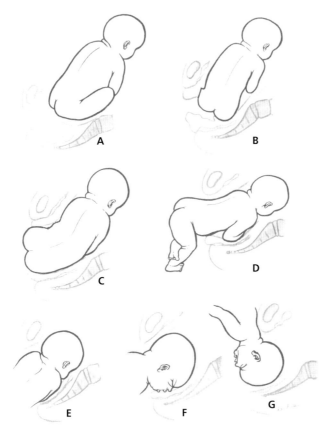

**Figure 8.4** Diagram of steps in the mechanism of labor in the breech presentation, left sacrum anterior position. **A**. Engagement of the breech in the oblique diameter high in the pelvis, where it may remain well into labor. **B**. Descent into the midplane with internal anterior rotation to left sacrum transverse position. **C**. Lateral flexion of the fetal lower trunk until delivered over the perineum. **D**. Delivery of the legs and the body to the umbilicus with rotation of the back anteriorly. **E**. Delivery of the shoulders. **F**. Beginning delivery of the head with the occiput anterior under the symphysis pubis. **G**. Delivery of the head over the perineum with the body supported.

from the right anterior quadrant of the pelvis and the sacrum points directly to the left side; the natal cleft now lies transversely.

Delivery involves continued lateral flexion as the anterior hip stems under the symphysis pubis; the posterior hip rolls over the perineum, and the whole fetal pelvis rises up over the pubis. *Restitution* and *external rotation* are not constant in breech presentation. Usually, the anterior hip returns to its original side and the sacrum comes to lie directly anterior. Sometimes, however, the back remains transverse and the shoulders are delivered in that position.

The movements of the shoulders are precisely the same as those of the breech. Descent occurs with the bisacromial diameter in the left oblique. If

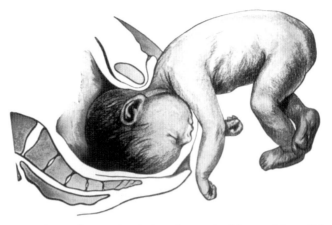

**Figure 8.5** Lateral view showing the ideal mechanism for delivery of the well-flexed aftercoming head. The occiput is anterior with the nape of the neck stemming just under the symphysis pubis. The face will be delivered over the perineum by further flexion.

no attempt is made to aid delivery by traction from below, the arms remain folded closely against the chest. The anterior shoulder rotates in the right anterior quadrant of the pelvis toward the pubis and stems behind it. A process of lateral flexion delivers the posterior shoulder and arm. Then the anterior shoulder appears from behind the pubis and, if no assistance is given, the body drops down so that the anterior neck is against the perineum and the nape of the neck is against the subpubic ligament. If the head is arrested high, restitution and external rotation of the shoulders take place, and the back again rotates to the side. If the head follows the body closely and drops into the pelvis, the fetal back may rotate anteriorly at once.

Under normal circumstances, the head enters the inlet when the shoulders are passing the vulva. The head then undergoes the expected mechanisms. Descent, flexion, and anterior rotation of the occiput occur in order. The sagittal suture enters in the right oblique as it does in LOA positions. When the chin has rotated to the hollow of the sacrum, flexion occurs (Fig. 8.5). The nape of the neck stems centrally under the symphysis pubis, and the chin, face, and forehead appear successively over the perineum. After this, the occiput escapes from behind the pubis. In sacrum posterior positions, the mechanism is nearly the same. In that case, the anterior buttock must rotate only 45 degrees to reach the pubis.

## Unusual mechanisms

Occasionally, after the breech emerges, the back overrotates beyond the pubis to the other side of the pelvis. Here the mechanism is similar to that of the shoulders in cephalic presentations. The fetus may thus be found with its back opposite to the position in which it was initially.

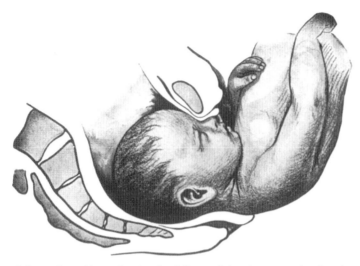

**Figure 8.6** Less favorable mechanism for delivery of the aftercoming head in the occiput posterior position. The bridge of the nose stems under the symphysis pubis and delivery of the head will take place by the occiput crossing the perineum. Compare with Fig. 8.5.

Excessive internal rotation of the breech may also occur, with the fetal abdomen facing toward the pubis. Subsequently, the shoulders enter in an oblique diameter and the proper mechanism is resumed. It is usually not possible to discover the cause of these irregular mechanisms.

A footling breech presentation undergoes the normal mechanism unless the posterior foot has prolapsed. In all labors, the construction of the forepelvis, the sacrosciatic ligaments, and the levator sling tend to direct the most caudad part of the fetus under the symphysis pubis. Thus, when the anterior leg has prolapsed, the breech glides along without difficulty. However, when the posterior leg has prolapsed, the breech is held higher, the anterior buttock impinges on—and sometimes above—the anterior ramus of the pubis, the posterior leg finds a path of least resistance on the other side of the pelvis, and often the back rotates to face the sacrum. The posterior limb now becomes the anterior one and follows out by the usual mechanism, but on the other side of the pelvis.

Abnormal rotation of the back is infrequent unless you apply traction to the trunk prematurely. If the back rotates to the posterior pelvis, the fetus descends with its abdomen facing upward toward the mother's pubis. Usually, the body will deliver in this position, but the aftercoming head may become stuck, with its occiput in the sacral hollow and the chin facing the pubis (Fig. 8.6).

One of three things may happen to the aftercoming posterior head under these circumstances. If the head is well flexed, with the chin applied to the fetal sternum, spontaneous anterior rotation of the occiput may occur just before delivery so that the head emerges optimally. If the head is relatively small and well flexed, it may deliver as an occiput posterior without great difficulty. If you gently lift the body of the child upward, you can facilitate this mode of delivery. Finally, if the head is extended, the chin may be caught on the pubic ramus above the inlet. In that case, lift the fetus upward, while slowly moving its chest against the symphysis. This makes the anterior neck the center of rotation, and will direct the occiput to pass over the perineum. Take special care here to avoid injuring the anterior neck structures. A generous episiotomy is important in such situations.

Delivery may also be complicated when one or both fetal arms leave the chest and are stretched up over the head (*extended arm*) or even cross behind the occiput to become located in the nape of the neck (*nuchal arm*). Management of these potentially serious complications is discussed below.

## Course of labor

The course of dilatation and descent in labor with breech presentation is essentially the same as with comparable vertex presentation, except that the breech tends to enter labor at a high station and to remain there until late in labor. The appearance of an abnormal pattern of dilatation or descent should alert you that fetopelvic disproportion may be present. If the labor curve patterns are not normal, it is generally wise to abandon a trial of labor in a breech presentation.

Premature rupture of membranes is common, as is escaping meconium-stained amniotic fluid. The latter is seen almost invariably in the second stage as the contents of the fetal bowel are extruded by pressure exerted on the abdomen during descent. Edema (equivalent to caput succedaneum) is found on the anterior hip, but may spread all over the buttock. The penis and scrotum or vulva may be extremely edematous and ecchymotic at birth. If a leg has been prolapsed for several hours, it will often be congested and swollen. Reassure the mother about these changes. They will all disappear within a week, and have no long-term consequences.

## Treatment

Three kinds of breech delivery can occur: (1) *spontaneous delivery*; (2) *assisted breech delivery (partial breech extraction)*; (3) *total breech extraction*.

### Spontaneous breech delivery

A spontaneous delivery proceeds according to the mechanism described above. Your role is simply to support the fetus as necessary, allowing the uterine contractions and the mother's bearing-down efforts to accomplish the delivery. This is the safest and least potentially traumatic way to accomplish the delivery. Be prepared to intervene if the spontaneous mechanism falters.

### Assisted breech delivery

In this technique, you will apply traction to the lower part of the body after the fetus has been extruded spontaneously as far as its umbilicus by the force of uterine contractions and maternal expulsive efforts. Use this technique if further bearing-down efforts do not elicit progress. It is necessary at this point to ensure that the rest of the delivery occurs smoothly and expeditiously, because pressure on the cord by the fetal body reduces oxygen delivery to the fetus. Do not, however, be tempted to rush through the delivery. Undue haste is counterproductive.

Anesthesia is desirable, although not always necessary. Local or pudendal block will often suffice, but if the patient has epidural anesthesia in effect, that will be ideal. Make a deep episiotomy as the breech crosses the perineum. It is more difficult to do so after the body has partially delivered. Episiotomy is useful to facilitate all the manipulations that may be required for the delivery. If the fetus is astride the cord, advance it and slip it over one thigh. If this fails, you might need to divide the cord and end the delivery promptly. Be sure the bladder is empty. If distended, it may interfere with delivery of the head.

The sequential maneuvers of assisted breech delivery include: (1) engaging the shoulders by traction on the fetal pelvis to deliver the scapulae while simultaneously rotating the body until the anterior shoulder stems under the symphysis; (2) delivering the shoulders by gently sweeping the anterior arm across the chest and then rotating the trunk in the opposite direction to move the posterior shoulder anteriorly where it can be readily delivered; (3) delivering the head (with its occiput now directed anteriorly) by flexing it over the perineum with combined suprapubic pressure and malar traction.

Once the fetus has delivered to the umbilicus, advance the cord so that it is not placed in tension as the fetus descends further. If it is a frank breech and the legs have not fully delivered, use the Pinard maneuver (see below) to free them from the birth canal. Grasp the pelvis with two hands (Fig. 8.7) and apply gentle downward traction until you see the anterior scapula clear the introitus. Now deliver the anterior arm by sweeping it across the chest (Fig. 8.8). Once you accomplish this, rotate the body so that the other arm is anterior and deliver it in the same manner. The rotation should be in the direction of the chest so that the undelivered arm remains well flexed. Do this by simply grasping the delivered arm, as if shaking hands, and rotating the fetus by gently pulling the free arm across the chest.

The fetal back is now facing up, and the occiput is anterior. Support the body of the fetus with your forearm, with its arms and legs straddling and

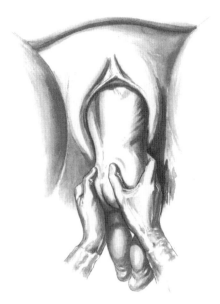

**Figure 8.7** Delivery from the umbilicus to the shoulder in assisted breech delivery. Take the breech in two hands with the thumbs over the back of the sacrum and the index fingers on the anterior superior iliac spines. Placing a dry towel around the lower trunk can help ensure your grip. Pull with gentle even traction in the direction of the axis of the inlet until the scapula of the anterior shoulder comes well under the symphysis pubis.

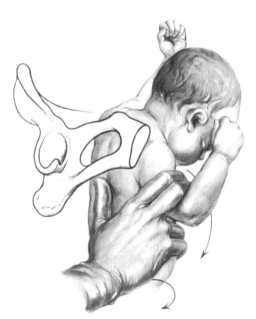

**Figure 8.8** To bring down the anterior arm, slip two fingers upward under the pubis over the fetal back and down to the elbow flexure. By flexing your fingers and rotating your wrist you can sweep the arm of the fetus over its chest and down and out.

with your hand in the vagina. As the head descends, raise your elbow, and deliver the head by flexion (Fig. 8.9). To do so, place the middle finger of your vaginal hand gently into the fetus's mouth or your first and third fingers over the malar eminences. In this way you can keep the chin flexed as you apply suprapubic pressure with your other hand to encourage delivery of the head (the Mauriceau-Smellie-Veit maneuver).

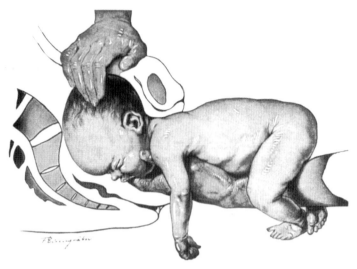

**Figure 8.9** This figure shows one method of delivering the aftercoming head. With the fetal body straddling your forearm, insert the hand into the vagina and pass an extended finger into the mouth. Use gentle pressure from above to bring the head into the pelvis, keeping the chin well flexed. While this technique works, there is danger of dislocating the jaw if your finger is flexed. It is preferable, therefore, to pass your fingers higher on the face and place them on the malar eminences. Pressure on this part of the face, combined with suprapubic pressure on the head will provide the necessary flexion for delivery.

### Total breech extraction

In this technique the obstetrician delivers the entire body of the fetus. It is a particularly hazardous procedure and should not be undertaken unless there are strong indications and no safer alternative is available. Examples would be a singleton breech or second twin presenting as a breech or transverse lie in which delivery is urgent and cannot await cesarean or further evolution of labor. This form of delivery is seldom used today. Do not attempt a total breech extraction unless you have developed the skills necessary to perform it and to deal with its associated complications.

Before proceeding, ensure that the cervix is fully dilated. The pelvis should be spacious and disproportion unlikely. The bladder and the rectum must be empty, and the mother given anesthesia. Sometimes, pharmacologic relaxation of the uterus is desirable for facilitating the manipulations that will be needed for the procedure.

The procedure has four parts: (1) bringing out the breech and legs; (2) delivering the shoulders; (3) disengaging the shoulder girdle; (4) delivering the aftercoming head. The last three are identical with the steps for assisted breech delivery.

It is essential that you first identify one of the fetal legs or preferably both. This will provide important information as to which leg is anterior in

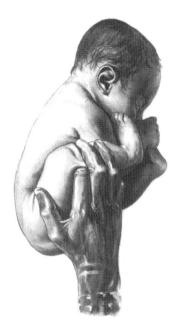

**Figure 8.10** Bringing down a foot with the Pinard maneuver in breech extraction. Pass your hand high into the uterus, avoiding the cord. Press the index finger into the popliteal fossa. This shortens the hamstring muscles and begins flexion of the leg. Slip the other three fingers over the knee to the ankle. Now slide the foot along the other thigh into the pelvis and out.

location. Doing your examination with the patient in deep Trendelenburg position may help in this regard. Select the anterior limb to deliver first, if possible, because doing so will help bring the fetal back under the maternal pubis.

In a frank breech presentation, it will be necessary to flex the extended fetal leg in order to grasp it for traction. Use the Pinard maneuver to accomplish this (Fig. 8.10). Slide a well-lubricated hand into the uterus between contractions. Insinuate your index finger into the popliteal space behind the knee and place your other fingers on the lower leg. Press the thigh and knee toward the fetal abdomen and flex the knee. This brings the foot down so it can be grasped. In a complete breech, the foot is already accessible. Be sure you are not pulling down a hand!

Pull gently on the leg, using your fingers to splint the long bones and deliver the anterior hip (Fig. 8.11). Flex the lower body laterally to deliver the other leg (Fig. 8.12). In a frank breech, another Pinard maneuver will be necessary to flex the posterior leg at the knee. At this point, the umbilicus has emerged. The remaining maneuvers are the same as described earlier for assisted breech delivery (see above).

### The modified Bracht method
The Bracht method (Fig. 8.13) is an alternative approach you can use to assist a breech delivery. It is a technique that supports the fetus through the normal mechanism of labor and vaginal delivery, and thereby minimizes

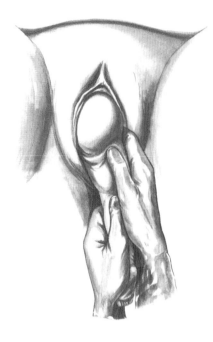

**Figure 8.11** Deliver the anterior hip by placing the thumbs parallel to the long bones and the fingers evenly over the rest of the limb. Pull downward in the axis of the inlet until the crest of the ilium has passed the arcuate ligament. Do not bend or twist the leg. The action must be even and smooth.

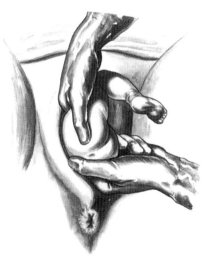

**Figure 8.12** Deliver the posterior hip. Pass the index finger of the other hand over the back along the crest of the ilium into the groin. With combined traction, the whole pelvis is brought out, following the usual lateroflexion mechanism. The second leg is allowed to drop out or is reduced by the Pinard maneuver.

the risk of trauma. Its basic principle is to mimic the natural vaginal breech delivery as if it were occurring with the patient upright, i.e., by correcting the misplaced gravitational pull that exists when the parturient is lying on her back or is in semi-sitting position. Furthermore, it ensures that the fetus will progress along the projected axis of the birth canal while it is being expelled over the perineum, rather than being pulled posteriorly by gravity.

The mother who bears down strongly at the same time as the uterus contracts supplies all the expulsive forces. For her to achieve optimal results in effecting the delivery, it is essential that she be in full control of her faculties, i.e., with minimal analgesia and only local perineal anesthesia.

In supporting her fetus during this maneuver, you will be required to elevate the fetal body progressively to follow the outward extension of the curve of the birth canal. In doing so, be sure not to hyperextend the fetal spine, most especially at the neck, while the body is being delivered. Having an assistant depress the perineum as the head emerges and another giving some suprapubic pressure to encourage flexion of the head can be useful.

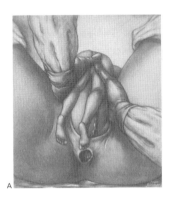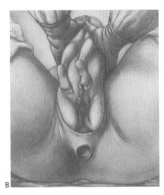

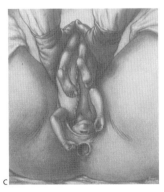

**Figure 8.13** Bracht method of delivering the breech to the umbilicus. **A**. Hold the body and legs together with your hands, merely supporting the breech and allowing it to move upward in the anteriorly curved external projection of the pelvic curve. **B**. Hold the baby with its back against the symphysis, but do not overextend the neck. This will result in spontaneous and simultaneous delivery of the elbows folded against the chest, followed by the arms and the shoulders in transverse position. Do not apply traction, but maintain the fetus in this position. **C**. The head delivers spontaneously, passing through the inlet in its most favorable diameter. Delivery is accomplished entirely by the mother's expulsive efforts alone.

---

**Box 8.4 Causes of extended or nuchal arms in breech delivery**

- Too early or too rapid traction on the body
- Small pelvis
- Fundal pressure during delivery
- Incompletely dilated cervix
- Presence of uterine contraction ring

---

## Complications during delivery

A host of complications can accompany breech delivery (Box 8.3). We will address here two of the most common serious problems: (1) extension of one or both arms; (2) entrapment of the aftercoming head in the uterus. The former is most often the result of traction being applied to the body too early in the course of the delivery. The latter may be a consequence of fetopelvic disproportion, malposition of the head, or delivery through an incompletely dilated cervix.

### Extended and nuchal arms

Normally the fetal arms lie crossed over the chest and, if nothing interferes, they are delivered in this position. The arms may sometimes be displaced up above the fetal head or actually come to rest behind the neck (Fig. 8.14). This is most likely to occur if traction is made on the body too soon, if the pelvis is small, or in other situations (Box 8.4). If one of these

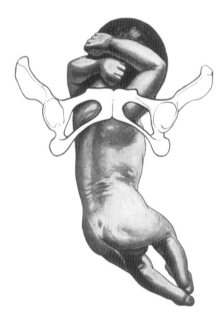

**Figure 8.14** Bilateral nuchal arms. Free the arms when they are in this position by rotating the body first 180 degrees in one direction (here counterclockwise in the direction the outer arm is facing) to dislodge one arm and then 180 degrees in the other direction to dislodge the other arm.

arm complications occurs in labor at or near term, further descent and atraumatic delivery will be impossible until it is resolved.

For the arm that is merely extended upward, pass four fingers high into the uterus, leaving the thumb outside, and glide them over the fetal back, shoulders, humerus, and elbow. Flex the elbow. Splint the humerus with your fingers and then slide the elbow across the face, and then down and out. First deliver the more accessible arm, usually the posterior one. You should cut a deep episiotomy in advance, if it has not already been done for the breech delivery, to provide space to facilitate your manipulation of the fetal arm.

Sometimes, it helps to push the fetus back into the birth canal a little to loosen the arms from the wedge-like impaction of the head. If it is too difficult to deliver the posterior arm, bring the anterior arm down from behind the pubis. If this fails, rotate the fetus toward its ventral surface. This should bring the anterior arm into the hollow of the sacrum. When this is done, liberate this arm first. Then rotate the trunk back in the opposite direction for access to the other arm.

You will recognize the more serious complication of nuchal arm (or arms) only when you insert your fingers to free the posterior arm. If you encounter this situation, rotate the body 180 degrees in the direction that the forearm is pointing while pushing the fetus back up slightly. Usually, this frees the nuchal arm and it can then be delivered as described above for the extended arm. If necessary, rotate the body back to its original position to free the other arm.

Be especially careful to do these maneuvers gently, as trauma may occur, including fractures and brachial plexus injury. Also, be sure of the orientation of the fetus before attempting any corrective action so that you do not attempt to bring the arm down over the back.

### Entrapment of the head

Few situations are as distressing as having successfully delivered the fetal body only to find that the head does not follow forthwith. Often, this is merely a matter of a relatively large head that does not promptly flex as it approaches the pelvic outlet. In this case, flex the head with a combination of suprapubic pressure and the Mauriceau maneuver. This will usually effect delivery. As an alternative, Piper forceps (see below) can be applied for delivery of the head. Above all, when the head does not deliver promptly for any reason, resist the temptation to place any traction on the body. To do so may stretch the neck, causing brachial plexus injury or, worse, spinal cord damage.

The most serious problems occur when the head arrests in the midpelvis or outlet. Quickly perform an examination to see if the cervix is incompletely dilated. If you feel a rim of cervix around the head, you can

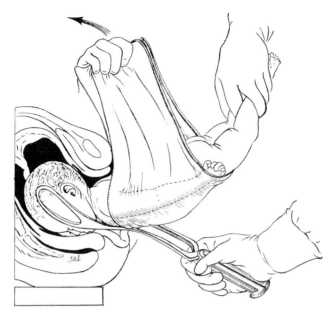

**Figure 8.15** Using Piper forceps to deliver the aftercoming head. The body and arms are elevated slightly with a sling made from a towel. Application of the forceps must be done from a kneeling position.

try to advance the rim by pushing it back over the head with your fingers. Usually, this is both difficult to do and potentially traumatic. Alternatively, put two or three right-angle retractors in the cervix to stretch it. This may work, but is also sometimes accompanied by cervical lacerations. It may be quite difficult to achieve full cervical dilatation, moreover, if the fetus is large. The last available option is to cut the cervix with bandage scissors at 12, 8, and 4 o'clock (Dührssen incisions). This is reserved for use only in those cases in which all else fails because it may be complicated by considerable bleeding, especially if the cervical incisions extend upward into the lower uterine segment.

When undertaking vaginal delivery of a fetus in breech presentation, Piper forceps should be available for immediate use at all times. They are especially useful for the aftercoming head because of the backward curving of the shanks, making it possible to apply them to the head from beneath the baby's body. Cradle the body and arms of the baby in a sling fashioned of a sterile towel (Fig. 8.15). Elevate the entire body slightly. Have the cradle held in place by an assistant. Then get down on one knee and apply the Piper forceps to the fetal head from below the body. Gentle traction and slow flexion of the head combined with gradual coordinated elevation of the fetal body bring the mouth and nose of the fetus into view over the perineum. In doing this procedure, guard constantly against overextension of the cervical spine.

If the aftercoming head cannot be delivered promptly after the body is out, it can be valuable to depress and retract the perineum with your hand or a broad speculum, wiping the vagina and oropharynx dry, thereby allowing the fetus to breathe with the head still in the pelvis. This will provide some additional time to effect controlled delivery of the head safely without exposing the fetus to continued hypoxia or to possible trauma from overly aggressive traction.

### Malrotation of the head

As noted above, sometimes the fetal back rotates so that the ventrum of the fetus passes under the symphysis. This orientation occurs more often in footling presentations when the posterior leg has come down, or during breech extraction when the obstetrician has inadvertently grasped the posterior leg for traction. Rarely, it may occur during an otherwise spontaneous breech labor.

The problem is almost always rectified spontaneously as the occiput turns from its posterior location a full 270 degrees past the promontory and through the other half of the maternal pelvis so that it comes to lie anteriorly and the abdomen faces posteriorly. The back thus rotates in the direction opposite from what you would expect. Be advised that you must not take any measures to counteract or resist this mechanism; doing so risks causing the back to remain posterior with the head facing up.

If such rotation does not occur, the chin remains anteriorly against the pubic ramus. In such cases, the head may still be deliverable vaginally, by either an extension or a flexion mechanism. Manual rotation of the head can be done, but it is a hazardous and difficult procedure. To assist the occiput posterior head to deliver, use gentle suprapubic pressure to the fetal forehead with one hand and lift the body with the other so that the fetal chest is applied to the mother's pubis. Be gentle, and do not place traction on the neck. Also, avoid undue compression of the anterior neck structures. Usually, the occiput will roll past the promontory into the hollow of the sacrum. It may then rotate anteriorly and then readily deliver by extension. If it does not, it can be delivered by flexion, as described above.

### External cephalic version

A strategy of attempting external cephalic version to convert breech to cephalic presentations in late pregnancy can reduce the prevalence of breech presentation in labor at term. Successful version occurs in about 50% of cases. Version can also be attempted during early labor, but the success rate then is probably less than 25%. Moreover, even those cases that are successfully

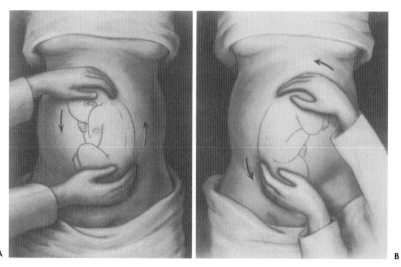

A                                                                                      B

**Figure 8.16** External cephalic version of breech to cephalic presentation. **A**. Push the breech away from the pelvic inlet with one hand and with the other, urge the head in the direction in which the face lies. **B**. Continually push the breech gently upward and away from the pelvic inlet while simultaneously pulling the head downward toward the pelvis. Use gentle pressure and rotate the fetus slowly.

converted still have a higher cesarean rate than do naturally-occurring vertex presentations. Complications of external cephalic version include placental abruption, uterine rupture, cord prolapse or entrapment, and fetal trauma. The risk of these complications is greatly reduced if the procedure is carried out gently and stopped if it does not proceed smoothly.

External version requires that the membranes are intact and the uterus relaxed. Epidural anesthesia can be helpful, but be mindful that anesthesia prevents the patient from alerting you that you are using excessive force. Properly done, a version will cause discomfort (usually described as strong pressure) as the fetus is rotated, but there should be little or no pain. Ensure that the fetal heart rate pattern is normal before attempting a version, and that there is no placenta previa or other abnormality that would make vaginal delivery inappropriate. The same technique can be used to attempt to convert a transverse lie to a longitudinal lie (see below).

Place the patient in moderate Trendelenburg position. This helps to move the breech away from the inlet and thus be more mobile. Use surgical lubricant (or ultrasound gel) liberally on the abdomen. Attempt the version between contractions or, preferably, give a short-acting uterine relaxant such as terbutaline. Use one hand to gently draw the breech out of the inlet into one iliac fossa while you press the head down into the opposite flank with your other hand (Fig. 8.16). Use alternate stroking and pushing movements, flexing the fetal trunk and neck as you attempt to roll the body forward. If resistance is met, attempt to turn it in the opposite direction. Once the head has been maneuvered over the inlet, hold the fetus in that position through at least several contractions. Monitor the fetal heart rate pattern continuously. If two attempts at version are not successful, abandon the procedure.

### Choosing a candidate for vaginal breech delivery

As noted, planned vaginal breech delivery has become uncommon, despite the evidence-based opinions of some experts that vaginal delivery is safe if used in selected cases by skilled practitioners. Appropriate cases are, of course, those with the lowest risk of complications (Fig. 8.17). Thus, the ideal candidate should have an estimated fetal weight neither very large nor very small; the presentation should be frank or complete breech; and there should be no complicating conditions (Box 8.5). Once labor is established, the patterns of cervical dilatation and fetal descent should be normal throughout the course of labor. If they are not, abandon the trial of labor. In general, we discourage the use of oxytocin in cases with breech presentation.

One solution to the relative lack of experience of many recently trained practitioners is to have the hospital create a "breech team" and to conduct "breech drills" to practice the steps in anticipation of the infrequent need to deal with vaginal breech births. The breech team consists of a group of experienced clinicians who could provide technical and cognitive expertise whenever a patient arrives in labor with a breech presentation and a vaginal delivery is planned or inevitable.

## Transverse lie

A *transverse lie* (also called a *shoulder presentation,* even though the shoulder may not be the part presenting over the inlet) is an error of fetal polarity in which the long axis of the fetus crosses the long axis of the mother. The fetal axis is not usually at a right angle to the mother's axis, but more obliquely oriented in relation to the mother's spine, most often with the breech nearer the pelvic inlet. An *oblique lie* is usually transitory in late pregnancy, and is thus characterized as an unstable lie. An oblique lie will generally convert to a longitudinal or transverse lie once labor begins. It is important for you to make the diagnosis of a transverse lie early in labor if you are to minimize fetal risk.

### Etiology

Transverse lie occurs about once in 300–400 deliveries. It is much more common in multiparas than in nulliparas and occurs more frequently in preterm labor than at term.

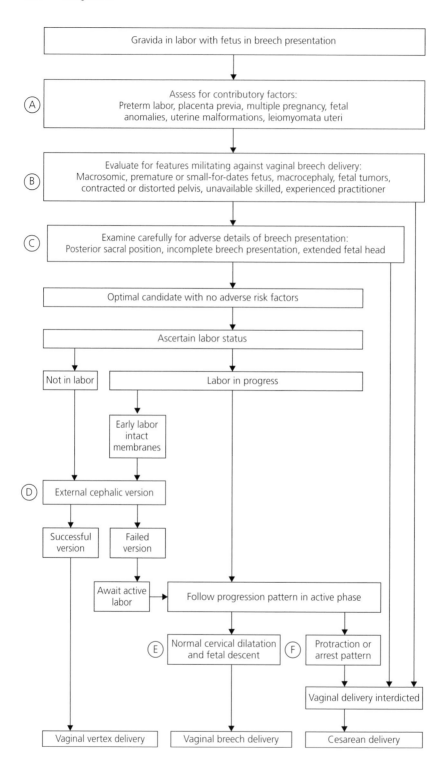

Anything in the pelvis that prevents engagement (e.g., inlet contraction, placenta previa, ovarian tumor, uterine leiomyoma) or that allows an unusual degree of fetal mobility (polyhydramnios, early gestational age) may result in a transverse lie. Multiple pregnancy and uterine or fetal anomalies are also commonly associated conditions.

### Box 8.5 Criteria favoring safe vaginal breech delivery

- Gestational age > 35 weeks
- Estimated fetal weight 2000–3800 g
- No hyperextension of fetal head
- Frank or complete breech
- Normal progress in dilatation and descent
- Normal fetal heart rate pattern
- Skilled obstetric practitioner available
- Absence of potentially complicating conditions
  - Placenta previa
  - Obstructing tumor
  - Uterine anomaly

**Figure 8.17** Algorithm for management of breech presentation.
**A**. Breech presentations are encountered relatively commonly in preterm labor; the rate diminishes toward term. Any anatomical distortion of the normally ovoid configuration of the uterine cavity may affect the presentation of the fetus, including placenta previa, uterine malformations and leiomyomata uteri. Fetal anomalies or neurological deficits in the fetus that prevent passive internal spatial accommodation may act in a similar manner. Seek out these problems as they may affect how management should be conducted.
**B**. Certain conditions are contraindications against vaginal breech delivery. They include fetuses less than 2500 g (because the head of a small fetus is relatively larger than the breech) or weighing more than 4000 g (because the maternal pelvis may be unable to accommodate it safely), and other conditions that are likely to be associated with fetopelvic disproportion, such as a small or distorted pelvis, or a fetus with a large head or a tumor. Cesarean delivery is preferable, moreover, if skilled, knowledgeable and experienced personnel are not at hand.
**C**. If essential criteria for safe vaginal breech delivery are not met, cesarean delivery is indicated. These include frank or complete breech, sacrum anterior mechanism, and a head that is not hyperextended. Absent these conditions, vaginal delivery is likely to fail, and the fetus may be seriously harmed if it is attempted.
**D**. If the gravida is not in labor or is in early labor with intact membranes, external cephalic version is a worthwhile consideration. If successful, it converts a potentially hazardous breech presentation to a safe cephalic presentation. Use a tocolytic agent to relax the uterus and monitor the fetal heart rate before and after.
**E**. If the labor patterns of cervical dilatation and fetal descent remain normal, proceed with vaginal breech delivery.
**F**. A protraction disorder (protracted active phase dilatation) or an arrest pattern (arrest of dilatation or of descent, prolonged deceleration or failure of descent) warrant intervention by cesarean delivery.

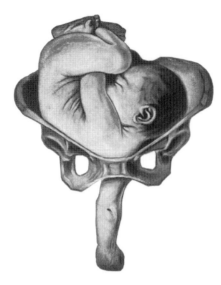

**Figure 8.18** Transverse lie in left acromion anterior position in advanced labor with prolapsed right arm, head in the left iliac ala, back down and anteriorly located.

Early in pregnancy, transverse lie is common. Even in the last month, especially in multiparas, it is found occasionally, but it nearly always corrects itself before labor begins by converting to a longitudinal lie. This process is called *spontaneous rectification*.

## Diagnosis

Prompt diagnosis is important because, except in unusual circumstances, cesarean delivery must be performed. Labor and vaginal delivery are associated with considerable risk.

As you begin the abdominal examination, you will first recognize that there is no longitudinal ovoid, but you can feel an ovoid that is more or less transverse instead. In addition, you will find that you cannot feel a fetal pole over the inlet or in the fundus. This may not be so obvious, especially if the fetal back is directed toward the fundus, where it is often mistaken for the breech. Your initial suspicions will be reinforced when you realize you cannot palpate the fetal back in either flank.

The point of reference for a transverse lie is the acromial process of the shoulder (Fig. 8.18). In left acromion anterior position (LAA) you can feel the large, round mass of the head low in the left flank. It is sometimes ballottable. The breech, which is deep and up high to the right, is difficult to palpate. You should be able to feel the small parts high in the uterus to the right of the midline.

In the right acromion posterior position (RAP), feel the head deep in the right flank. The breech is under the mother's spleen. The back cannot be outlined; instead, the area under the umbilicus seems filled with small parts.

When you suspect transverse lie, perform a vaginal examination for confirmation, having first ruled out placenta previa. If there is a transverse lie, you will find an empty vaginal vault. The cervix, if already softened and effaced, may hang down into the vagina like the cuff of a sleeve. If the cervix is dilated, the forewaters sometimes project through the cervix, filling the vagina. Any attempt to feel the fetus through the intact membranes may rupture them. This unfortunate occurrence should be avoided if possible, lest the cord or an arm prolapse. If labor has progressed for a while, the shoulder is more accessible and all the landmarks should become more discernible. Prolapse of the arm or elbow, while a potentially adverse event if neglected, does much to aid in diagnosis. Prolapse of the umbilical cord is also frequent, and obviously a cause for concern and immediate intervention.

After labor has been in progress for a long time, the presenting portions of the fetus may become so swollen that diagnosis will be difficult. Consider breech, face, and compound presentations in the differential diagnosis. Avoid confusion by searching carefully for the landmarks specific to each.

## Mechanism

There are mechanisms by which the transverse lie can deliver vaginally. We will not describe these here because they should never be observed in modern obstetrics, where cesarean delivery is almost always the only reasonable and safe route. The one exception in which vaginal delivery could be condoned would be that of an extremely premature dead fetus. Bear in mind, however, that even in that situation there is risk of obstructed labor and uterine rupture.

## Course of labor

You might someday be confronted with a patient who has been in labor for many hours with an undiagnosed transverse lie. If the membranes have ruptured early on with loss of most of the amniotic fluid, the uterus closely applies itself to the body of the uterus. If this occurs, cord compression may compromise the fetus, and manipulations during cesarean delivery may prove difficult and hazardous (see below). Once the diagnosis is confirmed, proceed to cesarean delivery.

If labor progresses with a transverse lie, intense uterine contractions force the shoulder into the pelvis. The fetus is folded together, the breech approaches the head, and the uterine ovoid becomes more globular. If the fetus is small or macerated and the pelvis is large enough, the uterus, aided by powerful maternal bearing-down efforts, may succeed in expelling the fetus by a process called *conduplicato corpora*. In this process, the fetus is folded upon itself and compressed sufficiently to permit the torso and the head to be delivered together vaginally. This type of delivery succeeds

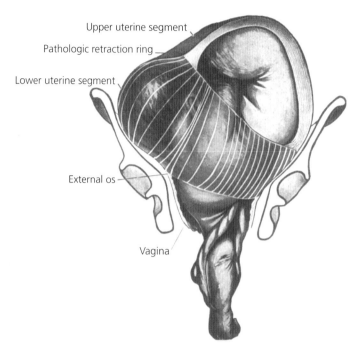

Upper uterine segment

Pathologic retraction ring

Lower uterine segment

External os

Vagina

**Figure 8.19** The appearance of a neglected shoulder presentation, right acromion anterior position, with prolapsed umbilical cord and prolapsed left arm. The shoulder is tightly wedged into the pelvis and the uterus is on the verge of rupture. The thick upper uterine segment has retracted over the fetus and is separated from the greatly overdistended and thinned lower segment by the pathologic (Bandl) retraction ring.

rarely, but it is fraught with risk of complications, including uterine rupture and severe cervical laceration, and is likely to result in a severely damaged or stillborn baby.

With obstructed labor, the uterus may be in a state of almost constant contraction. Your patient will complain of unremitting pain, and tenderness develops over the lower part of the uterus as it draws up over the fetus. The myometrium becomes thick in the upper segment and extremely thin in the lower segment. At the junction of these segments you might feel a groove or depression (Fig. 8.19), the ominous *pathologic contraction ring (Bandl ring)*. Above this groove, you can distinguish no fetal parts; below it, the fetus is easily felt. Fetal death may have already occurred from interruption of placental circulation and cord compression. Unless aid is given to effect cesarean delivery, the uterus will rupture and place the mother's life at risk as well. Undertaking cesarean delivery in the second stage, you may find the lower segment wall to be so thin that the introduction of your hand may rupture it. To avert such dire consequences, it is obvious that one must recognize transverse lie early and not allow it to evolve in this way.

## Prognosis

If the diagnosis is made early in labor, the outlook for mother and fetus is excellent. Labor may progress, however, because of the patient's failure to seek care or because diagnosis of the malpresentation is delayed. As already noted above, serious complications are common, but prognosis is considerably improved by expeditious termination of the labor by cesarean delivery as soon as a definitive diagnosis is made.

Sometimes a transverse lie will spontaneously convert to a longitudinal one prior to or during early labor. Once the active phase has been entered, however, such spontaneous conversion is much less common. If labor has not yet begun or is very early, external version to a longitudinal lie can be done in certain circumstances (see above).

## Treatment
### Cesarean delivery

Treatment of a gravida with a transverse lie identified during labor is almost always cesarean delivery. Before embarking on that procedure, search for a cause for the malpresentation, especially one that might influence your cesarean technique. If you know that a placenta previa exists, or that there is a neoplasm in the pelvis or a Müllerian anomaly, modify your surgical preparations and approach, and your choice of assistants accordingly. Under any circumstances, effecting cesarean delivery of a transverse lie can be challenging because intrauterine manipulation of the fetus is usually necessary. Intrauterine fetal death does not relieve you of concern for maternal risks. Because those risks persist even if the fetus is dead, cesarean delivery is still warranted for maternal reasons.

Perform the operation as early as possible in labor. A longitudinal skin incision is preferable, especially because a classical (vertical) uterine incision is likely to be necessary. You will generally find the lower uterine segment is not well developed unless the woman has been in labor for a long time. A classical incision is advantageous because it allows considerable space for manipulation of the fetus. Moreover, the incision can be lengthened if extensive maneuvering is needed to free a fetus impacted in the pelvis. Once the uterus is opened, grasp one or both of the fetus's feet and deliver the fetus through the uterine and the abdominal incisions by means of a combination of internal podalic version (grasping the foot or feet and rotating the fetus into a breech presentation) and breech extraction (see above).

The classical uterine incision has advantages in delivering the fetus in transverse lie, even though it is accompanied by increased morbidity compared to lower segment transverse uterine incisions: more blood loss, infection, bowel complications, and risk of rupture in subsequent pregnancies. The less preferable low transverse incision is an option here,

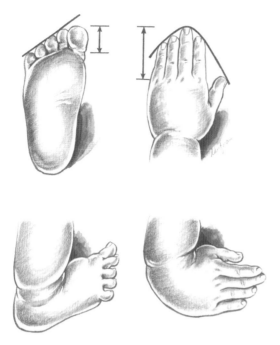

**Figure 8.20** Features helpful in distinguishing the fetal foot from the hand during vaginal examination. The straight line formed by the toes is different from the curve of the fingertips. The heel is sometimes recognizable as different from the wrist, although this is unreliable for differentiation.

especially if the fetal back is up. If used, make the transverse uterine incision generous, but curve its lateral aspects cephalad, so that an extension is less likely to be directed laterally into the uterine vascular bundle. Reach into the transverse incision and take hold of the fetal feet. This will usually be easy if the fetal back is up. If you are right-handed, stand on the patient's right side, using your dominant hand to identify the fetal parts. Pull the legs through the incision. This will begin to rotate the fetus into a longitudinal lie. Encourage this process by using your other hand to exert pressure to nudge the fetal head toward the fundus. If successful, follow through with a breech extraction (see above).

If the fetal back is down, you should proceed directly to cesarean delivery by way of a classical incision. If you discover the back is down after you have already made a transverse incision, however, you will need to advance your hand into the uterus past the fetal head to grasp the feet. This can be difficult, especially if the membranes have been previously ruptured and the uterus has closely applied itself to the fetal body. If you find yourself in this difficult situation, administer a uterine relaxant agent (nitroglycerine, terbutaline, or a halogenated inhalational drug if the patient is under general anesthesia) to enable you to perform the necessary manipulations more safely.

Remember, before pulling on an extremity for delivery, be sure you have grasped a foot, and not a hand! It can be surprisingly difficult to tell the difference, especially in a preterm fetus (Fig. 8.20). Feel for digits of equal length to confirm it is a foot. The fetal wrist can easily be mistaken for a heel when the hand is folded back or forward at the wrist. If you inadvertently pull an arm through the incision, it may be difficult to replace it and complete the delivery without having to extend the incision considerably.

### External cephalic version

Sometimes it is reasonable to attempt to convert a transverse lie to a cephalic presentation, using the same technique as described above for version of the breech.

Despite the shorter arc of rotation, success rates are lower than for breech presentations, perhaps because in a transverse lie the lower uterine segment is either occupied by something (placenta, tumor, etc.) or cannot reshape itself quickly to accommodate the fetal head. If you choose to attempt version of a transverse lie, be certain to exclude placenta previa or any obstructive masses first. Once you move the fetus to a longitudinal lie, hold it there for 30 minutes to allow the uterine wall to adjust to the new fetal polarity. If you are not successful in turning the fetus easily, or it returns promptly to its transverse orientation, do a cesarean delivery.

The transverse lie of a second twin is sometimes subjected to external or internal version. This circumstance is discussed in Chapter 12.

### Key points

- The course of dilatation and descent in labor with breech presentation is essentially the same as with comparable vertex presentation, except that the breech tends to enter labor at a high station and to remain there until late in labor.
- Three kinds of breech deliveries can occur: (1) spontaneous delivery; (2) assisted breech delivery (partial breech extraction); (3) total breech extraction.
- The Bracht method is an approach to assist a breech delivery. It supports the fetus through the normal mechanism of labor and delivery, minimizing the risk of trauma.
- During delivery of a fetus in breech presentation the arms may be extended above the fetal head or come to rest behind the neck. Extended or nuchal arms are most likely to occur if traction is made on the body too soon or if the pelvis is small.
- In breech cases, the Piper forceps should be available for immediate use at all times to apply to the aftercoming head, if needed.
- A *transverse lie* is an error of fetal polarity in which the long axis of the fetus crosses the long axis of the mother.
- The diagnosis of transverse lie is suggested by the presence of a transverse fetal ovoid, along with inability to identify the fetal head or

breech in the longitudinal poles of the uterus and the back or the small parts in its lateral aspects.

- If diagnosis is made early in labor, the outlook for mother and fetus is excellent. In cases in which the diagnosis is delayed until labor is advanced, serious complications are common.
- Transverse lie identified during labor almost always requires cesarean delivery. Before embarking on a delivery plan for transverse lie, search for a cause for the malpresentation.
- A classical incision is advantageous because it allows considerable space for manipulation of the fetus.
- Consider external cephalic version to convert the fetus to a longitudinal lie under certain circumstances.

## Further Reading

### Books and reviews

Novak-Antolic Z. Transverse lie, brow and face presentations. In: Kurjak A, Chervenak FA (eds) *Textbook of Perinatal Medicine*, 2nd edition. Informa Healthcare, London, 2006: 1912–17.

Foley M, Alarab M. Breech presentation. In: Kurjak A, Chervenak FA (eds) *Textbook of Perinatal Medicine*, 2nd edition. Informa Healthcare, London, 2006: 1918–27.

Mode of term singleton breech delivery. ACOG Committee Opinion No. 340 July 2006. American College of Obstetricians and Gynecologists, Washington, DC. Obstet Gynecol 2006;108:235–7.

Zhang J, Bowes WA Jr, Fortney JA. Efficacy of external cephalic version: a review. Obstet Gynecol 1993;82:306–12.

Vaginal delivery of breech presentation. Clinical Practice Guideline, Society of Obstetricians and Gynaecologists of Canada. No 226, June 2009.

### Primary sources

Ballas S, Toaff R, Jaffa AJ. Deflexion of the fetal head in breech presentation: incidence, management, and outcome. Obstet Gynecol 1978;52:653–5.

Duenhoelter JH, Wells E, Reisch JS, Santos-Ramos R, Jimenez JM. A paired controlled study of vaginal and abdominal delivery of the low birth weight breech fetus. Obstet Gynecol 1979;54:310–13.

Ferguson JE II, Armstrong MA, Dyson DC. Maternal and fetal factors affecting success of antepartum external cephalic version. Obstet Gynecol 1987:70:722–5.

Green JE, McLean F, Smith LP, Usher R. Has an increased cesarean section rate for term breech delivery reduced the incidence of birth asphyxia, trauma, and death? Am J Obstet Gynecol 1982;142:643–8.

Gimovsky ML, Wallace RL, Schifrin BS, Paul RH. Randomized management of the non-frank breech presentation at term. Am J Obstet Gynecol 1983;146:34–40.

Hannah ME, Hannah WJ, Hewson SA, Hodnett ED, Saigai S, Willan AR. Planned cesarean section versus planned vaginal birth for breech presentation at term: a randomized multicentre trial. Lancet 2000:356:1375–83.

Hofmeyr GJ. Effect of external cephalic version in late pregnancy on breech presentation and cesarean section rate: a controlled trial. Br J Obstet Gynaecol 1983;90:392–9.

Mazor M, Hagay ZJ, Leiberman JR, Biale Y, Insler V. Fetal malformations associated with breech delivery: implications for obstetric management. J Reprod Med 1985;30:884–6.

Pelosi MA, Apuzzio J, Fricchione D, Gowda VV. The "intra-abdominal version technique" for delivery of transverse lie by low-segment cesarean. Am J Obstet Gynecol 1979;135:1009–11.

Phelan JP, Boucher M, Mueller E, McCart D, Horenstein J, Clark SL. The nonlaboring transverse lie: a management dilemma. J Reprod Med 1986;31:184–6.

Sanchez-Ramos L, Wells TL, Adair CD, Arcelin G, Kaunitz AM, Wells DS. Route of breech delivery and maternal and neonatal outcomes. Int J Gynecol Obstet 2001;73:7–14.

## CHAPTER 9

# Avoiding and Managing Birth Canal Trauma

Many of your patients will suffer traumatic injuries to the birth canal. Most will be of little consequence, but some will carry serious risk of blood loss, infection, and discomfort. In addition, birth canal trauma can contribute to long-term disability in the form of fistulas, dyspareunia, pelvic floor relaxation, and urinary or fecal incontinence. For those reasons, you must make every effort to avoid or minimize such injuries and to repair them appropriately when they occur.

Much recent concern has arisen over the role of childbirth in degrading the long-term health of the pelvic floor and the surrounding structures. Such concerns have helped fuel the rising cesarean rate. There is no doubt that injury to the musculofascial supports of the lower genitourinary tract and anal continence mechanism can occur during vaginal delivery. Damage to the innervation of muscles involved in continence can also be caused or abetted by childbirth. The consequence of such injuries can be pelvic organ prolapse, as well as urinary and fecal incontinence. While vaginal delivery is often blamed for these problems, keep in mind that many factors other than parturitional trauma contribute to the prevalence of incontinence in our population (Fig. 9.1). Obesity and smoking, for example, are very important and quite prevalent risk factors, as is aging, independent of parity. Genetic factors are undoubtedly important as well. Moreover, if you accurately diagnose and properly manage injuries at the time of delivery, you will minimize their potential to cause serious long-term morbidity.

The anatomy of the birth canal and pelvic floor is complex, and precise repair of parturitional trauma can be daunting, even to the experienced surgeon. Too often, management of lacerations is relegated to the least experienced member of an obstetric team. The regrettable result may be a repair that looks respectable on the surface, but has flouted the requirement for accurate anatomic approximation beneath. Make yourself a

*Labor and Delivery Care: A Practical Guide*, First Edition. Wayne R. Cohen and Emanuel A. Friedman. © 2011 John Wiley & Sons, Ltd. Published 2011 by John Wiley & Sons, Ltd.

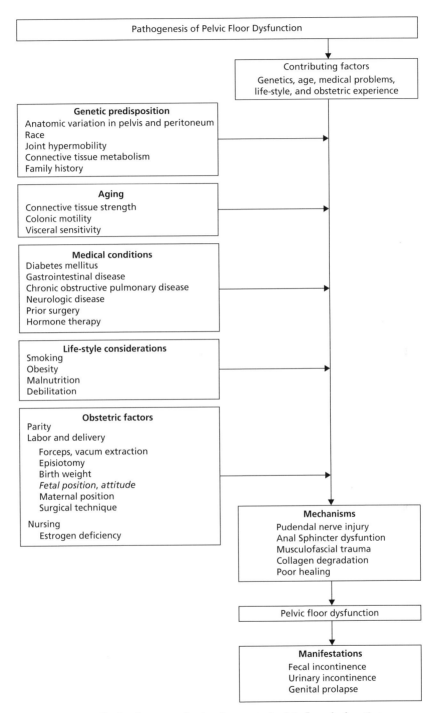

**Figure 9.1** Contributing factors to the development of pelvic floor dysfunction. (Adapted from Cohen WR, Romero R. Childbirth and the pelvic floor. In: Kurjak A, Chervenak FA (eds) *Textbook of Perinatal Medicine*, 2nd edition. Informa, London, 2006: 1979–88.)

student of pelvic anatomy and strive to master it; the effort will pay substantial dividends for you and your patients.

## Vulvar lacerations

The most frequent birth injury affects the vulvar orifice and the vagina. Fig. 9.2 shows the most common vulvar lacerations. They are usually superficial; however, significant hemorrhage may occur if a tear extends through the clitoris or deeply through the vulvar tissues.

Paraurethral lacerations occur frequently, especially in the nullipara, and have become more common as the use of episiotomy has declined. They result from pressure of the fetal head against the anterior vestibule and urethra during expulsion. An unyielding perineum forces the fetal head anteriorly as the occiput extends under the pubic arch. Most resulting tears are superficial, but the potential for complex and deep tissue injury exists.

Superficial wounds and simple splitting of the skin and mucosa seldom require suturing if they are not bleeding, as their edges usually appose when the mother's legs are brought together, and healing is rapid. If you repair deep tears, be sure to respect the anatomic structures beneath the skin. This is especially important if you encounter lacerations proximate to or transecting the urethra or clitoris, or if the tears extend into the

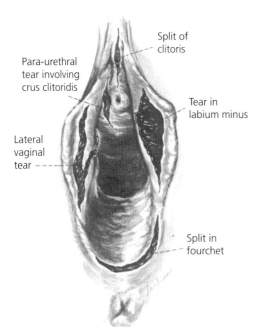

Para-urethral
tear involving
crus clitoridis

Split of
clitoris

Tear in
labium minus

Lateral
vaginal
tear

Split in
fourchet

**Figure 9.2** The vulvar structures showing the varieties of laceration that can be sustained during delivery.

erectile tissue (vestibular bulbs) in the labia majora. Always use the smallest caliber suture possible. Generally, size 4-0 absorbable suture is sufficient for these areas. Heavier suture may delay healing, damage tissue, facilitate infection, and cause discomfort.

## Perineal lacerations

The perineal body is composed of fat, connective tissue of the centrum tendineum, and rudimentary muscles. The external anal sphincter and, laterally, the sturdy arc of the levator ani muscle group coming down from the pubis are apparent on examination. The superficial transverse perinei muscles join at the midline, just below the fibers of the bulbospongiosus muscle that helps support the introitus. Lacerations of the perineal body (Fig. 9.3) occur in many first labors, but are less important than tears of the pelvic floor involving the levator ani muscles and investing fasciae. When the perineal body is torn and left unrepaired, the integrity of the urogenital diaphragm is breached. As a consequence, the anterior wall of the vagina sags, the posterior wall begins to roll out, and

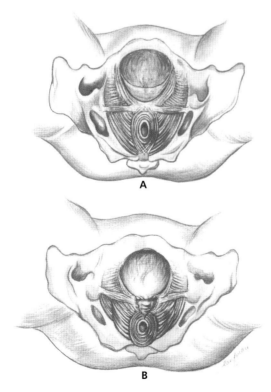

**A**

**B**

**Figure 9.3** Pelvic floor structures during delivery, illustrating damage done by the fetal head to unyielding maternal soft tissues: (**A**) distending the urogenital diaphragm; (**B**) lacerating the perineal body through the anal sphincters.

the vulva gapes permanently. If the tear is deeper, it may involve the anal sphincters or even extend up the rectal wall. If the anal sphincter mechanism is injured, incontinence of feces results unless proper steps are taken to correct the damage.

## Damage to the levator ani pillars

The levator ani muscles, with their superior and inferior fasciae, are often damaged in labor at term. The muscle suffers less actual injury than the fasciae. As the fetus descends, the presenting part stretches the pelvic floor radially and axially. The tissues in the path of the dilating wedge are forced downward as they are distended. The fasciae are stretched longitudinally from the cervix to the perineum. The two levator ani pillars are parted and the fasciae that hold the pillars in their relations to the rectum, the vagina, the perineum, and each other can be disrupted. This leads to diastasis of the pillars.

Tearing into the body of the levator ani muscle constitutes a continuation of the diastasis of the pillars. The two puborectalis bundles are pushed far apart, leaving a wide breach (Fig. 9.4). After healing has occurred, you can sometimes feel a thick muscle instead of a thin, flat, sling-like one; the disrupted muscle forms two pillars at the sides of a gaping introitus with the rectum often protruding between them.

Anatomically, in addition to the destruction of their supporting fasciae, the interlacing of the levator ani muscles with the sides of the rectum and anal sphincter may be severed. The tear may extend deeply into the ischioanal fossa. Levator pillar tears may be bilateral; usually, the tear on

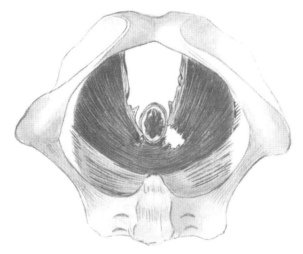

**Figure 9.4** Diagrammatic representation of pelvic floor structures showing separation of the levator pillars with tearing of the overlying fascia and, posterolateral to the rectum, lacerations into the body of the levator ani muscle group.

one side is deeper than the other. When this happens, the vagina and the perineum are always torn and sometimes the anal sphincter as well.

Sometimes the skin is intact after delivery, but all the deeper structures down to the rectum are torn; in such instances, superficial observation will not disclose the presence or the extent of the injury. If occult injury is suspected, it is necessary to incise the perineum in the midline to examine the external sphincter. A rectal examination, which you should do after every delivery, will help ensure the rectum is intact and might suggest the existence of an occult sphincter tear.

## Etiology

The most common cause of perineal lacerations is disproportion between the fetus and the soft parts of the birth canal. Either the head is too large or the canal is too small. The head may present unfavorable diameters to the passage, as in occiput posterior positions and brow presentations. Too rapid a delivery causes many tears by not giving the soft tissues time to dilate safely.

Not surprisingly, the most extensive injuries often occur during forceps or vacuum-assisted vaginal deliveries. Other predisposing factors are edema from long labor, excessive tissue rigidity in older nulliparas, or scars from previous injury. Sometimes a perineum tears readily with little apparent provocation, perhaps the result of inherently poor tissue integrity.

An important and generally unrecognized contributor to perineal tears is a narrow subpubic arch. Unless the head can occupy the space directly under the subpubic ligament, it is forced posteriorly toward the coccyx in the posterior aspect of the outlet near the end of the descent process, thus overstretching the levator ani muscles and the perineum. Extensive injuries can thus occur in women with a narrow subpubic arch or with a funnel pelvis. You should, therefore, evaluate the arch in advance of delivery. Knowing its shape will inform your delivery technique, enabling you to minimize trauma by ensuring against anterior pressure on the exiting head, avoiding instruments to aid vaginal delivery, and using episiotomy liberally and early. It may even help you to make timely decisions about the need for cesarean delivery.

Instrumental delivery can be particularly hazardous in a pelvis with a narrow subpubic arch, and even more so in a funnel pelvis. We strongly discourage use of delivery instruments in such patients. Forceps delivery may trap the vagina between the head and the pelvic bones. The vagina will then be forced or dragged downward and outward. If rotational movements are made with forceps at the same time, the vaginal walls may actually be torn from their pelvic attachments. If instrumental delivery is necessary, be sure you understand the pelvic type in which you are working so as to minimize injury.

Birth canal injury does not always occur in the form of visible lacerations. Occult problems abound, including a substantial number of anal sphincter injuries with intact overlying tissues. Pudendal and autonomic nerve injury can occur from overstretching or compression. Similarly, prolonged pressure on pelvic fasciae in an obstructed labor can result in pressure necrosis or can stretch tissues beyond their capacity to heal. Practicing good obstetrics will minimize the risk of such injuries.

## Treatment

Perineal lacerations are classified in four levels of severity. *First degree* tears are those in which the skin and mucosa are torn, but not the fascia or muscle beneath. *Second degree* tears involve the fascia and muscle between the vagina and the external anal sphincter. A *third degree* laceration is one in which the anal sphincter apparatus is torn, and a *fourth degree* tear extends through the wall of the rectum or the anus.

Preventive treatment is most valuable. Slow delivery to allow the elastic pelvic floor tissues to stretch safely is the secret for preventing tears in spontaneous and operative deliveries. Methods to minimize trauma are listed in Box 9.1.

Careful massage of the perineum and lower vagina, using sterile oils or water-soluble lubricant, can reduce shearing forces between the fetal head and the vagina and thus diminish the frequency and severity of perineal lacerations. If you position the patient during delivery so that her thighs are not abducted and flexed excessively, you will avoid stretching the perineal tissues. This will allow a greater degree of distension to occur safely, with a lower risk of trauma as the fetal head encounters the pelvic

---

**Box 9.1 Methods to protect the pelvic floor**

- Reduce risk with primary preventive care (weight loss, smoking cessation, exercise, etc.)
- Use clinical skills (labor curves, cephalopelvimetry, controlled pushing and delivery) to maximize likelihood of safe vaginal delivery
- Gradually massage ("iron out") the perineal tissues during the second stage
- Use episiotomy judiciously
- Lubricate the vagina liberally as the head crowns
- Consider open glottis pushing to promote gradual distension of perineal tissues
- Use alternative positions (e.g., lateral position, squatting, all-fours). When delivering a patient in modified lithotomy position, extend her hips somewhat as the head crosses the perineum
- Repair injuries carefully and anatomically
- Individualize management based on patient's preferences, pelvic anatomy, course of labor, length of perineum, fetal position, etc.

floor. When patients deliver in the semi-sitting position without stirrups, it is often helpful to extend the thighs slightly as the fetal head is delivered, rather than having them flexed tightly toward the abdomen, as is customary. This will relax the perineal structures somewhat and lessen the likelihood of trauma.

Of concern regarding both short- and long-term problems with incontinence is the duration of the second stage of labor. It is generally assumed that a long second stage predisposes to later pelvic relaxation, perhaps from overstretching of the fascial supports of the pelvic organs or factors relating to nerve injury or necrosis mentioned above. We emphasize that, although we advocate that the second stage not be terminated just because an arbitrary period of time has elapsed, delivery should be expedited for certain definable abnormalities of labor. Whenever maternal bearing-down efforts occur without some progress in fetal descent, the efforts result in descent of the entire uterus and potential damage to its supporting structures. Some labor abnormalities can be identified at the time of full cervical dilatation (failure of descent) or within 1 hour of it (arrest of descent) (Chapter 5). Continuing to have your patient push for an extra hour or two in order to meet a time standard will expose the connective tissue supports of the pelvic organs and the pelvic floor to unnecessary and potentially harmful mechanical stress.

The technical nuances that help maintain pelvic floor integrity are important. Equally critical is the need to manage labor intelligently and with keen judgment. Prompt identification and appropriate treatment of labor dysfunctions, keen attention to the mechanism of labor, and restrained use of oxytocin will minimize unnecessary time in the first and second stages of labor, and serve to identify patients in whom a safe vaginal delivery is unlikely.

### Episiotomy

Traditionally, episiotomy was thought to have an important role in preventing severe perineal (and fetal head) trauma. Its role in both respects has been questioned. Routine episiotomy for protection of the fetus is clearly not justifiable, and there is ample evidence that episiotomy increases the risk of severe perineal trauma in the form of third and fourth degree lacerations. Nevertheless, you will find episiotomy to be a valuable technique, if used selectively.

If danger to mother or fetus demands haste, a deep episiotomy can help expedite delivery. You can also use an episiotomy when the fetus is exceptionally large or when it presents with unfavorable diameters for passage of its head. A mediolateral episiotomy is preferable when space is expected to be a problem, but many obstetricians perform midline episiotomy routinely, and accept the fact that there is substantial risk of extension by laceration into the sphincter and the rectum. The median approach, even with extension, is generally associated with less bleeding and less postpartum pain. Mediolateral episiotomy is not only more difficult to repair, but it does not prevent sphincter laceration (although such laceration is encountered much less frequently than with median episiotomy).

The proper timing of episiotomy is of considerable importance. General practice is to make the incision as the fetal head is crowning when it becomes obvious that the alternative (delivery without episiotomy) will result in lacerations. This approach will certainly limit the number of episiotomies performed. But once the head is crowning and the vaginal tube is stretched maximally, most damage to the lower vaginal and perineal tissues has probably already occurred. Episiotomy prior to extreme distention of the perineum would likely have the greatest potential to reduce the likelihood of permanent damage. Your decision to use episiotomy should be individualized, based on the characteristics of the labor, the pelvis, and the fetus.

## Repair of perineal wounds

Perineal tears occasionally bleed profusely. Most lacerations, contrary to common belief, occur in the midline, and require the same technique for repair as would a median episiotomy. Staunch bleeding by compression with a sponge until the tissue can be approximated by suture. Do not begin the repair before the placenta has delivered because if you need to perform intrauterine manipulation for exploration or manual removal of the placenta, you might disrupt the repair and further damage the perineal tissues.

Perineal wounds that occur during parturition are remarkably resistant to infection, particularly considering the unavoidable contamination by rectal, vaginal or cutaneous organisms. Do not, however, allow the low infection rate to make you complacent about observing proper aseptic technique during repair. Perineal infection can be painful and debilitating; it can lead to fistula formation, scarring, and chronic dyspareunia; it can, albeit rarely, even lead to sepsis and death.

It is sensible first to cleanse the wound and adjoining surfaces with sterile saline. This is especially important if there has been gross fecal contamination of the perineum. Change to clean gloves, and take care not to touch the wound with anything unsterile. Use fresh sterile towels to isolate the field. Good exposure of the operative site is critical. Use good lighting. A dose of prophylactic antibiotics during the repair of third and fourth degree wounds is beneficial.

Have your assistant retract the anterior vaginal wall with a right-angle retractor. Without an assistant, self-retaining retractors can serve this

> **Box 9.2 Surgical principles for perineal repair**
>
> - Understand the regional anatomy
> - Obtain good exposure
> - Use appropriate anesthesia
> - Use fine, absorbable suture material
> - Do a layered anatomic closure
> - Avoid leaving dead space where hematomas or serous collections can form
> - Approximate tissue layers
> - Avoid excess compression of tissues
> - Avoid tension
> - Avoid sutures that penetrate the skin
> - Avoid sutures that penetrate the rectum

purpose. Before beginning the repair, carefully assess the extent and the depth of the anatomic structures involved. Whatever the nature of the laceration or episiotomy, the same set of surgical principles applies (Box 9.2). Above all, be sure you are familiar with the normal anatomy of the region; if you are not, you would obviously have difficulty carrying out a proper anatomic repair.

We believe midline episiotomy is the technique of choice unless a major extension seems inevitable because the perineum is very short, the subpubic arch narrow, or there is fetal malposition or macrosomia. A standard midline episiotomy traverses the perineal and vaginal skin, the portion of the bulbospongiosus muscle posterior to the vaginal introitus, the midline tendinous insertions of the superficial and deep transverse perinei muscles, and the levator ani muscles, as well as the urogenital diaphragm and the rectovaginal expanse of the endopelvic fascia.

Most obstetricians now use synthetic absorbable polygalactin sutures for episiotomy repair. These sutures are degraded at various rates. While some studies suggest less pain than with catgut sutures, the degree of postpartum pain probably depends more on the quality of repair technique, particularly on the tension of the sutures applied, and on the caliber of the suture than the material of which it is made. Use 3-0 or 4-0 sutures. Heavier material is only occasionally necessary, especially in midline repairs in which there will be little tension on the wound. Do not use suture that degrades slowly in the skin or subcuticular layers. You may find it persists there for many months and can cause discomfort. As a general rule, rapidly absorbing monofilament material is best. An exception would be the sutures used to reapproximate the anal sphincters, or situations in which some tension on the wound is inevitable, such as in a mediolateral episiotomy repair.

While there are many acceptable ways for you to repair an episiotomy or deep laceration, you should adhere to these principles (Box 9.2): each structure should be repaired anatomically with fine absorbable suture material, and each tissue layer should be approximated accurately with minimal tension. While repair of episiotomies and lacerations may seem simple, it is not always so. Few operative procedures that you carry out will have such potentially profound effects on your patient's future sexual, reproductive, and excretory function and general quality of life. Some technical suggestions follow.

1. Suture the vaginal mucosa and submucosa separately from the dense layer of endopelvic fascia found beneath it to maintain the normal separation of these tissue layers.

2. Recreate the fossa navicularis at the introitus with two or three vertically placed sutures (relative to the patient in lithotomy position) that include the very edge of the skin between the hymeneal ring and the distal edge of the posterior labial commissure, together with a substantially deeper and more lateral portion of the connective tissue and muscle beneath. These sutures reapproximate the bulbospongiosus muscle, support the vestibule, and recreate the shelf of tissue that normally exists external to the posterior part of the hymeneal ring.

3. If the wound is midline, you will generally not see the bellies of the transverse perinei muscles or the portions of the levator sling that meet there. However, know the expected position of these structures and place your sutures so as to reapproximate their midline attachments anatomically.

4. Avoid putting sutures in the skin. They hurt. Use a subcuticular closure or, even better, use superficial subcutaneous sutures to bring the skin to near-approximation. Once your patient's legs are down, the skin edges will appose and heal rapidly.

5. As with any surgical procedure, be sure anesthesia, exposure, and lighting are optimal.

In repairing a midline wound, remember that once the patient's legs are normally adducted, the wound edges will tend to fall together. Your job is to bring the appropriate layers into correct anatomic apposition so they will heal together. If you place sutures without undue tension, your patient will have minimal discomfort from the repair. Keep in mind the surgical aphorism: approximate, do not strangulate.

Suggestions for repairing third and fourth degree tears are summarized in Box 9.3. These injuries can challenge the most skillful surgeon, and should be approached with respect for their complexity and for the harm that attends improper repair. Of particular import is the need for you to repair the internal anal sphincter, a step often overlooked. There is little immediate effect of this shortcoming, but as women age, the resting tone of the internal sphincter takes on increasing importance in maintaining anal continence.

> **Box 9.3 Repair of third and fourth degree lacerations**
>
> - Adhere to general surgical principles (Box 9.2)
> - Close anorectal tissue with fine, absorbable monofilament suture
> - Always repair a torn internal anal sphincter
> - Suture the ends of the external anal sphincter together with minimal tension
> - Close the circumference of the external sphincter capsule with fine sutures
> - Approximate the connective tissue of the rectovaginal septum as a separate layer
> - Approximate the endopelvic fascia beneath the vagina as a discrete layer

The internal sphincter is much thinner and paler in color than the external sphincter. It extends further cephalad by about 2 cm, and can usually be distinguished from the surrounding connective tissue. Take special care to recognize when it is damaged and repair it with fine interrupted sutures.

## Vaginal lacerations

The vagina may tear during spontaneous delivery and, especially, during operative intervention for delivery. If the vagina is congenitally small or strictured or if it is rigid or scarred by previous lacerations or surgery, childbirth injury is particularly likely to occur. Precipitate delivery, forceps, and rapid breech extractions often cause vaginal tears as well. Occasionally, even an uneventful delivery will be associated with serious lacerations of the vagina and its surrounding tissues.

Tears that split the vaginal canal usually occur in the sulci anteriorly or posteriorly. In the worst cases, furthermore, extension of vaginal lacerations can open up the perivaginal spaces down to the pelvic bone. Hemorrhage in such patients is usually profuse, and obtaining hemostasis will undoubtedly tax your skills. Sometimes arterial embolization, balloon tamponade, or vaginal packing may be necessary to control bleeding from deep sulcus tears.

Anesthesia and adequate assistance for retraction and exposure are essential. Speed is required to staunch the blood loss. After suturing, you may sometimes find it necessary to use vaginal tamponade to prevent a hematoma in the loose paravaginal tissues. Tears around the base of the bladder require especially accurate repair, and even then cystocele may not always be prevented.

## Lacerations of pelvic fascia

Substantial damage to the retinaculum uteri of the endopelvic fascia, which invests the uterus, can lead to substantial long-term morbidity.

This type of injury most often occurs in the context of midcavity instrumental delivery or labor abnormalities that have not been managed optimally. Overstretching of the vagina and the underlying vesicovaginal fascia is responsible for most cystoceles. The retinaculum uteri is destroyed if the parametria are overstretched radially and pulled down. The cervix slides down toward the genital hiatus, the corpus falls into the axis of the vagina, and uterine prolapse may follow. The same result can occur if the uterosacral ligaments are injured during instrumental traction. Destruction of the posterior endopelvic fascia can result in a high rectocele.

Serious birth canal injuries are rarely seen today, the happy result primarily of the near-disappearance of difficult rotational forceps delivery and other invasive maneuvers from practice. Most contemporary practitioners will never see the urethra and the base of the bladder detached from the posterior wall of the pubis or the vagina torn from its fascial moorings, injuries that were not rare in the past. Occasionally, however, substantial injuries result from the action of natural forces alone or from errors in management of labor. For example, premature bearing-down efforts before second stage have the same effect as forced traction from below. For that reason, expulsive efforts should never be encouraged before the cervix is completely dilated and well retracted. Similarly, pushing for hours in a futile attempt to overcome cephalopelvic disproportion risks similar harm. To best preserve the pelvic fascia, you should allow the normal delivery process to evolve slowly and intervene promptly by cesarean delivery when the risk of injury is high.

## Hematomas of vulva and vagina

Blood vessels, particularly the veins in the perivaginal plexus, may tear during labor. A hematoma in the loose pelvic connective tissue results. Most commonly, such hematomas occur in the vulva, around the vagina, and in the broad ligaments. They tend to enlarge progressively, sometimes rapidly, and follow the cleavage planes of the fascial layers. If the hematoma begins below the levator ani muscle and the deep pelvic fascia, it distends the perineum and dislocates the rectum and the anus. If it extends around the vagina, it may fill the pelvis and displace the vagina to one side. Bleeding above the levator sling may extend up anteriorly into the false pelvis under the inguinal ligament. A hematoma that extends posteriorly may even dissect up to the kidney retroperitoneally. Hematomas may also form above lacerations or episiotomies that have been repaired. This occurs when you fail to achieve proper hemostasis by starting to suture the vaginal wound too low, that is, by not applying the first (topmost) suture above the upper angle of the laceration.

Although a hematoma begins to form at once, some time may pass before it becomes clinically manifest. Intense localized pain is the most prominent symptom of vulvar and vaginal hematomas. While the onset of the discomfort may be delayed, most women with a hematoma will complain of intolerable pain within an hour or two of delivery. You can easily recognize a vulvar collection. The skin is stretched over the expanding, tender mass and becomes reddish-blue. Vaginal hematomas most commonly cause intolerable pain and pressure in the rectum. They are less clinically obvious than vulvar hematomas, but an especially gentle vaginal examination will confirm their presence. They may be exquisitely tender to the touch. Less commonly, the hematoma will be anterior in location, and cause bladder or urethral pain. Hematomas that begin in the upper vagina and expand retroperitoneally are very uncommon, but dangerous. They may be asymptomatic until hypovolemia occurs, with cardiovascular instability from massive hidden bleeding.

Prompt diagnosis and treatment are important; delay means needless tissue destruction and blood loss. Uneventful recovery is the rule if the hematoma does not become infected. Secondary infections do occur, however, and it is, therefore, wise to observe your patient closely for signs and symptoms of infection.

You can leave small, stable hematomas to be absorbed spontaneously; but open and drain them at the first sign of infection. Expanding or markedly painful hematomas should be incised promptly. Under such circumstances, move your patient to a fully equipped operating room. Anesthesia is vital, as are proper exposure and good lighting. Open the hemorrhagic cavity broadly. Evacuate the clots and fluid. If discrete bleeding vessels are seen, ligate them. If no individual vessels are found, which is commonly the case, the wound should be carefully closed by suturing in layers to occlude any dead space and ensure hemostasis. The vaginal canal (not the hematoma cavity) is then firmly packed with gauze or a tamponade balloon. Continue to observe your patient carefully, lest continuing occult blood loss goes unnoticed. Remove the vaginal pack within 12 hours. Consider arterial embolization for vulvar or vaginal hematomas that cannot be controlled surgically.

## Cervical lacerations

Cervical injuries range from small nicks in the mucosa to deep rents extending through the cervix, the vaginal vault, and the parametrium. Rarely, they may extend into adjacent or distant areas, tracking under the peritoneal folds of the broad ligaments or into the peritoneal cavity. Nearly every labor is attended by some injury to the cervix, especially at

3 and 9 o'clock, accounting for the "fish mouth" appearance of the cervix right after delivery. Large tears result from excessively rapid or too forceful dilatation by the powers of labor or by the physician during an operative delivery. Healed scars from prior deliveries or operations, and fetal macrosomia or malpositions, are predisposing factors.

Bleeding is slight unless a large branch of the uterine artery or vein is torn. Small tears of the cervix heal without trouble, but larger ones, unless repaired, leave deforming scars. Perforating tears extending into the broad ligaments may be fatal. They require full institutional resources to assemble a surgical team for exploratory laparotomy.

Examine the cervix after every delivery. At the sides of the cervix there is less muscular and fibrous tissue and the tears occur most often in this location, producing the usual bilateral split (Fig. 9.5). If only the fibro-muscular part of the cervix tears, the overlying mucosa remains intact and a thin bridge of tissue, uniting the lateral margins of the anterior and posterior lips, is present. To repair such a laceration, cut the thin bridge and pull the fibromuscular tissue out of the deep recesses at each side. Omitting this important step will only bring the edges of the mucosa together, leaving the cervix vulnerable to repeat, and potentially more severe, lacerations in subsequent pregnancies.

When bleeding is profuse, it is not easy to suture the cervix because it is hidden in a pool of blood. Use ring forceps or vulsella to grasp the

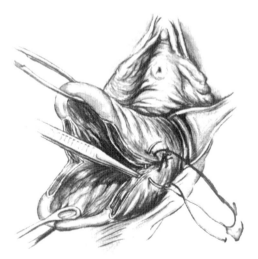

**Figure 9.5** Cervical lacerations. The typical cervical tear can be sutured with a continuous locking technique or with interrupted sutures. Suturing must be started above the apex of the wound. Be sure to include the fibromuscular substance of the cervix, which tends to retract. When the upper end of the tear is not easily visualized, put in interrupted sutures, using each for traction to bring the apex into view so it can be repaired under direct vision.

cervical lips and draw them down to the vulva. Pass a succession of interrupted stitches in the most accessible portion of the laceration, leaving the suture ends long. Once a few sutures are in place, exert steady gentle traction on them. This will usually bring the higher regions into view and within reach. You can thus place sutures successively higher and higher into the cervix. Be sure that you have repaired the uppermost portion of the laceration. Even the base of the broad ligament may be pulled into view in this way so that a spurting vessel that may have retracted can be ligated. Hemostasis in this area must be complete; otherwise, the bleeding may continue retroperitoneally and a hematoma will form. When placing sutures in this area, take great care to avoid introducing a suture into the bladder or around the ureter. Knowing the anatomy of the region, you will recognize that the ureters are located very close to the cervix at the base of the broad ligament, at which site they are especially vulnerable to being injured by a suture.

The most important suture is the one near the vaginal fornix, usually well above the upper angle of the laceration. This suture is intended to stop the hemorrhage from the large vessels at the apex and from those that may have retracted somewhat. You must place the highest suture in the cervical wound repair, analogous to the highest suture in a perineal laceration or episiotomy wound repair, beyond the uppermost part of the tear in order to be certain that a retracted vessel will not bleed later. Use a continuous locked suture, or interrupted sutures. The latter can be helpful when the laceration is difficult to visualize. Each tied suture can be used for traction to help expose the area for the next one. Since the ureter is nearby, as noted above, the needle for the first suture must be passed close to the uterus; the same principle applies for any suture placed in the lateral fornix.

## Uterine rupture

Rupture of the uterus during labor may be *spontaneous, traumatic,* or *postcesarean.* Uterine rupture in the context of a prior cesarean delivery is discussed in Chapter 11.

Spontaneous uterine rupture, i.e., without a predisposing previous hysterotomy, is rare, particularly if labor is managed appropriately. Predisposing risks include mechanical factors that obstruct advance of the fetus through the birth canal, such as cephalopelvic disproportion, shoulder dystocia, malpresentations, malpositions, and obstruction by maternal soft tissue tumors or by fetal hydrocephalus. In the presence of a mechanical obstruction in which timely delivery is not effected, even a normal uterine muscle may rupture eventually with strong contractions.

Excessive use of oxytocin may be particularly hazardous in this regard, especially in women of high parity. In addition, conditions that weaken the uterine wall may also promote rupture, including grand multiparity and pregnancy in an undeveloped horn of the uterus.

The mechanism of spontaneous rupture often involves attenuation of the lower uterine segment as labor progresses, particularly in the presence of insurmountable obstruction to descent. Allowing labor to continue in such circumstances progressively thins the lower segment to the point of disintegration. Spontaneous rupture of the lower uterine segment is usually longitudinal or oblique. At the height of a contraction, the thinned portion of the uterus tears open. This event is often associated with intense, acute pain. Sometimes, however, the separation of the fibers is gradual and the rupture is completed without producing alarming symptoms. The uterine contractions may force the fetus through the rupture. After the fetus is expelled through this new passage into the peritoneal cavity, the uterus contracts down alongside it. Characteristically, no further contractions are felt by the patient. Whenever contractions stop abruptly, you must assume rupture has occurred; however, be aware that contractions sometimes continue even after overt uterine rupture.

The edges of spontaneous ruptures are generally ragged. If the tear extends to the broad ligament, a massive hematoma may occur between its leaves. Blood loss can be rapid and extreme, and prompt surgical intervention is essential to preserve the mother's health and life.

Traumatic ruptures can occur with blunt or penetrating trauma at any time during pregnancy, particularly from vehicular accidents or acts of domestic violence. During labor, uterine rupture may occur when a forceps blade is thrust through the uterine wall or traction with forceps or vacuum extractor is attempted through an incompletely dilated cervix. Attempting to resolve a shoulder dystocia by introducing your hand alongside the fetus in the maximally distended lower segment may also cause such a tear.

## Fistulas

Genital fistulas related to childbearing are rare in the industrialized world, primarily because of improved obstetric techniques. In the developing world, however, they are still common causes of lifelong suffering and social ostracism. Always keep the third world experience in mind. It should serve to remind you that poorly managed or neglected labors can lead to considerable, sometimes irreparable, harm.

Various types of fistulas are encountered (Fig. 9.6). Most will require surgical repair. Vesicovaginal fistulas can result from direct trauma or,

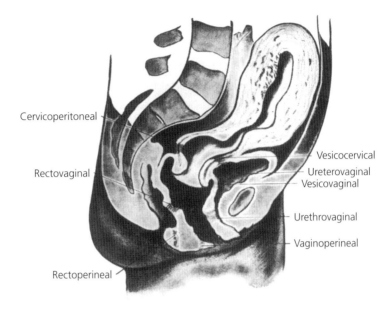

Cervicoperitoneal

Rectovaginal

Rectoperineal

Vesicocervical
Ureterovaginal
Vesicovaginal

Urethrovaginal

Vaginoperineal

**Figure 9.6** Common sites of genital fistulas of obstetric origin.

more commonly, from pressure necrosis of the bladder consequent to prolonged compression of the vesicovaginal septum between the fetal head and the maternal bony pelvis. The resulting ischemic tissue in bladder and vagina becomes necrotic, and a fistulous tract replaces it. Symptoms often begin in the first week of the puerperium, but may be delayed even longer. Urinary incontinence is usually the first indication of a problem.

Protect the bladder during delivery. It often empties itself while the patient is pushing in the second stage; occasionally, catheterization is advantageous to avoid the potential injury caused by having the head deliver past a full bladder. This is especially important if you plan to do an instrumental delivery.

Rectovaginal fistulas are more common than those involving the bladder. Usually, they are small and occur close to the anal verge. They may result from failure to recognize and repair a fourth degree laceration or from poor healing of such a laceration. A fistula may also occur if an errant suture is placed so that it enters the rectum during the repair of an episiotomy or a perineal laceration. Therefore, you should always do a rectal examination after any such repair to determine the presence of a penetrating suture. Corrected immediately, it rarely has consequences. Larger fistulas higher up in the vagina and the rectum are more problematic and difficult to repair. Usually, passage of stool or flatus from the vagina is the presenting symptom.

If your pregnant patient has had successful repair of a fistula previously, we strongly recommend that cesarean delivery be performed prior to labor. The trauma of another vaginal delivery can reopen the old wound and a repeat fistula operation may not be successful.

## Injuries to the bony pelvis

### Pathologic separation of the pelvic joints

Pregnancy increases the compliance of the ligaments and articular connective tissue that bind the pelvic bones, an adaptation that presumably eases the passage of the fetus through the pelvis. This acquired flexibility also makes the pelvic joints—highly stable structures in the nonpregnant state—vulnerable to injury.

Some degree of widening of the symphysis pubis is normal during pregnancy, and the sacroiliac joints become more mobile. The resulting slight instability causes the waddling gait your patients often have in the third trimester.

Occasionally, pathologic separation of the pelvic bones occurs during pregnancy or labor. This is most common in the pubic symphysis, but may also involve the sacroiliac joints. Although rare, complete rupture of a joint can occur. When pathologic separation occurs during labor, it is often in the context of a contracted pelvis, fetal macrosomia, or operative vaginal delivery. Indeed, improperly directed forceps traction, such as pulling upward too soon or too strongly, can rupture the pelvic ring. Most cases, however, occur in the absence of these risk factors. The cause of excessive weakening of the joints is unknown in these cases. It may have its origin in the genetics of connective tissue metabolism.

### Diagnosis and treatment

Your patient may have experienced pain in the symphysis pubis and the sacroiliac joints for several weeks prior to labor. She may notice that she has difficulty in rising from a sitting position, or that walking backward is more comfortable than going forward. These symptoms all suggest that some degree of pathologic pelvic joint separation is already present.

During spontaneous labor, further separation may occur gradually, or a frank rupture of the symphysis may be heard as a dull cracking sound at the moment that it occurs. Your patient may report that she felt something burst. Later, she will likely have pain, sometimes intense, over the affected joint, radiating down to the thighs. She will tend to lie in bed with the legs abducted and externally rotated. You will find tenderness over the pubis. Place two examining fingers in the vagina and press them against the pubic symphysis. Ask your patient to keep her hips and knees fixed, and have an assistant push up alternately on the patient's feet. You will sometimes be able to appreciate mobility of the pubic bones. Ultrasonographic or x-ray imaging may be used to help with the diagnosis, but the correlation between the degree of separation of the pubic bones and the patient's symptoms is not strong.

Recovery is usually spontaneous, but it may take 4–8 weeks before normal function returns. A supportive orthopedic girdle and non-steroidal antiinflammatory drugs will ease the discomfort. This can be quite a debilitating injury for a woman who needs to care for a new baby.

Sometimes the affected joint may not reunite, resulting in long-term disability. In such cases, the orthopedic procedure of wiring the pubic bones together can successfully resolve the problem.

Loosening of the sacrum from the innominate bones and small hemorrhages in the sacroiliac joints may result from labor. This probably explains many of the backaches that women experience after vaginal delivery. Pain and tenderness over the joints and abnormal mobility are diagnostic. Symptoms usually resolve spontaneously within 7–10 days after delivery. The treatment is antiinflammatory drugs, local application of heat, and sometimes a stabilizing girdle.

## Injury to the coccyx

During delivery the coccyx is often forced backward 2.5 cm or more. This excursion is permitted by a healthy sacrococcygeal joint. If the joint is ankylosed (usually the result of previous trauma), the bone itself may be fractured or the joint may separate. Chronic arthritis can result. The coccyx may be dislocated onto the anterior or posterior surface of the sacrum. Chronic pain can be the consequence of any of these injuries.

Fracture or dislocation of the coccyx during delivery causes obvious symptoms. Your patient may complain of tenderness, or of pain on defecation. She cannot sit comfortably, and pain centered in the coccygeal area often radiates up the back and down the thighs. She may have difficulty walking because of the pain. When she sits, she will rest the weight of her body on either trochanter. Examine her with a finger in the rectum and your thumb externally against the coccyx. You will find exquisite tenderness. You may be able to feel a dislocation or suspect a fracture. The latter is usually associated with crepitus. If there is doubt, a CT scan will confirm the diagnosis. Spontaneous recovery is the rule, but sometimes it takes 6 months or more for all symptoms to resolve. During recovery, heat can be helpful, and injection of the sacrococcygeal joint with a local anesthetic can provide symptomatic relief. In persistent cases, corticosteroid injections help some people, and in recalcitrant situations, coccygectomy, a major orthopedic procedure, can be performed.

An ankylosed sacrococcygeal joint may obstruct labor. Sometimes, one can hear the joint crack during a forceps operation or at a normal delivery. On rare occasions, the joint may have to be broken deliberately to allow delivery, but care must be taken not to injure the rectum. Rarely, the jutting bone may be so large and hard that it becomes necessary to undertake a cesarean delivery instead.

## Key points

- Birth canal trauma can cause blood loss, infection and discomfort. It can contribute to long-term disability in the form of fistulas, dyspareunia, pelvic floor relaxation and urinary or fecal incontinence.
- An important risk factor for perineal tears is a narrow subpubic arch.
- Repair all lacerations with a layered anatomic closure using fine absorbable suture material.
- Make yourself a student of pelvic anatomy; the effort will pay substantial dividends for you and your patients.
- Careful massage of the perineum and lower vagina using sterile oils or water-soluble lubricant can reduce shearing forces between the fetal head and the vagina and thus reduce the frequency and severity of perineal lacerations.
- Maternal bearing-down efforts without progress in fetal descent provoke descent of the entire uterus and potential damage to its supporting structures.
- A long second stage *per se* is not a strong risk factor for pelvic floor injury.
- Routine episiotomy for protection of the fetus is not justifiable, and episiotomy increases the risk of third and fourth degree lacerations.
- Instrumental vaginal delivery can be particularly hazardous in a pelvis with a narrow subpubic arch, and even more so in a funnel pelvis. We strongly discourage use of forceps or vacuum extractor in such patients.
- Consider arterial embolization for vulvar or vaginal hematomas that cannot be controlled surgically.
- If your pregnant patient has had successful repair of a fistula previously, we strongly recommend that cesarean delivery be done prior to labor.
- Pain and tenderness over the symphysis pubis, difficulty rising from a sitting position, and finding backward walking more comfortable than forward are symptoms of pathologic separation of the symphysis.
- Complaints of pain and tenderness in the coccygeal area when sitting or of pain on defecation after delivery suggest fracture or dislocation of the coccyx.

## Further Reading

### Books and reviews

American College of Obstetricians and Gynecologists. ACOG Practice Bulletin. Episiotomy. Clinical management guidelines for the obstetrician-gynecologist. Number 71. April 2006. Obstet Gynecol 2006;107:957–62.

Cleary-Goldman J, Robinson JN. The role of episiotomy in current obstetric practice. Seminars Perinatol 2003;27:3–12.

Cohen WR, Romero R. Childbirth and the pelvic floor. In: Kurjak A, Chervenak F (eds) *Textbook of Perinatal Medicine*, 2nd edition. Informa, London, 2006: 1979–88.

Renfrew MJ, Hannah W, Albers L, Floyd E. Practices that minimize trauma to the genital tract in childbirth: a systematic review of the literature. Birth 1998;25:143–60.

### Primary sources

Danforth KN, Townsend MK, Lifford K, Curhan GC, Resnick NM, Grodstein F. Risk factors for urinary incontinence among middle-aged women. Am J Obstet Gynecol 2006;194:339–45.

De Leeuw JW, de Wit C, Kuijken JP, Bruinse HW. Mediolateral episiotomy reduces the risk for anal sphincter injury during operative vaginal delivery. BJOG 2008;115:104–8.

Duggal N, Mercado C, Daniels K, Bujor A, Caughey AB, El-Sayed YY. Antibiotic prophylaxis for prevention of post-partum perineal wound complications: a randomized controlled trial. Obstet Gynecol 2008;111:1268–73.

Frudinger A, Halligan S, Spencer JAD, Bartram CI, Kamm MA, Winter R. Influence of the subpubic arch angle on anal sphincter trauma and anal incontinence following childbirth. BJOG 2002;109:1207–12.

Rustamova S, Predanic M, Cohen WR. Changes in symphysis pubis width during labor. J Perinat Med 2009;37:370–3.

Sultan AH, Kamm MA, Hudson CN, Bartram CI. Third degree obstetric anal sphincter tears: risk factors and outcome of primary repair. BMJ 1994;308:887–91.

Sultan AH, Kamm MA, Hudson CN, Thomas JM, Bartram CI. Anal sphincter disruption during vaginal delivery. N Engl J Med 1999;341:1709–14.

Thorp JM Jr, Bowes WA Jr, Brame RG, Cefalo R. Selected use of midline episiotomy: effect on perineal trauma. Obstet Gynecol 1987;70:260–2.

# CHAPTER 10

# Inducing Labor

*Induction* of labor is a process for initiating labor by pharmacologic or mechanical means. If labor has already begun, measures used to enhance contractions are designated *augmentation* of labor instead (Chapter 5). Both are commonly practiced. In some institutions, more than half of all gravidas are subjected to induction or augmentation of labor. Complications of induction and augmentation, although infrequent in occurrence, may be severe and sometimes become manifest without forewarning. The latter makes it difficult to ensure maternal and fetal well-being. Therefore, you should undertake induction and augmentation only for clearly defined reasons. Moreover, the intervention should be done under optimal circumstances to help minimize risks. Whenever considering induction or augmentation of labor, you must evaluate risks against benefits and demonstrate that the latter outweigh the former. It is prudent, furthermore, to document the details of this evaluation in the medical record.

Clinical situations in which induction of labor is carried out, particularly for those cases in which conditions are not favorable, often involve two distinct phases, a period of *priming* followed by the induction proper. Priming, also called *ripening*, consists of efforts to prepare the cervix and lower uterine segment to facilitate later labor induction. Labor sometimes begins during the priming phase, rendering a subsequent separate induction phase unnecessary. As with labor induction, priming is not without risk and, like induction, should not be embarked upon without detailed consideration of its potential harms and benefits.

## Indications

A number of conditions preexist or develop anew in late pregnancy that are intrinsically hazardous to mother or fetus. Ample support for

*Labor and Delivery Care: A Practical Guide*, First Edition. Wayne R. Cohen and Emanuel A. Friedman. © 2011 John Wiley & Sons, Ltd. Published 2011 by John Wiley & Sons, Ltd.

## Box 10.1 Indications for induction of labor

- Urgent indications
  - Severe pregnancy-induced hypertension
  - Chorioamnionitis
- Non-urgent indications
  - Fetal compromise
  - Oligohydramnios
  - Intrauterine growth restriction
  - Preterm premature rupture of membranes
  - Postterm pregnancy
  - Chronic hypertensive disease
  - Diabetes mellitus, especially if poorly controlled
  - Maternal cardiac, renal, or pulmonary disease
  - Abruptio placentae
  - Rh alloimmunization
  - Fetal death
- Prophylactic indications (dubious indications)
  - Prevent fetal macrosomia
  - Prevent postterm pregnancy
- Elective or logistic indications (seldom acceptable indications)
  - Maternal desire or demand
  - Prevent uncontrolled delivery outside hospital
  - Gravida lives remote from hospital
  - History of short labor
  - Organize family and work responsibilities
  - Prevent anesthesia accidents (e.g., aspiration)
  - Assure constant physician attendance
  - Maintain orderly hospital occupancy
  - Psychosocial reasons

intervention can be said to exist if the risks of the priming and induction processes, plus the risks of the delivery and the fetal risks of prematurity, are quantitatively less than those of continuing the pregnancy.

Conditions that warrant labor induction include a variety of maternal and fetal disorders, as listed in Box 10.1. Be aware, however, that the mere presence of one or more of these conditions does not automatically require you to proceed with an induction of labor. Only when the problem progresses in severity to become a real present threat to the health of mother or fetus (in contradistinction to a future threat that may or may not eventuate) can the induction be justified. This applies especially if the pregnancy is not far enough advanced to ensure against the neonatal risks of premature birth.

Indications are divisible into four distinct groups (Box 10.1): (1) urgent problems requiring prompt intervention due to a current threat to maternal or fetal health; (2) nonurgent issues with potential adverse impact not yet overtly manifest, but with a high probability of becoming manifest in the near future; (3) prophylactic indications that constitute worrisome problems that might arise in the future; (4) elective or logistic indications, which seldom warrant exposing mother and fetus to the risks of priming and induction.

Urgent problems are few in number, but are often so severe when they arise that they clearly justify expeditious induction. Nonurgent indications are much more common, but seldom develop to a sufficient degree of severity to constitute actual threats. Prophylactic indications, by and large, have not been shown to be beneficial and we do not recommend them. Elective inductions are those performed without medical or obstetric justification. They are very common, but are not appropriate except under the most unusual of circumstances.

## Contraindications

As an obvious guiding principle, anything that contraindicates labor and vaginal delivery has to be considered a contraindication to inducing labor. Identifiable maternal and fetal contraindications are listed in Box 10.2. Principal among them are uterine scars, whether from prior cesarean delivery, metroplasty, or penetrating myomectomy. The presence of such a scar places the gravida at risk of possible catastrophic complications of uterine rupture during labor. Of special concern in this regard is the use of prostaglandin for the priming process, which carries the greatest risk of uterine rupture. The collagen-degrading activity of prostaglandin, which works to great advantage in changing the integrity and consistency of the cervix to make it more favorable for successful induction, may weaken a cesarean scar in the lower uterine segment and make it vulnerable to rupture. Oxytocin also appears to increase the risk of rupture, albeit less so than prostaglandin, perhaps directly related to its effect in causing the uterus to contract more forcibly than is likely to occur in unstimulated labor. Both agents are, therefore, best avoided for priming or induction of a gravida with a scarred uterus.

Similarly, if vaginal delivery cannot occur because of some obstructive factor, you should not undertake induction. Anticipate that vaginal delivery is unlikely to be safely achievable, for example, if the maternal pelvis is contracted or misshapen. In addition, even if the pelvis is of ample size and has normal architecture, it may not be adequate to accommodate a large fetus, so you should remain alert at all times to indicators of cephalopelvic disproportion (Chapters 4 and 5).

> ## Box 10.2 Contraindications against induction of labor
>
> - Maternal contraindications
>   - Prior cesarean delivery
>   - Prior myomectomy in which the incision entered the endometrial cavity
>   - Prior hysterotomy
>   - Prior uterine reconstructive surgery
>   - Placenta previa
>   - Cephalopelvic disproportion
>   - Distorted or contracted pelvic architecture
>   - Uterine hypercontractility
>   - Uterine overdistention
>     - Polyhydramnios
>     - Multiple pregnancy
>   - Umbilical cord prolapse
>   - Active genital herpesvirus infection
>   - Invasive carcinoma of cervix
> - Fetal contraindications
>   - Prematurity
>   - Macrosomia
>   - Malpresentation
>   - Hydrocephalus
>   - Nonreassuring fetal status
>   - Multifetal pregnancy

## Risks

As previously stated, priming of the cervix and induction and augmentation of labor carry risks. While those risks are not common, they can be serious. Because they are sometimes severe when they arise, you have to be mindful of them and weigh them in the balance of your risk–benefit considerations before undertaking a labor induction. Most of those risks, listed in Box 10.3, result from excessive stimulation of uterine activity.

The gravid uterus becomes increasingly sensitive to oxytocin as pregnancy advances toward term. Moreover, the response of a given uterus to oxytocin in late pregnancy is highly variable and unpredictable. To make matters worse, there is no reliable test to determine in advance how the uterus will react to a particular dose of the drugs used for priming and induction. That is why it is so important for you to administer those agents with extreme caution, to use them only when the benefits are clearly greater than the risks, and if you do use them, to monitor the uterine contractions continuously to detect changes and to determine whether the fetus is reacting adversely to those contractions.

Uterine hypercontractility may take the form of contractions that are too long (uterine tetany), too frequent (uterine tachysystole), coupled

> **Box 10.3 Risks of induction of labor**
>
> - Maternal
>   - Uterine hypercontractility
>   - Failed induction (cesarean delivery)
>   - Chorioamnionitis
>   - Uterine atony
>   - Postpartum hemorrhage
>   - Prolonged labor
>   - Abruptio placentae
>   - Cervical laceration
>   - Uterine rupture
>   - Cesarean hysterectomy
>   - Amniotic fluid embolism
>   - Drug hypersensitivity reaction
>   - Water intoxication (from oxytocin)
> - Fetal
>   - Prematurity
>   - Precipitate dilatation, descent, and delivery
>   - Birth trauma
>   - Intracranial hemorrhage
>   - Hypoxia
>   - Umbilical cord prolapse

(two or more contractions with intervals of relaxation between them too short to permit placental–fetal reoxygenation), polysystole (a sequence of contractions without full relaxation between them), or hypertonus (excess resting tone between contractions). Singly or in combination, these patterns not only risk maternal damage, such as cervical lacerations, uterine rupture, and postpartum hemorrhage (from tears or uterine atony), but fetal harm as well by impeding uterine blood flow, thereby causing fetal hypoxia. This serious fetal problem may be further compounded by abruptio placentae.

Additionally, precipitate labor—in which there is abnormally rapid dilatation, descent, and delivery—may result from the tumultuous contractions that sometimes occur in response to the uterotonic agents used for priming and induction. Precipitate labor adds a further dimension to the risk of maternal soft tissue damage and potentially causes rapid compression–decompression injury to the fetus during the delivery process, contributing to intracranial injury.

Among the most common of the deleterious outcomes of labor induction is failure to achieve its objective of effecting vaginal delivery. By itself, this is not a serious issue, i.e., it is not inherently harmful. It becomes a complication with potential harm because of what healthcare providers do in response to it. There is a mindset among many obstetricians that interprets induction failure, even after a single brief attempt, as reflexively justifying cesarean delivery. This is not to suggest that induction attempts should be repeated more than a day or two in sequence, but to declare it a failure after a brief trial without some strong indication to intervene is inappropriate. There is no controversy over proceeding with cesarean delivery if the original indication for the induction warranted intervention at the outset and the indication still pertains (or has worsened) after a single failed trial induction. However, if the indication for the induction was marginal or insubstantial in the first place, then cesarean delivery is not automatically necessary if the attempt to induce labor failed. A better alternative is to reconsider allowing the pregnancy to proceed without any further attempts to induce the labor before it starts spontaneously. The hard part of that strategy of course is explaining to the patient why you undertook her labor induction in the first place. You can readily avoid this difficult problem by not undertaking any labor induction without a strong indication.

Another risk, water intoxication, applies to the use of oxytocin only. Although it is rarely encountered, it can be particularly devastating. When it becomes necessary to administer an oxytocin infusion at a high rate, the antidiuretic effect of this agent will be become evident. This applies most often when the rate exceeds 40 mU/min, particularly when given in conjunction with a large volume of intravenous fluid. Generalized fluid retention and hyponatremia result. Neurologic manifestations are headache and confusion progressing, if uncorrected, to encephalopathy, convulsions, coma, and death. Water intoxication is avoidable by using the minimum necessary dose rate and avoiding extended infusions. Dilute the drug in an electrolyte solution, and when large amounts are required to produce effective uterine contractions, doubling the concentration of oxytocin in solution (and reducing the rate of infusion accordingly) will help reduce the risk.

The risk of prematurity from induction falls into two categories: one is related to intentional preterm birth associated with induction for substantive indications before term; the other is associated with inductions done ostensibly at term for marginal indications or electively. Prematurity from the former is expected and understood. Prematurity from the latter, however, is an adverse consequence of undertaking labor induction without clear confirmation of gestational age. You can reduce the chances of this occurring by doing inductions only when clearly indicated and by verifying fetal pulmonary maturity when necessary prior to attempting labor induction (Box 10.3).

In regard to the selection of the timing of induction, it is often possible to postpone the process even for a brief period of time to diminish the likelihood of prematurity. There are advantages to delaying delivery, when safe and feasible, in the interest of enhancing neonatal well-being among babies born even during the last few weeks of pregnancy. Thus, if at all possible, you should carefully consider whether it is feasible to hold off any induction, unless clearly indicated by some threatening maternal or fetal condition, until at least 39 weeks.

## Prerequisites

Since any uterotonic agent used for priming, induction, or augmentation of labor carries the aforementioned risks, your objective should be to avoid using them indiscriminately and, when it is necessary to administer them, to take special precautions. A valuable approach in this regard is for you to ensure the environment in which the uterine stimulation is done is optimal, the personnel are skilled and knowledgeable, and to select patient candidates who fulfill essential prerequisites (Box 10.4). We strongly recommend against using any ripening or induction agent other than in a fully-equipped labor unit. Every labor and delivery unit should have a protocol that strictly governs the administration of oxytocin in order to minimize its risks.

Critical to a good outcome is preparing your patient so she will be emotionally and physically ready to undergo the rigors of the process and be willing to embark upon it. She must understand why it is being done, what alternatives exist, including doing nothing until spontaneous labor begins on its own, and the relative benefits and risks of each of these various

---

**Box 10.4 Prerequisites for induction of labor**

- Presence of personnel
  - Trained, skilled, knowledgeable professionals
  - Readily available and physically present when needed
  - Obstetric attendant, nursing, anesthesia, pediatrics at all times
  - Able to recognize and deal with complications
- Suitable facilities
  - Immediately available, fully equipped operating room
  - Blood bank
  - Laboratory
- Prepared patient
  - Emotionally and physically prepared
  - Counseled fully and informed about issues
    - Indications, risks, alternatives, methods, possible failure, consequences
- Optimal conditions
  - Patient at or near term
  - Absence of contraindications
  - Favorable Bishop score

options. You must inform her about what will be done to her in the priming and the induction sequence and what the prospects are for success or failure. Information about how long it will probably take is useful as well, freely acknowledging that prediction is difficult. Keep her—and her support persons, with her prior approval—advised of progress, or lack of progress, with periodic words of support and encouragement. Such details are important for her to know so she will be able to participate actively with you in making informed decisions as the process evolves.

Inductions should optimally take place in a facility where an operating room is immediately available in the event a severe complication requires aggressive intervention (e.g., ruptured uterus, prolapsed cord, or refractory postpartum hemorrhage). When minutes count, the difference between having a fully-staffed, open, functional operating room and one that has to be set up first by personnel summoned from outside the hospital can mean the difference between health and harm or even life and death. The same applies for having the ability to obtain adequate amounts of blood and blood products quickly when it is necessary to deal with an acute hemorrhage. Blood bank facilities, therefore, are essential. Laboratory back-up is similarly critical.

The requisite knowledgeable and skilled personnel for these services must be available on the premises at all times. In addition to the obstetric team, consisting of the primary obstetrician, an able assistant, and nurses who can function in both the labor unit and the operating room, an anesthesiologist and pediatric staff are needed at minimum. Being on call is insufficient for optimal safety. They must all be in the labor unit or close by and available to recognize problems as they arise and to deal with them expeditiously.

Our discussion of the prerequisites for priming and induction would not be complete without emphasis on selection criteria that you can use to advantage to enhance your ability to choose candidates whose induction is likely to succeed. More important, those criteria provide you with information to help you make logical decisions about how to manage gravidas who have strong indications to deliver, but who are not the best candidates for labor induction. Your sequential decision making (see below, under Management) is affected by whether the attempt to induce labor is likely to fail or evidence of progression toward success can be shown.

Of relevance among the features you should address in this regard is the duration of the pregnancy. As earlier stated, the closer the fetus is to term, the better its outcome will be. Important in respect to choosing when to intervene is the balance between the positive aspect of encouraging intrauterine maturation and the negative one of exposing the fetus to whatever adverse influence is imposed on it by its intrauterine environment. You will often find it difficult to identify when that balance is reached.

To find it, you will need frequent periodic assessments of fetal status, allowing pregnancy to continue as long as the fetus remains in good condition, and intervening when new objective evidence shows that the fetus needs to be delivered. Once the choice to intervene has been made, determine whether there are any contraindications against priming or induction. If there are, you should proceed to cesarean delivery. If no contraindications exist, evaluate the mother for the various component factors that make up the Bishop score (detailed below). The score has been shown to be especially useful for predicting success or failure of an induction. It will often prove valuable to you in helping you tailor your management plans to the special needs of your patient and her fetus.

## Bishop score

A particularly utilitarian tool you should familiarize yourself with and regularly employ before priming and induction of labor is the Bishop score (Table 10.1). It is based on simple clinical evaluations of four maternal features and one fetal feature. Each is easily and accurately determined by vaginal examination. Collectively, these features are influential in determining whether labor induction is likely to be successful. The features are: (1) cervical dilatation; (2) cervical effacement; (3) cervical consistency; (4) cervical position relative to the axis of the vagina; (5) fetal station.

Each is separately assessed and scored according to characteristics representing their normal advancing development as pregnancy reaches term before the onset of labor. It is clinically recognized that labor is most likely to begin spontaneously when the cervix is soft, well dilated and effaced, and axial in position, and the fetal head is well engaged. The more favorable each of the component features, the higher the score. Poor characteristics are scored zero; the best attributes are scored either 2 or 3. The scores are added together to provide the overall Bishop score, ranging from zero to 13.

**Table 10.1** Bishop Score for assessing inducibility

| Factor | Score 0 | Score 1 | Score 2 | Score 3 |
| --- | --- | --- | --- | --- |
| Cervical dilatation, cm | Closed | 1–2 | 3–4 | 5 + |
| Cervical effacement, % | 0–30 | 40–50 | 60–70 | 80 + |
| Cervical consistency | Firm | Medium | Soft | |
| Cervical position | Posterior | Axial | Anterior | |
| Fetal station | −3 | −2 | −1, 0 | +1, +2 |

Modified from Bishop EH. Obstet Gynecol 1964;24:266–8.

While the component parts of the Bishop score are given equal weight in reaching the total score, they are not actually equal with regard to their ability to predict the success of an induction. Cervical dilatation, for example, carries the greatest influence; fetal station the least; the other three fall between. In fact, some obstetricians assess inducibility using dilatation alone.

Inductions done in gravidas with scores of 9 or more succeed consistently; those with middling scores of 5 to 8 fail in about 5%; while those with particularly unfavorable scores of 4 or lower can be expected to fail in at least 20%. Although priming improves success rates because it advances the Bishop score, it cannot be fully relied upon to do so.

## Management

### Preinduction priming

Preinduction priming methods fall into two groups, mechanical means and pharmacologic agents. Some are part of our obstetric heritage and others are innovations; some have been shown to be effective and others much less so. Mechanical measures (Box 10.5) tend to yield inconsistent results, although successes are reported. They include amniotomy, stripping of membranes, balloon dilators, hygroscopic laminaria, and extraovular saline infusion by transcervical catheter. Pharmacologic agents (Box 10.6) used for priming include prostaglandin E2 and prostaglandin E1. A variety of other potentially useful priming agents are also currently under study.

### Mechanical means

Amniotomy, rupturing the membranes artificially to induce labor, has a long and checkered history. It works especially well in initiating labor in gravidas who are ready for labor, i.e., those who have a high Bishop score. Rupturing membranes, however, runs the risk of chorioamnionitis developing. The latent period from amniotomy to onset of labor is highly variable. When there is considerable delay, infection may develop.

Amniotomy performed when the fetal head is not engaged risks prolapsed cord. Even if the head is already engaged, a loop of cord may become compressed after amniotomy. Therefore, it is an important safeguard to assess the fetal heart rate pattern before and after rupturing the membranes. Since this risk is not possible to predict or avoid, it follows that amniotomy must be undertaken in a labor unit where the problem can be detected at once and dealt with promptly to prevent fetal harm.

The common practice of "stripping membranes" is inconsistent in its ability to induce labor and appears to be somewhat less likely to be associated with labor onset in the near future than amniotomy. This perhaps

> ### Box 10.5 Mechanical means for preinduction priming
>
> - Amniotomy
>   - Effective if cervix favorable
>   - Long and variable latent period to onset of labor
>   - Risks chorioamnionitis and cord prolapse
> - Stripping membranes
>   - Inconsistent benefit for priming
>   - Risks infection, bleeding, rupture of membranes
> - Laminaria
>   - Apparently effective for priming
>   - Risk of infection, found in the past, may no longer be relevant
> - Transcervical balloon catheter
>   - Effective for priming
>   - Best results with large balloon
>   - Low risk and low cost
> - Extraovular saline infusion
>   - Inconsistently effective when used alone
>   - Enhances effectiveness of other methods
>   - Low risk

reflects that providers may undertake it in less favorable cases. To strip the membranes, insert your examining finger into the cervical canal beyond the internal os. Then sweep your finger around the circumference of the lower uterine segment, separating the membranes from their tenuous attachment there. In theory, this procedure can promote infection, rupture of the membranes, and bleeding, but it is widely used, and probably associated with little risk.

Laminaria (or a synthetic equivalent) placed into the cervix will absorb fluid by hygroscopic action and thus swell gradually to cause the cervix to dilate. Laminaria are used effectively for termination of pregnancy during early gestation. They have been reported to have some success in altering the cervix in late pregnancy as well, improving the Bishop score and facilitating the action of oxytocin given subsequently to initiate labor. Infection, which was a common complication of the use of laminaria in the past, seems to be less of an issue with modern materials.

Placing a balloon catheter transcervically into the lower uterine segment also dilates the cervix and makes the uterus more amenable to the uterotonic effects of oxytocin administered later. A large Foley catheter, or a commercially available catheter designed specifically for this purpose, is inserted and its balloon inflated. The larger the balloon, the more effective the device in priming the cervix. Slight constant downward traction is applied to bring the balloon in contact with the internal cervical os, where the pressure is maintained to enhance its ability to prime the cervix. The external part of the catheter is taped to the patient's thigh for this purpose. In 8–12 hours, the balloon is generally expelled because the cervix has dilated. Effacement may not be achieved concomitantly. Administering oxytocin at this point can be expected to initiate labor in most cases. Reports of favorable results using this method, unassociated with increased numbers of adverse consequences, make it worth considering as an inexpensive, low-risk technique. Compared with pharmacologic agents, it has the additional advantage of not causing uterine hypercontractility.

Extraovular saline infusion is popular in some areas as a means to prime the cervix. It is usually administered in conjunction with other methods. Sterile saline, prewarmed to body temperature, is infused at a rate of 30–40 mL per hour. Although reported results are not entirely consistent, combining saline infusion with another method, such as transcervical catheter or prostaglandin, may enhance the value of that method for priming. Saline infusion does not seem to augment the risk of infection when used in conjunction with a balloon catheter.

### Pharmacologic agents

Prostaglandins are the mainstay of the currently available drugs for preinduction priming (Box 10.6). They work by breaking down collagen in tissues (by promoting matrix metalloproteinase enzyme activity), changing the consistency and integrity of the cervix to make it more amenable to the influence of uterine contractions. The two principal varieties are prostaglandins E2 and E1. Prostaglandin E2, generic name dinoprostone, is commercially distributed in two different forms for clinical application: a gel for intracervical administration and a wafer designed for slow release intravaginally. The other prostaglandin in current use, generic name misoprostol, is a synthetic analog of prostaglandin E1. It comes in tablet form, approved as a medication to prevent peptic ulcers due to nonsteroidal antiinflammatory drugs. It is readily available and inexpensive, but its use for preinduction priming is "off label" in the US.

Both forms of prostaglandins are quite effective, and about equally so, for preparing the cervix for later induction. When they are given, labor often begins during the priming process, precluding the need to proceed with oxytocin induction. Both are associated with a number of adverse side effects, also in about equal frequencies. The most important of these is uterine hyperstimulation, which may result in fetal hypoxia. In addition, they can cause nausea, vomiting, diarrhea, and fever. You should not give this drug to a woman who has asthma or glaucoma. Further, prostaglandins should not be administered if the membranes are ruptured or you anticipate rupturing the membranes.

The gel form of prostaglandin E2 is administered intracervically in a dose of 0.5 mg from a prefilled 2.5 mL syringe. Allow it to come to room

> **Box 10.6 Prostaglandin preparations for use in preinduction priming**
>
> - Prostaglandin E2 (dinoprostone)
>   - Effective for preinduction priming
>   - Administered as gel intracervically (Prepidil®) or as wafer in carrier device intravaginally (Cervidil®)
>   - Risks uterine hypercontractility and fetal compromise
>   - High cost per application
> - Prostaglandin E1 (misoprostol)
>   - Effective for preinduction priming
>   - Not formally approved for use in priming (off-label use)
>   - Administered in tablet form intravaginally (Cytotec®)
>   - Risks uterine hypercontractility and fetal compromise
>   - Low cost

temperature before administering. It comes with two short endocervical attachments to help guide the gel into the proper location within the cervical canal near the internal os: The short, 10 mm extension is intended for a cervix that is at least 50% effaced; the longer, 20 mm extension is for an uneffaced cervix. With the patient in lithotomy position, expose the cervix with a speculum. Choose the endocervical extension appropriate for her degree of effacement. Attach it to the syringe. Fill the extension with gel by pressing on the plunger assembly, expelling the air. Then gently insert the extension into the cervix and administer the gel high in the cervical canal. Keep the gravida in supine position for 15–30 minutes to minimize leakage. With effective priming, but no labor onset, initiate oxytocin induction (see below), but not sooner than 6–12 hours. If priming is ineffective, you can repeat the dose at 6-hour intervals for up to three doses.

The other form of prostaglandin E2 (proprietary name Cervidil®) is administered intravaginally in a slow-release delivery system consisting of a drug-containing polymer slab within a polyester pouch with an attached tail to facilitate removal. The device, which contains 10 mg of dinoprostone, is designed to release the drug at a rate of 0.3 mg per hour over a 12-hour period. Kept frozen prior to use, the device is inserted without warming it first. With the gravida in lithotomy position, expose the cervix with a speculum. Lay the device transversely in the posterior vaginal fornix. Instruct the patient to remain supine for at least 2 hours after placement. You can insert it without a speculum. Do not contaminate the insert with surgical lubricant, as it can interfere with release of the drug. Remove it after 12 hours if labor has not begun; or sooner, if it has, or if some adverse event makes it advisable to do so. If labor has not begun and you wish to proceed with induction, do not institute oxytocin until at least 30 minutes after the device has been removed.

Because misoprostol is not approved for use as a preinduction priming agent by the Food and Drug Administration, there are no formal recommendations for its administration. Clinical experience has shown that a regimen of 25 μg intravaginally, repeated at 3–6 hours as needed, is safe and effective. Using doses of 50 μg or greater is associated with unacceptably high rates of uterine hypercontractility and fetal compromise. The drug comes in tablets containing 100 μg and 200 μg, which can be divided by your pharmacist to provide the correct dosage. Controlled studies demonstrate that a 25 μg regimen of misoprostol reduces the average time from induction to delivery and requires fewer cesarean deliveries compared to either form of dinoprostone. In addition to these advantages, misoprostol is considerably less expensive than dinoprostone.

## Induction with oxytocin

After priming, proceed with an oxytocin regimen for labor induction under the following circumstances: if labor does not begin during the cervical priming process; if the indication for induction is still appropriate (i.e., if its benefits outweigh its risks); if there are no contraindications; and if the cervix has become favorable.

Oxytocin is a naturally-occurring nonapeptide produced in the hypothalamus and stored in the posterior lobe of the pituitary gland, from which it is released periodically in tiny amounts. It is involved, by a complex mechanism that is not fully understood, in initiating and supporting the progress of labor in human pregnancy. A synthetic form of oxytocin is commercially available for induction or augmentation of labor.

You have to be constantly mindful that oxytocin is a very powerful pharmacologic agent, capable of producing uterine contractions that are far in excess of what is needed for safe, effective labor. Those excessive contractions are capable of diminishing fetal oxygenation, causing placental separation or rupturing the uterus, and as a consequence inflicting severe harm on mother and fetus. To avoid these serious complications, you must take special precautions to administer oxytocin in very dilute solutions by carefully-controlled intravenous pump infusion. The rate of infusion has to be titrated according to the uterine response to the drug. Titration means adjusting the rate of administration by increasing it slowly over time to achieve a desired contractility pattern and not exceeding that uterine response. Further, even after this contractility pattern is established, periodic readjustments of the infusion rate may be necessary based on changing uterine response to the agent. To comply with this admonition, it is necessary for you to ensure that your patient's uterine contractions are monitored frequently for their intensity, frequency, and duration and that the fetus's reaction to those contractions is assessed often for any evidence of adverse impact. Because complications demanding rapid intervention can arise rapidly and without forewarning during labor induction, the application of continuous electronic uterine contraction and fetal heart rate monitoring has become the de facto standard of care whenever oxytocin is being given. It also follows logically that attentive, knowledgeable personnel must be constantly in attendance to ensure that developing problems are recognized and addressed promptly. Nurses involved with ongoing assessment of gravidas receiving oxytocin for labor induction appreciate (or soon learn to appreciate) how important their role is in detecting those problems, astutely designating oxytocin as a "high-alert medication."

Dilute the contents of an ampule of oxytocin, which contains a total of 10 units of the drug, in 1000 mL of Ringer's lactate solution. When mixed, 1 mL of this solution contains 1 mU of oxytocin. (Obviously, other concentrations can be used, so long as the dose rate is not different.) First, begin a separate intravenous infusion of Ringer's lactate without the drug. Then set up the oxytocin infusion to "piggy-back" into the initial line, in a port as close as possible to your patient. Use an electronic infusion pump to regulate the administration rate. The piggy-back arrangement is essential to prevent inadvertent bolus administration if flow in the primary intravenous line is increased. Delivering oxytocin very rapidly can have devastating results.

A conservative program for safe administration is to begin the infusion at a rate of 0.5–1.0 mU of oxytocin per minute. It is prudent to use a checklist before beginning to be sure that all criteria for administration of the drug are met.

Observe the effect on uterine activity and fetal heart rate over the next 15–30 minutes. Increase the pump infusion rate in small increments of 1–2 mL per minute at 15- to 30-minute intervals until the desired contractility pattern is reached. Aim to simulate strong, active labor with contractions of moderate intensity (i.e., between easily indentible and firm to palpation, the equivalent of 40–60 mmHg if measured by internal strain gauge), lasting 40–60 seconds and recurring every 2–4 minutes.

At any time that excessive uterine contractions develop or an abnormal fetal heart rate pattern occurs in response to those contractions, stop the infusion at once. The half-life of oxytocin in the circulation is 3 minutes, so the level drops rapidly over a relatively brief time. The uterine effect, however, takes longer to dissipate, often up to 40 minutes. The excessive contractions may, therefore, persist for some time. Usually, the adverse fetal effect, if any, will subside quickly. If the hypercontractility continues and the fetus does not recover quickly, administer an intravenous bolus of 100–200 µg of nitroglycerin, which is a safe, effective, rapidly-acting tocolytic agent. Its effect in reducing or stopping contractions can usually be seen within 1–2 minutes. Repeat it, if necessary, in 3 minutes. This is another "off label" not approved by the Food and Drug Administration, but supported by published reports. Much higher doses have also been administered in refractory cases with good results, but they should be given only with great caution. Because nitroglycerin is a powerful vasodilator, do not administer it to an unstable hypovolemic gravida in whom it can cause severe hypotension. Alternatively, terbutaline may be used to diminish uterine hypercontractility, although it is somewhat slower to take effect than nitroglycerin.

The uterus at or near term can be exquisitely sensitive to the effect of exogenous oxytocin. Giving oxytocin, even in the careful way just described, may result in unexpected hypercontractility and adverse fetal impact. The conservative regimen outlined here, starting at a low infusion rate and increasing it in small increments at relatively long intervals, is recommended as a means to minimize those hazards. Some advocate a more "active management" approach, beginning with infusion rates as high as 6 mU per minute and increasing the rate rapidly in increments of up to 6 mU per minute at intervals of 20–40 minutes. The objective is to reach effective contractions sooner with more rapidly progressive labor. Results are about as good as the more conservative regimen, although its risks, while infrequent, are potentially greater. Given that safety has to be a foremost consideration in the risk–benefit assessment, therefore, we cannot recommend adoption for general use.

## Decision-making issues

Managing patients who are under consideration for induction of labor or whose labor is being induced can be difficult. It involves a series of complex decisions. Making those decisions is facilitated if you approach them in a logical sequence (Fig. 10.1). Your overview is simplified considerably by separately and serially addressing issues in five distinct areas: (1) choosing whether or not to induce labor based on risk–benefit evaluation; (2) ascertaining the degree of urgency for delivery; (3) determining the best time to undertake intervention based on dynamic assessment of changing risk–benefit relations; (4) carrying out preinduction priming, if called for; (5) dealing with the induction per se.

### To induce or not

Assemble the objective facts that will determine, first and foremost, whether an induction is truly indicated. If not, the procedure must be

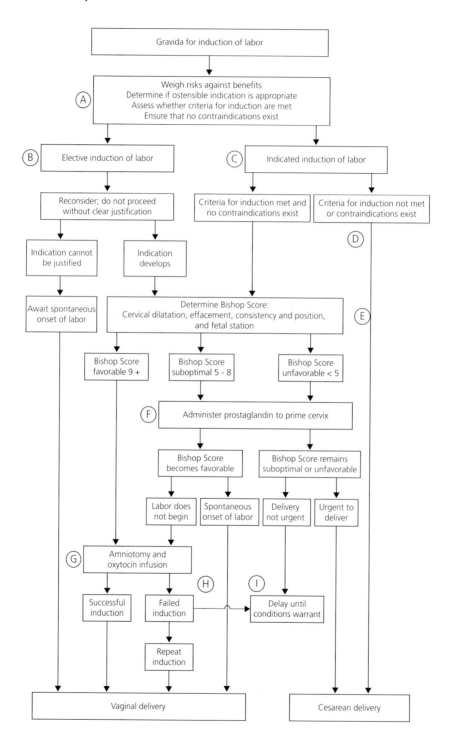

considered elective, i.e., without any medical or obstetric justification. That principle applies no matter how small those risks are in terms of frequency of occurrence and severity. If no sound indication for induction exists, desist. Await the spontaneous onset of labor. If a true indication should develop before labor begins on its own, you can reconsider inducing the labor.

**Figure 10.1** Algorithm for priming and induction of labor (see text for details).
**A**. Evaluate maternal and fetal status. Identify and document the indication for induction. Determine whether the indication is a current threat to mother or fetus. Be sure the criteria for induction are met and no contraindications to induction or vaginal delivery exist.
**B**. In the absence of a medical or an obstetric indication that poses an actual risk to mother or fetus, the induction must be considered elective. Except in rare instances, elective inductions cannot be condoned because the risks of the induction, no matter how infrequent or how small those risks might be, outweigh nonexistent benefits.
**C**. If there is a legitimate prevailing indication, proceed with the induction unless criteria have not been met or contraindications interdict it.
**D**. If safe vaginal delivery is not likely and there is clear rationale to deliver in the interest of maternal or fetal well-being, proceed with cesarean delivery instead.
**E**. Determining the Bishop score will provide utilitarian information about the probability that induction of labor will succeed and help in deciding whether preinduction priming is necessary.
**F**. If the Bishop score is less than optimally favorable (less than 9), undertake priming first. Priming with prostaglandin often results in rapid modification of the cervix so the subsequent induction will go easily. Alternatively, induction may not be needed at all if labor begins spontaneously during the priming phase.
**G**. Priming is unnecessary if the Bishop score is in the favorable range (9 or more). Proceed with labor induction using carefully titrated pump infusion of dilute oxytocin, constantly monitoring uterine contractility response and fetal reaction to those contractions. Be sure skilled personnel are in attendance so that complications are recognized immediately and dealt with expeditiously.
**H**. Failed induction should not be interpreted as an indication for cesarean delivery. The exception is the situation in which the original indication for the induction was so strong that it constituted a good reason for such intervention in the first place. If urgency dictates intervention but permits additional time for further attempts to induce, a second induction may be undertaken after a suitable period of overnight rest.
**I**. An induction that fails after one or two attempts, in the absence of strong indications for prompt delivery, warrants reassessment of the original indication to determine how severe it really is and the degree of urgency, if any, it imposes to effect delivery. For the case in which the risk is remote and potential, rather than immediate and actual, delivery is not urgent. It is preferable under these circumstances to desist altogether. Send the patient home and follow her and her fetus carefully with serial testing. As long as everything is going well, wait for spontaneous onset of labor. If the underlying condition worsens, however, intervene either by another induction or by cesarean delivery, as called for by the developments that arise.

## Assessing urgency

If an acceptable indication is present, your next objective is to determine if its existence means there is urgency to effect delivery. Often, the problem is not yet so severe that it requires you to intervene at that time. A valuable alternative is to follow the case with sequential testing of maternal and fetal status. This will allow the fetus to mature in utero and the mother's soft tissues to become more favorable so that, when conditions warrant, an induction can be carried out more quickly and with greater likelihood of successfully effecting safe vaginal delivery.

If there is urgency, mobilize the personnel who will be needed. Assess whether conditions are favorable for induction. Rule out contraindications against vaginal delivery. There may be a great urgency to effect delivery. If so, there may not be enough time to attempt a long priming-induction process, particularly if conditions for induction are unfavorable. Under such circumstances, prudence and good sense would dictate undertaking cesarean delivery instead.

Usually, however, the degree of urgency is not pressing. If so, gather additional information to help you plan ahead. Ascertain whether the fetus is mature. This may not weigh heavily in your decision to proceed if the risks to the fetus of remaining in utero are greater than those of being born prematurely. Nonetheless, advising the neonatology team that the fetus is immature will serve them well in making suitable preparations for the resuscitation and intensive care that the infant may require at birth and subsequently. If your institution does not have the necessary facilities to handle the special needs of such an infant when it is born, seriously consider moving the patient to a tertiary care institution where the induction can be carried out to deliver the neonate directly to a team able to take optimal care of it at once. The benefits of such predelivery transport are substantial, with well-documented improvements in morbidity and mortality. Also be sure to prepare your patient so that she is fully informed and consents to the transfer.

## Timing the induction

Choosing the best time to induce labor is your next order of business. It involves finding the proper balance between the progressively increasing risk from a maternal or a fetal condition and the diminishing risk of prematurity as pregnancy advances toward term. This is never easy. It requires what is called a process of "dynamic decision making" that addresses a moving target of risk–benefit evaluation. It is very different from the more common and much easier "static decision making" in which one weighs risks and

benefits at a given moment in time, and then makes an appropriate decision to act on that evaluation.

The dynamism alluded to in the term "dynamic decision making" refers
to serially reevaluating the risk–benefit equation during pregnancy to
try to determine the time when the risks of continuing the pregnancy
begin to exceed the risks of the induction process. If that time can be
determined objectively, it will constitute the optimal moment to switch
your management attitude from conservative watchful waiting to aggressive intervention.

## To prime or not

With a strong indication, no contraindication, all prerequisites met, and
everything in readiness in the event of a complication, you and your
patient are in a good position to proceed. For those cases in which the
cervix is middling (Bishop score 5–8) to overtly unfavorable for induction
(Bishop score less than 5), preinduction priming with a prostaglandin or
a balloon catheter will ordinarily be your initial approach.

## Managing the induction

If the cervix is favorable (Bishop score 9 or more), preinduction priming is
unnecessary. Skip directly to oxytocin induction. Begin oxytocin infusion
with carefully titrated dilute solution regulated by an infusion pump in
the manner detailed above. You can perform amniotomy simultaneously,
if there are no contraindications. Ordinarily, you can expect labor to begin
and to progress normally over the next few hours. As long as both maternal and fetal status remain good, as determined by monitoring their condition continuously, and the labor course progresses normally, safe vaginal
delivery can be expected. Conduct the management of an abnormal labor
pattern, if it should arise, as described in Chapter 5, opting for cesarean
delivery when it is clearly indicated for obstetric reasons.

Another possible development, not uncommon if induction is undertaken with less-than-optimal conditions, is one in which the condition for
which the induction was being undertaken worsens, yet vaginal delivery
is still remote. If it happens, reconsider whether it is appropriate to stop
the trial of labor and proceed with cesarean delivery instead so as not to
unduly jeopardize mother or fetus.

## Dealing with failure

Oxytocin infusion causes the uterus to contract regularly, usually within
minutes after you initiate the infusion. Those uterine contractions can

be expected to yield objective changes in cervical dilatation within a few hours. Induction has to be deemed a failure if the cervix has not changed after an interval of 8 hours of oxytocin infusion. While this is admittedly an arbitrary limit, continuing much beyond 8 hours is not likely to be associated with any further labor progress; moreover, it will probably exhaust the patient. Therefore, stop the infusion after 8 hours if there is no clinical evidence of cervical change.

The options that are available for you to pursue at this point are: (1) to continue with the induction despite the likelihood that it will not benefit the patient; (2) to proceed directly with cesarean delivery, assuming the failure to be the indication for the operative delivery; (3) to desist for a while, allow the patient to rest overnight, and then begin again the next morning; or (4) to stop the induction, rest the patient, reconsider whether the induction is truly indicated, and realizing belatedly that the risks of continuing the pregnancy are actually less than persisting in trying to induce the labor, explain the situation to the patient, and allow her to go home until labor begins or until maternal or fetal conditions worsen sufficiently to warrant another attempt to induce labor or, failing induction, to perform a cesarean delivery.

The first of these options, continuing reflexively, is not sensible because it is unlikely to be of any benefit. The second, undertaking cesarean delivery, is a regrettably common practice based on the mistaken perception that the failure of the induction by itself becomes a justification for cesarean delivery. This would depend on the urgency of the need to deliver the fetus. If the indication for the induction was not strong enough to warrant cesarean delivery when the induction was started, you must clearly understand that it does not become an indication that demands cesarean delivery merely because the induction fails.

Repeating the induction the next day is an option that is worth pursuing only if a special set of conditions warrant it. Those conditions include a strong indication and a cervix that is at least moderately favorable (Bishop score 5 or more). If there is a weak indication and a less-than-favorable cervix, which is the situation that prevails for many inductions of labor, it is just not prudent to persist with repetitive induction attempts.

## Key points
- Induction of labor can only be justified if the risk of continuing the pregnancy exceeds the risk of the induction.
- The presence of an adverse condition is not, by itself, an indication for induction unless that condition is sufficiently severe to constitute a current risk to mother or fetus, particularly if the induction is not likely to be successful.

- Optimal timing of an induction requires repetitive reevaluation of fetal status to determine when the fetal risk of remaining in utero exceeds the risk of its being delivered prematurely.
- Never induce labor if vaginal delivery is contraindicated.
- Uterine hyperstimulation, a potential cause of harm to mother and fetus, is the primary risk of preinduction priming and induction of labor.
- Because uterine hyperstimulation and its adverse consequences can develop without forewarning during priming and induction, these processes must be undertaken with great care and continuous surveillance by skilled personnel who are able to detect the problem as it arises and to deal with it expeditiously, and who are actually in attendance.
- Continuous monitoring of uterine contractions and fetal status is essential during priming and induction.
- If the indication is strong and there are no contraindications, but the cervix is unfavorable based on a low Bishop score, preinduction priming should be done with a prostaglandin preparation or mechanical means, such as an indwelling balloon catheter.
- In the presence of an indication that threatens maternal or fetal well-being and a favorable cervix, proceed directly to labor induction, administering oxytocin by infusion pump with or without amniotomy.
- Failure of induction is not, by itself, an indication for cesarean delivery unless the original indication for the induction justified cesarean delivery.

## Further Reading

### Books and reviews

American College of Obstetricians and Gynecologists. Induction of labor. Practice Bulletin, No. 10, November 1999.

American College of Obstetricians and Gynecologists. Vaginal birth after cesarean delivery. Practice Bulletin, No. 54, July 2004.

Caughey AB, Sundaram V, Kaimal AJ, Gienger A, Cheng YW, McDonald KM, et al. Systematic review: elective induction of labor versus expectant management of pregnancy. Ann Intern Med 2009;151:252–63.

### Primary sources

Axemo P, Fu X, Lindberg B, Ulmsten U, Wessen A. Intravenous nitroglycerin for rapid uterine relaxation. Acta Obstet Gynecol Scand 1998;77:50–3.

Bailit JL, Gregory KD, Reddy UM, Laughon SK, Branch DW, Burkman R, et al. Maternal and neonatal outcomes by labor onset type and gestational age. Am J Obstet Gynecol 2010;202:245:e1–12.

Bishop EH. Pelvic scoring for elective induction. Obstet Gynecol 1964;24:266–8.

Clark SL, Miller DD, Belfort MA, Dildy GA, Frye DK, Meyers JA. Neonatal and maternal outcomes associated with elective term delivery. Am J Obstet Gynecol 2009;200: 156.e1–4.

Dunne C, Da Silva O,Schmidt G, Natale R. Outcomes of elective labour induction and elective cesarean section in low-risk pregnancies between 37 and 41 weeks' gestation. J Obstet Gynaecol Can 2009;31:1124–30.

Ehrenthal DB, Jiang X, Strobino DM. Labor induction and the risk of a cesarean delivery among nulliparous women at term. Obstet Gynecol 2010;116:35–42.

Friedman EA, Niswander KR, Bayonet-Rivera NP, Sachtleben MR: Relation of prelabor evaluation to inducibility and the course of labor. Obstet Gynecol 1966;28:495–501.

Friedman EA, Niswander KR, Bayonet-Rivera NP, Sachtleben MR: Prelabor status evaluation: II. Weighted score. Obstet Gynecol 1967;29:539–44.

Gelber S, Sciscione A. Mechanical methods of cervical ripening and labor induction. Clin Obstet Gynecol 2006;49:642–57.

Lydon-Rochelle M, Holt VL, Easterling TR, Martin DP. Risk of uterine rupture during labor among women with a prior cesarean delivery. New Engl J Med 2001;345:3–8.

Martin VA, Hamilton BE, Sutton PD, et al. Birth: final data for 2006. National Vital Statistics Reports 2009;57:1.

Niswander KR, Friedman EA, Bayonet-Rivera NP. Prelabor pelvic score as a predictor of birth weight. Obstet Gynecol 1967;29: 256–9.

Simpson KR, Knox GE. Oxytocin as a high alert medication: implications for perinatal patient safety. MCN Am J Matern Child Nurs 2009;34:8–15.

# CHAPTER 11

# Cesarean Delivery

The use of cesarean delivery has increased steadily in most of the industrialized world over the last several decades. The cesarean delivery rate in the United States has reached about 32%, and the rise shows no signs of abating. Although our ability to deliver a baby by a relatively safe abdominal operation is an enormous and undeniable benefit to the health of women and children, cesarean delivery is not a procedure free of hazard. Like all surgical operations, it should be used only when its risks are clearly outweighed by its potential benefits.

Unfortunately, there are practitioners who resort to cesarean delivery whenever they are confronted with a vexing obstetric problem. Although some of these operations are appropriate, many are not. Cesarean delivery is a major surgical procedure that always requires serious consideration of its justification. Reserve cesarean delivery for those patients in whom vaginal delivery cannot, in your considered judgment, be accomplished without jeopardizing fetal or maternal life and health. If you cannot document those risks objectively, and are unable to demonstrate that the risks of continuing the pregnancy exceed those of intervening operatively, then you do not have ample support for proceeding with cesarean delivery and thereby exposing the mother to the hazards of the surgery.

## Indications for cesarean delivery

Potential indications for cesarean delivery are listed in Box 11.1. The most common are previous cesarean delivery, dysfunctional labor or cephalopelvic disproportion, abnormal fetal heart rate patterns, and malpresentations. We have addressed many of these problems, including the role of cesarean delivery in their management, in Chapters 4, 5, 7, and 8. Interpretation of fetal heart rate patterns is not in the scope of this volume.

*Labor and Delivery Care: A Practical Guide*, First Edition. Wayne R. Cohen and Emanuel A. Friedman. © 2011 John Wiley & Sons, Ltd. Published 2011 by John Wiley & Sons, Ltd

> **Box 11.1 Indications for cesarean delivery**
>
> - Maternal factors
>   - Prior hysterotomy (e.g., cesarean delivery, myomectomy)
>   - Prior uterine rupture
>   - Prior repair of genital prolapse or fistula
>   - Mechanical obstruction of birth canal (tumors, bony deformities)
>   - Active phase or second stage dysfunction unresponsive to or inappropriate for oxytocin stimulation
>   - Cephalopelvic disproportion
>   - Maternal infections (e.g., HIV, active genital herpes simplex lesions)
>   - Maternal medical disorders that could be compromised by labor or vaginal delivery (e.g., some cerebrovascular disorders)
>   - Patient request
> - Fetal and placental factors
>   - Placenta previa
>   - Vasa previa
>   - Malpresentation (breech, transverse lie)
>   - Umbilical cord prolapse
>   - High risk of Erb palsy
>   - Acute fetal oxygen deprivation
>   - Multifetal pregnancy
>   - Congenital malformations (e.g., osteogenesis imperfecta type III, hydrocephalus with macrocephaly)

Disproportion between the fetal head and the pelvis warrants cesarean delivery, but you can seldom identify this with confidence until your patient has been in labor. Thorough cephalopelvimetry is a valuable guide in this regard, but only when interpreted in conjunction with the evolving cervical dilatation and fetal descent patterns and, when appropriate, with the response to oxytocin augmentation of uterine contractility. This concept holds equally for nulliparas and multiparas. Just because your patient delivered a term-size baby previously does not insure her against cephalopelvic disproportion in a subsequent pregnancy.

Cesarean delivery may sometimes be contraindicated temporarily by the mother's general condition. If feasible, the procedure should be delayed until her status is more optimal to withstand the anesthesia and the operative strain. Examples include the eclamptic patient during and shortly following a seizure, or the patient with decompensated congestive heart failure, ketoacidosis, or an acute painful sickle cell crisis. Waiting until the mother is stable is almost always feasible, even when fetal indications exist. The intrauterine environment will usually improve rapidly to benefit the fetal status while the mother's condition is being corrected.

Generally, you should not carry out a cesarean delivery if the fetus is dead unless there is a serious problem threatening the mother's well-being.

For a woman whose pregnancy is complicated by placenta previa, for example, you will need to empty the uterus abdominally in order to avoid serious maternal hemorrhage. Similarly, in some severe instances of placental abruption, cesarean delivery is needed when the mother's life is threatened by hemorrhage and coagulopathy. Insurmountable cephalopelvic disproportion, neglected malpresentation, obstruction of the birth canal by tumors, and conjoined twins all warrant cesarean delivery, even if the fetus is no longer alive.

## Types of cesarean delivery

There are two primary methods of cesarean delivery: the lower segment operation, in which an incision is made either transversely or, much less often, vertically in the lower uterine segment; and the classical cesarean delivery, for which a vertical incision is made in the upper uterine segment.

The most common method is the transverse lower segment incision. The advantages of this approach over the classical uterine incision are reduced hemorrhage (because the lower segment is thinner and has more connective tissue—and is therefore less vascular—than the corpus), easier repair, lower risk of subsequent rupture, and less postoperative adhesion formation. The only relative disadvantages are the additional time it takes to develop the peritoneal flap and advance the bladder, and the possibility of lacerating the uterine vessels if the incision extends laterally. The speed and ease of the classical incision are its main advantages. It is primarily useful when the lower segment is inaccessible because of adhesions or leiomyomas. Some prefer the classical incision in cases of placenta previa or if there is a transverse lie with the fetal back down. The counterbalancing disadvantage of the classical incision is the need to cut through the considerable thickness of the upper segment myometrium, potentially causing hemorrhage, hematoma formation, febrile morbidity, poor healing, and greater risk of rupture in a future pregnancy. In addition, a classical incision tends to be more difficult to repair and more likely to cause postoperative adhesions, resulting in a greater incidence of bowel obstruction.

The vertical lower segment incision is of no value in term pregnancies. It is useful primarily in very preterm cases. Because the lower segment is not fully developed, and thus very narrow, until near term, a transverse incision can readily extend laterally into the uterine vessels as the fetal head is delivered, causing severe hemorrhage. A vertical incision can be safely fit into this narrow strip of the lower uterus without inviting this risk. In addition, a vertical incision can theoretically allow atraumatic delivery without incurring the high risk of subsequent rupture of the classical incision, provided it does not extend upward into the thick, vascular upper myometrium. Unfortunately, despite the best efforts of the surgeon, the low vertical incision often intrudes on the upper uterine segment, thus negating its putative advantage in diminishing the risk of rupture. Also, extension of the lower pole may injure the bladder. In general, therefore, the risk of a vertical low segment incision exceeds its benefit.

## Surgical techniques

### Preoperative preparation

The patient's blood should be typed and screened for antibodies by the blood bank prior to beginning a cesarean delivery. This will save considerable time, should transfusion become necessary. Have cross-matched blood available when you anticipate excessive blood loss, such as in the presence of placenta previa.

Shaving the skin incision site is optional. If you choose to shave, do so in the operating room just prior to cleansing the abdominal surface.

Most obstetricians put an indwelling Foley catheter in the mother's bladder before surgery. As an option, you can empty the bladder when necessary with an 18-gauge needle inserted through the anterior wall of the bladder during the case. If you use a catheter, remove it as soon as possible after surgery so as to minimize the associated risk of urinary tract infection.

Place the patient supine on the operating table, which should be tilted 15 degrees to the patient's left side to prevent aortocaval compression by the uterus. As an alternative, keep the table horizontal and place a wedge under her right hip. A single intraoperative dose of prophylactic antibiotics reduces the chance of postpartum uterine infection.

### Transverse lower uterine incision

You can approach the lower uterus through a number of different abdominal incisions. The most commonly used is a Pfannenstiel incision. It can be accomplished rapidly and has the advantages of minimal postoperative interference with respiratory function and great resistance to dehiscence. It also provides a good aesthetic appearance and is generally less painful during recuperation than a vertical skin incision.

Avoid making the Pfannenstiel incision in the skin crease above the mons pubis. If you do, the scar may retract as it heals, giving a less-than-ideal cosmetic result. If you make the incision 1 cm above the crease, the resulting scar will be less apparent. Another reason to incise some distance above the mons is to decrease the chance of bladder injury as you enter the peritoneal cavity.

Rather than truly transverse, i.e., straight across the lower abdomen, make the incision curved, with its convexity inferior, like a smile. This reduces the risk of severing segmental nerves of the abdominal wall, which sweep inferiorly and medially as they traverse the anterior abdominal wall. Also, remember that the skin incision generally needs to be only about 14 cm long. If you extend the incision too far laterally, you risk injury to the iliohypogastric or ilioinguinal nerves. When necessary, these nerves should be identified and protected.

With your patient prone and tilted laterally, her abdominal skin may be distorted by having been stretched to one side, making it difficult to place the incision symmetrically on her abdomen. While an uneven skin incision is of no medical importance, your patient will likely prefer an even, cosmetically-appealing, smile-shaped scar to one that more resembles a smirk. If you take pride in your work, so will you. To avoid this pitfall, push the uterus to the midline before you make the incision so the abdominal wall is in its normal position. After you incise the skin, allow the uterus to return to its skewed orientation.

Another means to ensure a symmetric skin incision is to scratch superficial vertical marks, using the back of your scalpel tip, in the midline and at measured points every 2 cm or so up to 5–7 cm to either side of it. Use these light scratches, which heal without a trace, to guide you in making the incision so that its lateral ends are equidistant from the midline. In addition, these marks facilitate precise reapproximation of the skin edges without tension during closure.

The Pfannenstiel technique involves transverse incisions in the skin and in the anterior rectus fascia. That fascia is then separated from its midline attachment to the linea alba between the umbilicus and the pubic symphysis. Before dividing this attachment, insinuate an index finger just lateral to the midline between the rectus muscle and the anterior sheath. Use your right finger if you are on your patient's right side. Have your assistant do the same thing on the other side of the midline, i.e., between the left rectus muscle and its anterior sheath. Rotate your finger while keeping it against the linea alba to establish a space on both sides of the midline. This space serves to facilitate cutting the fascia off the linea alba without damaging the fascial integrity.

Be careful not to sweep your finger laterally, because doing so may injure the perforating branches of the inferior epigastric vessels. When cut or torn, they tend to retract into the rectus muscle, making hemostasis difficult to achieve. The resulting hematoma can become quite large, and may not be clinically evident for many hours postoperatively. Cut the anterior rectus fascia free from the linea alba in the superior and inferior aspects of the incision. Then, separate the bellies of the rectus abdominis and pyramidalis muscles in the midline. To enter the peritoneal cavity, vertically incise the transversalis fascia and peritoneum together.

Take care to avoid damaging the urinary bladder as you enter the peritoneal cavity. It is vulnerable at this stage, especially if your patient has had previous pelvic surgery that might have distorted its normal anatomic relations. Expose the lower uterine segment with retractors. Make a transverse curvilinear incision with its convexity downward in the vesicouterine fold of the visceral peritoneum for about 5 cm on each side of the midline. Then use sharp dissection under direct vision to separate the bladder from the uterus, taking special care to stay in the avascular space between posterior wall of the bladder dome and anterior wall of the uterus. Avoid cutting into the bladder wall, which is usually quite vascular. Insert a wide retractor to displace the bladder behind the symphysis pubis and out of the operative field and to expose the lower uterine segment.

Use a scalpel to make a 1–2 cm incision transversely across the midline of the lower segment down to the fetal membranes. If possible, avoid rupturing them until you are ready to deliver the fetus. Insert bandage scissors into the small opening and complete the lower segment hysterotomy, curving the incision upward at its lateral ends. In that way, if your incision should extend as the fetal head emerges, the tear will be less likely to extend laterally into the uterine vessels. Be very careful not to injure the fetus when you make the uterine incision.

Some obstetricians extend the initial incision in the lower segment by inserting the index finger of each hand in the midline opening and pulling the uterine wall apart laterally. This works well if the lower uterine segment has been considerably thinned by the labor process. While this technique obviates the risk of fetal injury from scissors, overzealous stretching can easily extend the incision into the broad ligament and the uterine vessels. Because of the potentially serious hemorrhagic risk from uncontrolled lateral digital force, using scissors is preferable to extend the transverse incision in the lower segment.

The abdominal wall and uterine incisions should be made large enough so you can deliver the fetal head without undue effort. Any limitations to the available space in a Pfannenstiel incision is mostly related to how completely you free the midline of the anterior fascia, described above, and your ability to retract the rectus abdominis muscles laterally. No matter how wide you make the transverse incision in skin and fascia, failure to free up under the anterior fascia vertically, both cephalad and caudad, may constrain the space needed to effect delivery of the fetus. If necessary, you can create more space by cutting through each rectus muscle belly transversely about halfway from the midline. Be sure to stop well short of the inferior epigastric vessel bundle, which is usually situated under the lateral half of the rectus muscle. The bleeding caused by cutting into these vessels will be considerable and difficult to control.

Inexperienced surgeons tend to make the uterine incision too small. Experience, if you learn from its lessons, readily demonstrates that doing so has substantive disadvantages. In addition to making the delivery difficult and exerting unnecessary compressive force on the fetal head, an inadequate incision increases the chance that uterine lacerations will occur during the struggle to effect delivery of the fetus.

After you have made the uterine incision, insinuate one hand inside the lower portion of the uterus with your palm facing the fetal head and your fingers directed toward the cervix. Remove all abdominal retractors, determine the position of the head, and then gently guide the occiput anteriorly into the uterine wound. Pull the head slowly and gently upward into the incision while you or your assistant applies transabdominal pressure on the uterine fundus. In this combined manner, you can deliver the head readily in most cases. You can facilitate delivery through the uterine incision if you keep the fetal head well flexed, hence the importance of knowing its position. If the head is in an OP position, flexion and rotation to OT—or better still, OA if that is possible—prior to extraction will ease the delivery. If rotation to OT or OA cannot be done easily, do not persist. Ensure the incision is large enough to accommodate the deflexed head and then deliver it in the OP position. Once the head is delivered, you will usually find it a simple matter to deliver the shoulders slowly one at a time, analogous to how they would be expected to emerge vaginally.

Occasionally, it will be necessary to use instruments, such as forceps or a vacuum extractor, to assist with delivery of the fetal head from the uterus. Sometimes, a single forceps blade, used as a *vectis*, can be helpful (Chapter 14). In that case, use the instrument to guide the head into the incision. Never use it as a lever or exert force against the head with it. To do so exposes the fetal head and maternal tissues to potential trauma.

If the head is deep and tightly wedged in the pelvis, transvaginal pressure on the fetal skull applied from below by an assistant can help to dislodge it. Deliver such pressure with great care, using the palm of the hand or the flat portions of your fingers to distribute force over as large an area of the skull as possible. Using fingertips alone to apply pressure concentrates a large force in a very small area and is, therefore, fraught with danger of traumatizing the skull and its contents. Verify that the individual applying the pressure is knowledgeable about this principle; if not, instruct him or her in advance to ensure against inflicting harm.

Rarely, you may find that delivery is impeded by a contracted uterus. In this situation, and indeed any other in which the fetal head is not readily delivered, it is important that you remain calm and resist the temptation to use excessive force to accomplish the delivery. Sometimes simply waiting for the contraction to abate will resolve the problem. If it does not, give a rapidly-acting tocolytic drug such as nitroglycerin after discussion with the anesthesiologist. A dose of 100–200 µg intravenously will usually suffice.

Once the baby is delivered, administer oxytocin intravenously at a rate of at least 50 mU/min to stimulate uterine contraction in the interest of accelerating the process of placental separation, and thus aiding in hemostasis. Meanwhile, either await placental separation, or use your hand to fully develop the plane between the placenta and the uterine wall, and then extract the placenta manually. Once you have removed the placenta, carefully examine the decidual surface of the uterus. If necessary, wipe it clean of any residual membranes using a laparotomy pad wrapped around your fingers. If the cervix had not dilated before the cesarean delivery, probe the cervical canal with a finger to ensure there will be adequate postoperative lochial drainage. Change your glove after this procedure if your finger has entered the vagina.

Repair the uterine wound with two layers of continuous absorbable suture, taking great pains to secure accurate apposition of the myometrium, especially at the angles of the uterine incision. It does not matter whether or not endometrium is included in the first layer of sutures. Lock the first layer suture to help with hemostasis. Use a continuous imbricating stitch for the second layer. Some prefer interrupted sutures for one or both layers because they provide additional assurance of hemostasis. When you have finished, there should be no visible portion of the cut edge of the uterine wall. Avoid doing a one-layer closure of the uterus. While it saves time, the resulting scar may be more likely to rupture in a subsequent pregnancy.

Before proceeding to close the abdominal wall, inspect and manually explore the abdominal cavity to be sure there is no occult abnormality. Exploration of the upper abdomen will necessarily be somewhat limited by the location of the incision, and, if neuraxial anesthesia is used, by patient discomfort. Nevertheless, if you minimize stretching of the peritoneum, you will usually be able to palpate structures in the upper abdomen and, if necessary, visualize them.

Use warm saline lavage to remove accumulated blood and amniotic fluid from the abdominal cavity. Then exchange the soiled towels you placed around the incision site at the beginning of the case with clean ones. Closing the visceral peritoneum of the bladder flap and the parietal peritoneum of the abdominal wall is optional. We suggest that you take the time to do so. This step may reduce adhesion formation between the anterior surface of the uterus and the abdominal wall. Such adhesions can be nettlesome problems in a subsequent cesarean delivery. Moreover, repairing the transversalis fascia is appropriate to restore the anatomic integrity of the abdominal wall. Close the anterior rectus fascia with a continuous suture of strong, nonabsorbable or delayed-absorbable synthetic suture. Place the sutures at least 1 cm from the wound edge and space them about 1 cm apart. Interrupted sutures are a reasonable alternative.

After the fascia has been closed, irrigate the subcutaneous tissue with warm saline. This removes tissue debris and blood clots, and reduces the bacterial count, lessening the chance of wound infection.

Suturing the subcutaneous layers (fasciae of Camper and Scarpa) is optional. The key is to avoid leaving dead space in this area, because that would encourage serum collections and bacterial growth. These layers should always be reapproximated in obese women. To get the best cosmetic result, close the skin with staples or, preferably, a continuous subcuticular suture. Apply adhesive strips to reduce tension on the skin edges during healing.

An abdominal incision in a morbidly obese woman presents special problems, particularly if she has a large pendulous abdominal panniculus. Transverse incisions in obese women confer lower risk of postoperative respiratory morbidity, wound infection and separation, and hernia formation, but they may take more time, be more difficult to accomplish, and provide less satisfactory exposure than vertical incisions. For cesarean delivery, we generally recommend a transverse approach, but this choice must be individualized depending on the situation and the woman's anatomy.

For a transverse incision in the lower abdomen of very obese patients you have the choice of locating it in the skin beneath the panniculus or above it. Making the incision below the heavy abdominal fat pad is generally easier, and we prefer it; however, it requires a means to retract the panniculus away from the operative field during the procedure. This can be accomplished in various ways. Taping it and anchoring the tape to the table usually works. Bear in mind, however, that retracting a large panniculus can compromise respiratory and cardiac function considerably. Both require careful monitoring. Also, special postoperative attention is required to keep the wound and surrounding skin clean and dry. Making the incision above the panniculus is acceptable, and is technically easier. It allows easier postoperative evaluation of the incision, and avoids the need for special attention to the skin beneath the panniculus. If you use this approach, plan carefully. The skin incision needs to be generous. Long instruments will be necessary. If you make the incision too high on the abdominal wall, exposure of the lower uterus may be challenging; if you make it too low you might find your incision emerge in the subpannicular fold on the posterior side of the pendulous portion of the abdominal wall skin, a discomfiting development.

## Classical incision

For a classical cesarean delivery, a midline abdominal wall incision from the level of the pubic symphysis to just below the umbilicus is ideal. After the

peritoneal cavity is open, examine the uterus to determine its axial rotation. The uterus is commonly dextrorotated; less often, it is levorotated.
Correct the rotation and make a midline longitudinal incision 11–12 cm
long through the thickness of the uterine wall down to the amniotic membranes. As with any cesarean incision, take time and care not to cut the
fetus, especially if the membranes have been previously ruptured.

It is common to encounter the placenta, which is frequently implanted
on the anterior surface of the uterine cavity. In such cases, it is best if
you dissect quickly with the flat of your hand along the cleavage plane
to the edge of the placenta, where you can puncture the membranes and
enter the amniotic sac. It is less preferable to cut through the placenta
because considerable fetal hemorrhage may result. In either case the procedure should be carried out expeditiously to minimize fetal blood loss
and hypoxia. If you know the location of the placenta from prior imaging, use this information to plan the location of the incision so as to avoid
the placenta, or at least to approach its edge rather than its center.

Once you have entered the amniotic cavity, insert your hand to identify
and grasp one foot or, preferably, both. Do a gentle breech extraction to
deliver the fetus through the uterine and abdominal wounds (Chapter 8).
Deliver the aftercoming head with care to avoid traction on the neck from
pulling on the body or the shoulders. Traction risks damage to the cervical spinal cord. This is especially important if the head is hyperextended,
as in a face presentation.

Close the classical incision with at least three layers of interrupted absorbable suture, carefully apposing the myometrium and closing all dead space.
The first row approximates the edges of the deep portion of the myometrium; the second closes dead space, apposes most of the remaining thickness of the uterine wall, and ensures hemostasis; and the third secures the
superficial myometrium and edges of the visceral peritoneum.

## Vertical lower uterine incision

This approach is similar to that of the transverse lower segment incision
already described, except for the direction of the incision. Create a peritoneal flap and separate the bladder from the uterus in the same manner,
using a transverse peritoneal incision. Here, however, the upper peritoneum requires considerably more dissection. Make an initial small incision vertically in the lower segment and extend it with bandage scissors
downward toward the bladder and upward to just short of the thick myometrium of the upper uterine segment. If your patient has been in labor
for some time, the lower segment will probably be stretched, thinned out,
and elongated so that it is sometimes possible to make the entire incision
in this region. Closure requires two layers of continuous sutures. Be careful during closure of the visceral peritoneum not to advance the bladder

too far up the uterine wall, as this can cause considerable difficulty in a subsequent cesarean delivery.

## The patient with a prior cesarean delivery

In the first half of the 20th century, most cesarean deliveries were done with the classical incision, and the rate of rupture in subsequent pregnancies, often associated with catastrophic bleeding, was unacceptably high. Moreover, blood bank technology was primitive by today's standards. The prevailing opinion that all women with a cesarean scar should be delivered by a planned repeat cesarean delivery prior to term was, therefore, quite reasonable. The more recent preference for the low segment transverse incision, which carries a much lower risk of rupture during a subsequent pregnancy, has made attempts at a later vaginal birth more acceptable. In addition, advances in medical and surgical care have dramatically improved our ability to manage uterine rupture and its serious consequences. The generally good results of labor and delivery in women with previous cesarean delivery leaves you and your patient with difficult choices in what is essentially a low-risk, high-stakes enterprise. That is to say, the frequency of complications during labor in a pregnancy with a low transverse cesarean scar is low, but the potential consequences of uterine rupture are great, and include maternal and fetal death in the worst instances.

There is much controversy concerning the management of patients who had a prior cesarean delivery (or other form of hysterotomy) and the advisability of allowing a trial of labor in subsequent pregnancies. This is obviously an issue of great consequence for your individual patient. It is also one with weighty public health importance, because the principal contributor to the burgeoning national cesarean rate is repeat cesarean delivery. Recent trends among obstetricians in the industrialized world have strongly favored repeat cesarean delivery over attempts at vaginal delivery.

The inclination to eschew trials of labor has been growing for several reasons. Obstetricians and patients have legitimate concerns about the risk of uterine rupture and its potentially catastrophic complications. Physicians' concerns about legal liability in the event of a uterine rupture have certainly played a role as well. The admonition that trials of labor should be permitted only in hospitals able to perform immediate emergency delivery and with the staff and expertise to deal expeditiously with severe hemorrhage has (understandably and appropriately) discouraged many physicians and institutions from allowing attempts at vaginal birth. An unfortunate consequence of this trend is that many women with a prior cesarean delivery who would readily accept the risks of a trial of labor are denied the option of doing so.

The advantages of a successful vaginal birth are evident. It involves less time in hospital, easier recuperation, and adds no risk to future pregnancies. For the baby, there is considerably less respiratory morbidity, and probably other advantages related to enhanced immune function.

Factors that reduce the probability of a successful trial of labor are listed in Box 11.2. The ideal candidate for successful vaginal birth would be a woman less than 40 years old who had one or two prior low transverse cesarean deliveries at term, and who enters spontaneous labor with a favorable cervix. It is of further benefit if she has had a previous vaginal delivery, and if the indication for her first cesarean delivery is no longer applicable in her current pregnancy. Such nonrecurring indications include conditions such as placenta previa, breech presentation, or severe preeclampsia.

You should generally encourage women with multiple conditions associated with reduced likelihood of success to have a repeat cesarean delivery. The rate of successful vaginal delivery after trials of labor in favorable candidates is quite good, about 70–80%. The risk of uterine rupture is at most between 0.5% and 1.0% in appropriately selected patients with prior low transverse incisions. The risk of rupture of a classical incision scar is much higher, variously reported as 4–9%.

---

**Box 11.2 Factors predisposing to a failed trial of labor after prior cesarean delivery**

- Prenatal factors
  - Multiple gestation
  - Maternal obesity
  - Prior dysfunctional labor
  - Prior fetal macrosomia
  - Unfavorable pelvic architecture
  - Uterine anomaly
  - More than two previous cesarean deliveries
  - Prior vertical uterine incision, especially classical incision
  - Prior uterine rupture
  - Prior inverted T- or J-shaped scar
  - Prior lateral extension of incision into uterine pedicle
- Intrapartum factors
  - Fetal macrosomia
  - Fetal malpresentation or malposition
  - Floating fetal head at labor onset in nullipara
  - Unripe cervix at labor onset
  - Gestational age >40 weeks
  - Induction or augmentation of labor
  - Abnormal cervical dilatation or fetal descent
  - Fetal malposition

There are distinct advantages to a planned repeat cesarean delivery. Among them are that the patient will have an empty stomach and, therefore, a lower anesthesia risk. Also, the risk of uterine rupture prior to a repeat cesarean delivery is very small. Nevertheless, it is important to remember that some uterine ruptures occur prior to labor, especially those associated with classical incisions, but sometimes with transverse uterine incisions as well. Some patients find a psychosocial advantage in the opportunity to plan the delivery date in advance, and in avoiding the pain of labor.

The disadvantages of repeat cesarean delivery, compared to a successful trial of labor, relate to the risk of iatrogenic prematurity if gestational age has been incorrectly calculated, higher cost, longer hospitalization and recuperation, and excess neonatal and maternal morbidity. In addition, there are morbidity and mortality risks that accrue to subsequent pregnancies, in addition to those relating to uterine rupture as just discussed. These risks occur in the form of more difficult surgery because of intraabdominal adhesions, placenta previa, and placenta accreta.

Scheduled repeat cesarean deliveries should not be done prior to 39 weeks of pregnancy in women with low transverse scars. Earlier cesarean delivery (at 36–37 weeks) is appropriate if your patient has a classical cesarean scar, because these rupture with greater frequency in late pregnancy prior to labor.

To obviate the chance of unintentional preterm delivery at a cesarean planned for 39 weeks of pregnancy, the American College of Obstetricians and Gynecologists has published clinical guidelines for minimizing the chance of inadvertent preterm birth (Box 11.3). If you feel you must deviate from these requirements, document the reasons thoroughly in your patient's record. Be sure you can objectively substantiate that the risks of proceeding to deliver prior to 39 weeks' gestational age exceed the risks of waiting until the fetus is more mature or labor begins spontaneously.

---

**Box 11.3 Fetal maturity requirements for a planned cesarean delivery**

Gestational age of at least 39 weeks should be documented by one or more of the following:

- Fetal ultrasonographic imaging at < 20 weeks was consistent with menstrual dates
- Fetal heart activity was first detected by Doppler ultrasound at least 36 weeks previously
- It has been at least 36 weeks since hCG was detected in the patient's urine or blood

(modified from ACOG Practice Bulletin Number 97, September 2008. Fetal lung maturity. American College of Obstetricians and Gynecologists, Washington, DC, 2008)

Biochemical confirmation of fetal lung maturity can be a valuable adjunct to this analysis when uncertainty exists about gestational age. We caution, however, against using lung maturity determinants as the sole indication that the fetus is ready for delivery. Organ maturation occurs at varying rates in different systems. The best evidence that a term fetus has reached optimal maturity and is ready for delivery is the onset of spontaneous labor. It may be best to await labor if you have doubts about fetal maturity.

### Determining who is a candidate for a trial of labor

An approach to determining whether your patient is an apt candidate for a trial of labor is presented in Fig. 11.1. In this context, an appropriate candidate is one whose risk of uterine rupture during labor is judged to be low, based on her obstetric history and on risk factors identified during prenatal care. A low risk is what would be expected in optimal circumstances, i.e., less than 1%.

Remember that risk assessment in these cases is not a static process. It should be updated whenever new information arises. For example, a woman who has a low risk based on her history and prenatal course might reconsider continuing a trial of labor (i.e., choose to have a cesarean delivery instead) if an arrest of dilatation occurs in the presence of a malposition and a large estimated fetal weight. Also, it is important to respect your patient's wishes. Your job is to be sure she understands the level and the nature of the risks she will incur. You may make a recommendation based on your best medical judgment, but she should be the arbiter of the decision about planned cesarean delivery versus a trial of labor. In that regard, we recommend you use a dedicated consent form for these cases. This helps provide specific risk information for your patient to review, serves to stimulate questions from her, and codifies the decision.

Many aspects of risk assessment in these situations remain unsettled. Data are limited, and few prospective trials exist, so we must make our best judgments based on the available data. We are uncertain, for example, about how the chance of uterine rupture changes with the number of prior cesarean deliveries. Most authorities feel comfortable allowing women with one or two previous cesarean deliveries to have a trial of labor. The risks with three or more previous cesarean deliveries are uncertain, but may very well be higher than with just one or two. If called for, judicious use of oxytocin during a trial of labor seems safe, but take care not to cause uterine hypercontractility. The presence of twins or of a macrosomic fetus, being postterm, or having diabetes mellitus may inflate the need for repeat cesarean delivery, but probably not the risk of uterine rupture.

## Managing the trial of labor

While safety of a trial of labor cannot be guaranteed, adopting a strategy of close surveillance and early intervention in the event of abnormal labor or suspicion of rupture of the scar can minimize risk. You and the hospital staff should be prepared to intervene promptly if uterine rupture is suspected. You should also be prepared to deal with a placenta accreta, because the presence of a uterine scar seems to predispose to both placenta previa and placenta accreta.

If all of your patient's prior deliveries were by cesarean, the progress of her trial of labor should be judged using criteria for nulliparas (Chapter 3). For unknown reasons, there is a higher frequency of arrest and protraction disorders in women laboring with a hysterotomy scar. Whether these disorders reflect the presence of cephalopelvic disproportion or a deficit in contractility because of the scarred uterus is unknown. Whatever the reason, it raises the question of whether it is safe to use oxytocin in patients with a uterine scar. Unfortunately, we do not have a definitive answer to that question.

Most of the studies in which the issue has been examined have not found increased risk but, intuitively, it seems that the more forceful the uterine contractility imposed on the scar, the greater would be the chance of it being pulled apart. The best approach is cautious conservatism.

Avoid labor induction in patients with a hysterotomy scar, unless there is a truly compelling reason to initiate labor. If you do induce labor, choose candidates who do not require extensive cervical ripening. Labor dysfunctions that would prompt oxytocin stimulation in other circumstances should preferably be resolved by repeat cesarean delivery when they occur in a gravida undergoing a trial of labor after a prior cesarean. If you choose to use oxytocin in a particular situation, use a low-dose infusion regimen and take precautions to prevent uterine hyperstimulation.

While it was once thought that the use of an epidural anesthetic would mask the symptoms of uterine rupture, considerable experience suggests that this is probably not the case. It is reasonable, therefore, to use epidural anesthesia if the patient desires it. Many lower segment scars separate without pain. Patients in whom pain is a significant symptom will usually feel it despite the analgesia. Often uterine rupture is associated with vaginal bleeding or abrupt changes in the fetal heart rate pattern, both of which are as useful and important to monitor as is pain.

Current evidence supports the safety of a trial of labor with a low transverse scar in twin and in postterm pregnancies. If the previous scar is unknown, a trial of labor is reasonable if you can infer from the situation that the previous cesarean delivery was done through a low transverse route. For example, a woman with a transverse skin scar in whom the cesarean delivery was done during labor at or near term in the developed

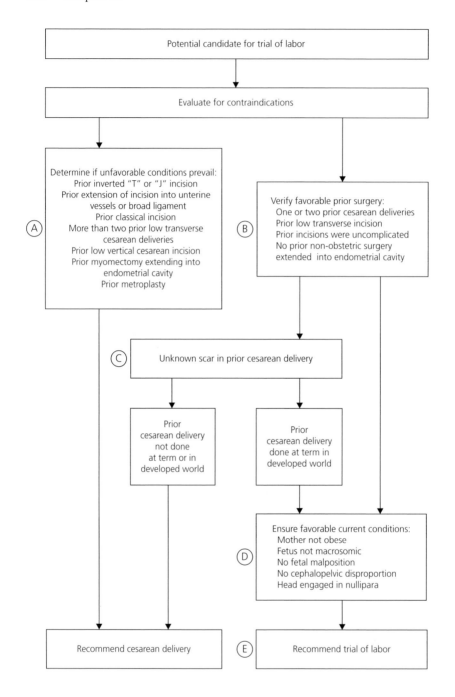

Potential candidate for trial of labor

Evaluate for contraindications

(A) Determine if unfavorable conditions prevail:
Prior inverted "T" or "J" incision
Prior extension of incision into unterine vessels or broad ligament
Prior classical incision
More than two prior low transverse cesarean deliveries
Prior low vertical cesarean incision
Prior myomectomy extending into endometrial cavity
Prior metroplasty

(B) Verify favorable prior surgery:
One or two prior cesarean deliveries
Prior low transverse incision
Prior incisions were uncomplicated
No prior non-obstetric surgery extended into endometrial cavity

(C) Unknown scar in prior cesarean delivery

Prior cesarean delivery not done at term or in developed world

Prior cesarean delivery done at term in developed world

(D) Ensure favorable current conditions:
Mother not obese
Fetus not macrosomic
No fetal malposition
No cephalopelvic disproportion
Head engaged in nullipara

Recommend cesarean delivery

(E) Recommend trial of labor

world is unlikely to have had a classical cesarean delivery. By contrast, if the patient has a vertical skin scar, and the procedure was done preterm, prior to labor, or in the developing world (where there may be limited access to trained obstetricians), she is more likely to have had a vertical uterine incision.

Women who had a previous cesarean delivery that required an inverted "T" or an extended "J-shaped" uterine incision, who had a uterine rupture in a previous pregnancy, or whose incision extended laterally into the uterine vessels should be counseled against a trial of labor. The same is true of those with prior transfundal surgery. Their risk of uterine rupture in a subsequent pregnancy is just too great to warrant a trial of labor.

Information about the safety of labor after a low vertical incision is scant. The risks probably lie between those of the low transverse and classical incisions. As noted above, low vertical incisions often include part of the uterine corpus. We counsel against a trial of labor in women with low vertical scars.

As a general guideline, we suggest you take a liberal approach to supporting trials of labor in women with a low transverse uterine scar. We emphasize, however, that these labors require close surveillance and cautious intervention (Fig. 11.2). As with any medical procedure, do not

**Figure 11.1** Selecting a candidate for a trial of labor.
**A**. To ensure that the gravida is a suitable candidate, first rule out any contraindications against labor. Evaluate the information available about the prior delivery to determine the nature of the incision. Be wary of a vertical incision or one in which healing is suspect because of an extension, either of which exposes the uterus to increased risk of rupture in a subsequent pregnancy. A history of more than two prior cesarean deliveries is also of concern, as is myomectomy or other uterine surgery extending full-thickness through the uterine wall. A trial of labor under these circumstances is not recommended.
**B**. If the prior incision is likely to withstand a trial of labor with minimal risk of rupture, continue your evaluation by next determining if current pregnancy conditions are favorable.
**C**. It is appropriate to consider trial of labor if the status of the prior incision is unknown, provided the earlier cesarean delivery was done at term in an industrialized nation because almost all cesareans in those areas are done through a low transverse incision.
**D**. Before making a final recommendation for a trial of labor review the current condition of mother and fetus to rule out any unfavorable issues that increase the risks. Among the most important of these are maternal obesity, fetal macrosomia and malposition, and cephalopelvic disproportion.
**E**. It is the patient who makes the ultimate decision about a trial of labor, but her decision must be based on a thorough understanding of the risks and benefits. Be sure to document the details of that informed consent interchange.

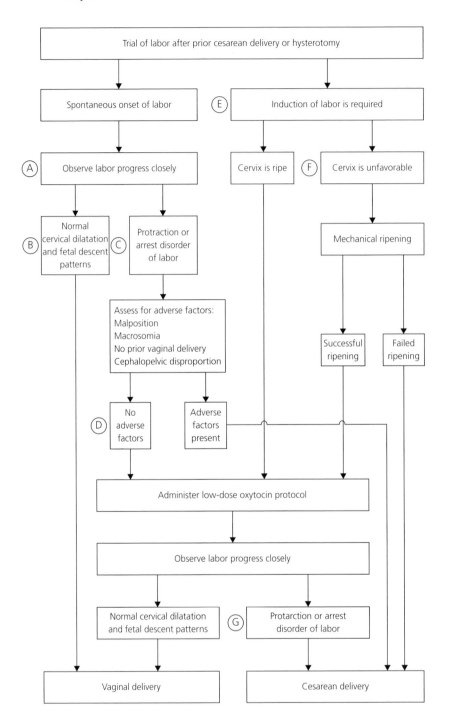

oversee a trial of labor in a woman who has had a prior cesarean delivery unless you feel confident in your ability to manage complications and have an available team of physicians and nurses skilled in responding to acute obstetric and surgical emergencies. Do not introduce any unnecessary risks. Be judicious about the use of oxytocin and circumspect about abiding very long labors. Provide and document comprehensive informed consent. Expect a good outcome, but always be prepared to deal with the worst.

## Patient-request cesarean delivery

A new expression has recently entered our lexicon: *patient-request cesarean*. It refers to cesarean delivery done purely on an elective basis, i.e., without any medical or obstetric indication. The patient often requests this, but some obstetricians now offer it as an option for delivery to women with a normal pregnancy. In some communities, elective cesarean delivery at term is becoming an increasingly common mode of delivery. In this regard, it is pertinent to wonder how much of this nascent trend is truly patient-driven, and how much the medical establishment has influenced patient demand in various ways.

The disturbing affinity for elective cesarean delivery has been fueled by several factors. These include women's fears that labor and vaginal delivery will cause pelvic floor damage, leading to sexual dysfunction or to incontinence later in life. Patients and physicians express concern that vaginal

**Figure 11.2** Management of a trial of labor.
**A**. Spontaneous labor at term is associated with a higher vaginal delivery rate than induced labor.
**B**. If labor progress is normal, and cephalopelvimetry is favorable, there is a high likelihood of safe vaginal delivery.
**C**. The presence of a dysfunctional labor pattern reduces the chance of success. If factors militate against a likely safe vaginal birth, it is generally best to opt for cesarean delivery. Examples of such factors include the discovery of unfavorable cephalopelvic relations, a malposition, or a large estimated fetal weight. If the mother is very obese or has never had a vaginal delivery, these factors also weigh against success.
**D**. More favorable extant conditions warrant continuing the labor trial. If the fetal position is normal, its weight not excessive, and cephalopelvimetry shows that sufficient space exists, allow labor to continue. For a protraction disorder, no oxytocin is generally necessary. For an arrest disorder, consider a low-dose oxytocin infusion.
**E**. Induction of labor is feasible for patients with a transverse uterine scar. Success is most likely if the cervix has already ripened. Use a low-dose oxytocin infusion.
**F**. If cervical ripening is necessary, do not use prostaglandins; rely instead on a balloon catheter.
**G**. If a protraction or arrest disorder is documented while the patient is receiving oxytocin, recommend cesarean delivery.

delivery is more likely to result in fetal birth injury or asphyxia. Many obstetricians believe they are far less likely to be sued if they perform a cesarean delivery than if they countenance labor and vaginal delivery. The latter is a correct generalization, but the situation will undoubtedly change as more cesarean deliveries are performed and more of their immediate and long-term complications occur.

Some (but not all) polls of women have shown that a substantial minority would prefer elective cesarean delivery to normal labor and vaginal delivery. To justify their preference, they cite the fears noted above about injury to themselves or to their fetus, and view labor as more painful and distressing than surgical delivery. Some women also value the social conveniences of choosing the delivery date of their child, and appreciate the control over the birth process that elective cesarean delivery affords them.

Many obstetricians have succumbed to the lure of elective cesarean delivery. It is more convenient for them, reduces sleep deprivation, mitigates the risk of legal accusations of negligence, and satisfies certain patients.

There is an important ethical facet of this issue you need to confront. Most of us are comfortable with respecting a patient's medical choices when she declines care we suggest. If, for example, we recommend a blood transfusion to a patient and she refuses it on religious grounds, we would respect her right to make this choice and do our best to manage her without transfusion. Our role would be passive acceptance of the patient's desire for autonomy. Responding to an affirmative patient request is, however, a different matter. Acquiescing to a woman's wish for medically unindicated surgery requires you to take an action you may not agree is appropriate.

Ethics committees of some organizations have concluded that patient-choice cesarean delivery is justifiable if it is viewed to be in the best interests of the woman's general health and welfare. You must decide where you stand on this contentious issue.

To be sure, there would be measurable benefits of a policy of universal elective cesarean delivery. It will reduce the frequency of birth trauma, fetal asphyxia, vertical transmission of several serious infections, and obviously, intrapartum fetal death. It might also eliminate the burden of pelvic floor dysfunction attributable to vaginal birth. At what cost, however, would these appealing advantages accrue?

Cesarean delivery, even under the ideal circumstances of a planned elective procedure, has risks that more than outweigh its presumed benefits. If the cesarean rate were to grow higher, maternal morbidity and mortality would increase due to anesthesia accidents, surgical misadventures, or other complications. The risk of severe postpartum hemorrhage, for example, is about ten-fold higher in cesarean delivery as compared to vaginal delivery. Cesarean delivery also confers substantially higher risk of postpartum endometritis and pneumonia. Furthermore, the harms of cesarean delivery continue into future pregnancies in the form of uterine rupture, placenta previa, and placenta accreta. For the baby delivered by elective cesarean delivery, there is a 10- to 30-fold higher incidence of respiratory morbidity. Recent data suggest that vaginal birth may provide babies with better early immune function and resistance to infection than cesarean delivery. It is not certain to what degree the prevalence of pelvic floor pathology will be affected by an increase in cesarean deliveries, because many genetic, behavioral, and medical factors other than delivery mode influence a woman's risk of incontinence (Chapter 9). Sound and attentive management of labor and delivery will serve to minimize risks of injury to the fetus and to the birth canal without the need to resort to major surgery of dubious value. In our view, the virtues of good obstetric care with selective cesarean delivery would trump the putative benefits of widespread elective cesarean delivery.

The matter of elective, or patient-choice, cesarean delivery is obviously a complex one. It has medical, economic, ethical, and social implications that we have only begun to unravel. Given the prevailing controversies and uncertainties swirling about this issue, how should you deal with it?

Begin by seriously considering the option of cesarean delivery without medical indication in the context of your own value system. Decide whether it is something that you are comfortable with medically and ethically. Once you have done so, you will be in the best position to discuss this issue with your patient. Do what you think is right in this regard, not what is most expedient. That approach will give you the most personal satisfaction and the least anxiety when you need to confront this issue in your office or clinic.

## Key points

- Reserve cesarean delivery for those patients in whom vaginal delivery cannot be accomplished without jeopardizing fetal or maternal life and health.
- The most common indications for cesarean delivery are previous cesarean delivery, dysfunctional labor or cephalopelvic disproportion, abnormal fetal heart rate patterns, and malpresentations.
- The most common abdominal incision for cesarean delivery is a Pfannenstiel incision. It can be done rapidly, causes minimal postoperative interference with respiratory function, resists dehiscence, and provides a good aesthetic appearance.

- Abdominal incision in a morbidly obese woman presents special problems, especially if she has a large abdominal panniculus. Generally, transverse incisions are preferable to vertical ones with regard to respiratory function and wound integrity.
- The advantages of the lower uterine segment incision over the classical uterine incision are reduced hemorrhage, easier repair, lower risk of subsequent rupture, and less postoperative adhesion formation.
- To assist with cesarean delivery of a head wedged deep in the pelvis, an assistant should use the palm or the flat portions of her fingers to dislodge the head by pressure applied transvaginally.
- Take a liberal approach to supporting trials of labor in women with a low transverse uterine scar. These labors require close surveillance and an available team of physicians and nurses skilled in responding to acute obstetric and surgical emergencies.
- The ideal candidate for successful vaginal birth after previous cesarean delivery is less than 40 years old, had one prior low transverse term cesarean delivery for a nonrecurring indication, enters spontaneous labor with a favorable cervix, and had a previous vaginal delivery.
- During a trial of labor after prior cesarean delivery be judicious about the use of oxytocin and avoid very long labors.
- The matter of elective, or patient-choice, cesarean delivery has complex medical, economic, ethical, and social implications. Decide whether it is something that you are comfortable with medically and ethically.

## Further Reading

### Books and reviews

ACOG Practice Bulletin Number 97, September 2008. Fetal lung maturity. American College of Obstetricians and Gynecologists, Washington, DC, 2008.

ACOG Practice Bulletin Number 115, August 2010. Vaginal birth after previous cesarean delivery. American College of Obstetricians and Gynecologists, Washington, DC, 2010.

Evaluation of cesarean delivery. American College of Obstetricians and Gynecologists, Washington, DC, 2000.

Guise JM, Denman MA, Emeis C, Marshall N, Walker M, Fu R, et al. Vaginal birth after cesarean: new insights on maternal and neonatal outcomes. Obstet Gynecol 2010; 115:1267–78.

Hawkins JL. Epidural analgesia for labor and delivery. N Engl J Med 2010;362: 1503–10.

Smith GCS. Delivery after caesarean section. In: Studd J, Tan SL, Chervenak FA (eds) *Progress in Obstetrics and Gynaecology*. Churchill Livingstone, Edinburgh 2006; 17:245–63.

Steer PJ, Modi N. Elective caesarean sections: risks to the infant. Lancet 2009;374: 675–6.

## Primary sources

Caughey AB, Shipp TD, Repke JT, Zelop CM, Cohen A, Lieberman E. Rate of uterine rupture in women with one or two prior cesarean deliveries. Am J Obstet Gynecol 1999;181:872–6.

Chazotte C, Cohen WR. Catastrophic complications of previous cesarean. Am J Obstet Gynecol 1990;163:738–42.

Chazotte C, Madden R, Cohen WR. Labor patterns in women with previous cesareans. Obstet Gynecol 1990;75:350–5.

Guise JM, Denman MA, Emeis C, Marshall N, Walker M, Fu R, et al. Vaginal birth after cesarean: new insights on maternal and neonatal outcomes. Obstet Gynecol 2010;115:1267–78.

Hansen AK, Wisborg K, Uldbjerg N, Henriksen TB. Cesarean delivery and respiratory morbidity in term infants. BMJ 2008;336:85–7.

Hershkowitz R, Fraser D, Mazor M, Lieberman JR. One or multiple cesarean sections are associated with similar increased frequency of placenta previa. Eur J Obstet Gynecol Reprod Biol 1995;62:185–8.

Lydon-Rochelle M, Holt VL, Easterling TR, Martin DP. Risk of uterine rupture during labor among women with a prior cesarean delivery. N Engl J Med 2001;345:3–8.

Macones GA, Peipert J, Nelson DB, Odibo A, Stevens EJ, Stamilio DM, et al. Maternal complications with vaginal birth after cesarean delivery: a multicenter study. Am J Obstet Gynecol 2005;193:1656–62.

Main EK. Reducing cesarean birth rates with data-driven quality improvement activities. Pediatrics 1999;103:374–83.

Nelson RL, Furner SE, Westercamp M, Farquhar C. Cesarean delivery for the prevention of anal incontinence. Cochrane Database Syst Rev 2010;2:CD006756.

Silver RM, Landon MB, Rouse DJ, Leveno KJ, Spong CY, Thom, EA, et al. Maternal morbidity associated with multiple repeat cesarean deliveries. Obstet Gynecol 2006;107:1226–32.

Socol ML, Peaceman AM. Vaginal birth after cesarean: an appraisal of fetal risk. Obstet Gynecol 1999;93:674–9.

Tita ATN, Landon MB, Spong CY, Lai Y, Leveno KJ, Varner MW, et al. Timing of elective repeat cesarean delivery at term and neonatal outcomes. N Engl J Med 2009;360:111–20.

Wang F, Shen X, Guo X, Peng Y, Gu X. Epidural analgesia in the latent phase of labor and the risk of cesarean delivery: a five-year randomized controlled trial. Anesthesiology 2009;111:871–80.

Wong CA, Scavone BM, Peaceman AM, McCarthy RJ, Sullivan JT, Diaz NT, et al. The risk of cesarean delivery with neuraxial analgesia given early versus late in labor. N Engl J Med 2005;352:655–65.

Zhang J, Yancey MK, Klebanoff MA, Schwarz J, Schweitzer D. Does epidural analgesia prolong labor and increase risk of cesarean delivery? A natural experiment. Am J Obstet Gynecol 2001;185:128–34.

# CHAPTER 12

# Delivering Twins

A pregnancy associated with more than one fetus is at increased risk of both maternal and fetal complications. The greater the number of fetuses, the higher the risk (Table 12.1). Multiple pregnancy is managed quite differently from singleton pregnancy, both in the antepartum course and during labor and delivery. Caring for the gravida with twins requires you to be alert to early diagnosis, knowledgeable about the problems that are likely to arise, and insightful in your role as healthcare provider who can act appropriately to reduce those risks.

The frequency of multiple pregnancies has risen considerably in recent decades (Table 12.2). This increase is the consequence of two principal factors: assisted reproductive technology and an aging population of gravidas. Women who choose to delay conception until an advanced age are more likely to have twins than those conceiving earlier (Table 12.3). The four-fold increase in twinning from the teen years to the mid-30s, and more than double again for conceptions in the late 40s, is probably due to rising levels of follicle-stimulating hormone in older women. Infertile women whose conceptions result from the implantation of several embryos or who are given agents that stimulate ovulation, such as clomiphene citrate or gonadotropins, are also likely to have twins or triplets or higher-order multifetal pregnancy.

**Table 12.1** Morbidity and mortality in multiple pregnancy as related to the number of fetuses

|  | Singletons | Twins | Triplets and higher |
| --- | --- | --- | --- |
| Infant death, per 1000 (first year) | 11.2 | 66.4 | 190.4 |
| Neonatal death, per 1000 (first month) | 7.8 | 55.9 | 168.8 |

*From Oleszczuk JJ, Oleszczuk AK, Keith LG. Twin and triplet birth: facts, figures, and costs. Female Patient 2003;28:11–16.

*Labor and Delivery Care: A Practical Guide*, First Edition. Wayne R. Cohen and Emanuel A. Friedman. © 2011 John Wiley & Sons, Ltd. Published 2011 by John Wiley & Sons, Ltd.

While the nuances of prenatal care are beyond the scope of this book, remember that antepartum considerations weigh heavily in the care required during labor and delivery. You should, therefore, be aware of the need for special attention to certain details of clinical investigation early in gestation that will help tailor management later in pregnancy. These include determining gestational age accurately, detecting twinning as early in the pregnancy as possible, and differentiating chorionicity, all of which are best done in the first or early second trimester. In addition, you must serially assess fetal growth (of both fetuses relative to gestational age) and growth discordance (of each fetus relative to its co-twin). The latter is an important indicator of presence of twin-twin transfusion syndrome (see below). Further, you have to be alert to identify the death of one sibling and the presence of congenital anomalies and conjoined twins. In the third trimester, look for subtle signs of approaching premature labor because it is an all-too-common complicating feature

**Table 12.2** Trends in multiple pregnancy over time

| Year | Twins | Triplets | Quadruplets | Quintuplets + |
|------|-------|----------|-------------|---------------|
| 2005 | 133,122 | 6,208 | 418 | 68 |
| 2003 | 128,665 | 7,110 | 468 | 85 |
| 2001 | 121,246 | 6,885 | 501 | 85 |
| 1999 | 114,307 | 6,742 | 512 | 67 |
| 1997 | 104,137 | 6,148 | 510 | 79 |
| 1995 | 96,736 | 4,551 | 365 | 57 |
| 1990 | 93,865 | 2,830 | 185 | 13 |

*From Martin JA, Hamilton BE, Sutton PD, Ventura SJ, et al. Births: final data for 2005. Nat Vital Stat Reports 2007;56:24–5.

**Table 12.3** Multiple pregnancy by maternal age

| Maternal age, y | All multiple births, per 1000 | Twins, per 1000 | Triplets +, per 1000 |
|-----------------|-------------------------------|-----------------|----------------------|
| Total | 33.8 | 32.2 | 1.6 |
| < 15 | 11.6 | 11.6 | — |
| 15–19 | 16.8 | 16.6 | 0.2 |
| 20–24 | 22.9 | 22.4 | 0.5 |
| 25–29 | 32.0 | 30.6 | 1.4 |
| 30–34 | 42.6 | 40.0 | 2.6 |
| 35–39 | 51.4 | 48.0 | 3.4 |
| 40–44 | 57.7 | 54.4 | 3.3 |
| 45+ | 215.6 | 197.2 | 18.4 |

*From Martin JA, Hamilton BE, Sutton PD, Ventura SJ, et al. Births: final data for 2005. Nat Vital Stat Reports 2007;56:24–5.

of multiple pregnancies. Preterm delivery often occurs spontaneously or is indicated on the basis of maternal or fetal complications.

## Maternal considerations

While most of the risk associated with multiple pregnancy is fetal, the mother is not free of hazard. Twinning affects the hemodynamic status of the gravida by increasing her blood volume an average of 20% over the 50% increase ordinarily encountered in singleton pregnancy; if she is carrying triplets, the increase is still greater. Anemia is quite common due to the great increase in plasma volume, and is often further compounded by iron deficiency. Decreasing colloid osmotic pressure predisposes to edema. While these effects are usually tolerated, congestive heart failure with pulmonary edema may result in women with concurrent heart disease or those given a beta-adrenergic agent as a tocolytic to try to stop premature labor.

Both gestational hypertension and pregnancy-induced hypertension are twice as likely to occur in women with twin pregnancy as those carrying a singleton fetus. Moreover, pregnancy-induced hypertension, when it develops in gravidas with multiple pregnancy, will probably arise earlier and be more severe. Further, the special variant of severe hypertensive disease, the HELLP syndrome (featuring hemolysis, liver dysfunction, and thrombocytopenia), is more common among women with twins, as is the sometimes fatal complication of acute fatty liver. This knowledge should serve to alert you to the need for careful evaluation of your patients with twins for early detection and prompt treatment of these conditions.

The risks of venous thromboembolic disease can be expected to be increased as well. Be alert for signs of this complication, and if your patient has other risk factors (bed rest, thrombophilia, obesity, etc.), prophylactic anticoagulant drugs should be considered.

Bed rest is commonly recommended routinely for women carrying multiple fetuses in the mistaken belief that it will help prolong the pregnancy and prevent preterm labor and delivery. Exposing the mother to the risk of thrombophlebitis cannot be condoned when the ostensible benefit of bed rest to the fetuses is not objectively verified.

Hydramnios is a common occurrence in twin pregnancies. Often arising without apparent reason in twins, it is sometimes the result of twin-twin transfusion syndrome. If the latter, it primarily serves as an indicator of diminishing fetal well-being. However, it can also contribute adversely to the gravida's condition. The uterus, already enlarged by the multiple fetuses, is further overdistended by the large volume of amniotic fluid. The huge uterus elevates the diaphragm, thereby compressing the lungs and restricting ventilatory excursion. At minimum, this makes the gravida quite uncomfortable; in due course, she may experience severe respiratory distress. In the latter instance, periodic amniocentesis to reduce uterine volume may offer temporary relief. Amnioreduction has to be done slowly to avoid placental abruption. Moreover, the amniotic fluid volume is usually rapidly restored, so symptoms return quickly. It may thus become necessary to interrupt the pregnancy prematurely in the interest of maternal well-being.

Hydramnios also aggravates supine hypotension. This condition, not unusual in singleton pregnancies, occurs more often, sooner, and with considerably greater intensity in multiple pregnancies. It is ordinarily encountered when the mother lies on her back. With a markedly over-distended uterus, however, it can even develop when the gravida is in a sitting or semi-sitting position or reclining on her side; if so, position change will not serve to correct it as it does effectively in singleton pregnancies.

Uterine overdistention by twins is commonly associated with uterine atony after delivery. This in turn causes potentially severe postpartum hemorrhage, sometimes resistant to uterotonic agents. Always be prepared to deal with uterine atony after a twin delivery.

## Fetal considerations

There are many intrauterine risks to being a twin. The risk of death of one or both twins is much higher than for singleton fetuses (Table 12.4). That risk begins soon after conception and continues throughout pregnancy and beyond. Survivors are also at risk of long-term morbidity. Twinning can be diagnosed reliably by ultrasonographic imaging quite early in pregnancy. Among cases diagnosed prior to 7 weeks' gestational age, one twin dies in 27%, a sequence called "vanishing twin." In another 9%, both twins die. Furthermore, among twins carried to viability, the overall neonatal mortality is more than 7–10 times higher than it is in singleton fetuses.

**Table 12.4** Effect of chorionicity on morbidity and mortality of co-twin after death of one twin*

|  | Monochorionic twins | Dichorionic twins |
| --- | --- | --- |
| Preterm birth, % | 68 | 57 |
| Death in utero, % | 12 | 4 |
| Neurodevelopmental defect, % | 18 | 1 |

*From Ong SS, Zamora J, Khan KS, Kilby MD. Prognosis for the co-twin following single-twin death: a systematic review. Br J Obstet Gynaecol 2006;113:992–8.

In higher-order multifetal pregnancies (triplets or more), the rate of neo-natal death is more than 20 times greater. Premature birth is the leading cause of perinatal death of twins, but other complications, as reviewed below, have deleterious impact as well.

## Prematurity

It is worth repeating that the major cause of mortality and morbidity for the fetuses in multiple gestation is premature birth. Pregnancy duration averages 39 weeks with a singleton fetus, but only 35 weeks with twins, 32 weeks with triplets, and 29 weeks with quadruplets or more (Table 12.5). Nearly two-thirds of twins deliver before 37 weeks' gestational age, and one in five are born prior to 32 weeks. Thus far, nothing in our obstetric armamentarium seems able to improve this situation for the fetuses in multiple pregnancy.

## Malpresentations

Fetal malpresentations of twins are commonplace, occurring in 13% of first twins and 58% of second twins (Table 12.6). When malpresenta-tions occur in singleton gestations, they are difficult enough to manage

**Table 12.5** Prematurity and low birth weights in multiple pregnancy by number of fetuses

|  | Singletons | Twins | Triplets | Quadruplets | Quintuplets + |
|---|---|---|---|---|---|
| Gestational age, wk | 38.7 | 35.2 | 32.0 | 29.3 | 29.4 |
| Birth weight, g | 3298 | 2323 | 1655 | 1225 | 1147 |
| Preterm < 37 wk, % | 11.1 | 60.4 | 92.6 | 94.9 | 89.6 |
| Very preterm < 32 wk, % | 1.0 | 12.1 | 36.3 | 79.2 | 79.1 |
| Low birth weight, < 2500 g, % | 6.5 | 57.5 | 95.4 | 98.0 | 95.5 |
| Very low birth weight, < 1500 g, % | 1.1 | 10.2 | 34.8 | 73.4 | 84.8 |

*From Martin JA, Hamilton BE, Sutton PD, Ventura SJ, et al. Births: final data for 2005. Nat Vital Stat Reports 2007;56:24–5.

**Table 12.6** Fetal presentations in first and second twins

| Presentation of fetuses (First-Second) | Frequency, % |
|---|---|
| Cephalic-Cephalic | 42 |
| Cephalic-Breech | 27 |
| Cephalic-Transverse | 18 |
| Breech-Breech | 5 |
| Other combinations | 8 |

*From Divon MY, Marin MJ, Pollack RN, Katz NT, et al. Twin gestation: fetal presentation as a function of gestational age. Am J Obstet Gynecol 1993;168:1500–2.

(Chapter 8). When they occur in multiple pregnancies, those difficulties are magnified. As a consequence, clinical management of their labor is often resolved by resorting reflexively to cesarean delivery whenever a malpresentation is discovered, suspected, or even just possible, i.e., when conditions are such that a malpresentation is likely to develop.

This kind of oversimplification of decision making is usually inappropriate because it violates the general principle that requires you to individualize the care of every patient according to her specific needs. However, it can frequently be justified in the management of twins by the fact that the risks associated with their cesarean delivery may be less than the risks of failing to diagnose a fetal malpresentation or, worse still, of managing it imperfectly. Moreover, it is increasingly probable that healthcare providers will have less and less opportunity to acquire the special expertise needed for the management of the problem. This is the very same trend as the diminishing experience and level of skill among practitioners called upon to provide the care necessary to effect safe vaginal delivery of the singleton fetus in breech presentation.

Cephalic presentation is encountered among most first twins, but about half of them are associated with malpresentation in the second twin. In deciding how to deliver a first twin with a malpresentation, the answer is essentially the same as it is for singleton fetuses in malpresentation. There is no argument with regard to transverse or oblique lie, which require cesarean delivery if they occur in a first twin.

For managing breech presentation of the first twin, you have two options. If you ordinarily do cesarean delivery of all singleton fetuses with a breech presentation, a common practice today, it should logically follow that you apply the same policy to the management of the malpresentation in first twins. There is thus ample justification for you to undertake cesarean delivery for both transverse lie and breech presentation. This is particularly so if you do not have the experience, knowledge, and skill to manage them safely or cannot secure the services of someone who does. The alternative of allowing labor and vaginal breech delivery is applicable provided such expertise is available and the fully-informed patient agrees.

The same simple solution of routine cesarean delivery, however, does not apply to the remaining large majority of cases in which the first twin is cephalic in presentation. Nearly all of these fetuses, if allowed to proceed to labor and vaginal delivery, will have a good outcome. Indeed, the results are essentially the same as for singleton fetuses with cephalic presentation, compared on a weight-for-weight basis. In theory then, the decision to allow labor and vaginal delivery of most first twins ought to be straightforward. However, it is not. The reason reflects the fact that second twins are frequently found with a malpresentation.

As noted above, many cases in which the first twin is in cephalic presentation will have the second twin in either longitudinal lie as a breech or a transverse lie. These lies are often unstable, i.e., the second fetus will not necessarily remain in its original orientation during the labor or following the birth of the first twin. Considerable instability, with great likelihood that the presentation will change, occurs if the twins are small, the amount of amniotic fluid is relatively great, and the patient's parity is high. It may change to a favorable cephalic presentation, but it is much more likely that the malpresentation of the second twin will persist or worsen (i.e., a breech presentation may spontaneously convert to a transverse lie). If it persists, the choices for managing the second twin are either cesarean delivery or some form of difficult and potentially hazardous procedure leading to vaginal delivery. These latter options include breech extraction, internal podalic version to breech presentation followed by breech extraction, or external cephalic version to cephalic presentation (Chapter 8) followed by additional labor and vaginal vertex delivery . Undertaking any of them demands competence based on experience—and even in experienced hands, the risks are high. In addition to maternal and fetal trauma from these procedures, cord prolapse and abruptio placentae may further complicate them.

If the second twin is known to be in malpresentation, therefore, allowing the first twin to deliver vaginally would unnecessarily place the second fetus at risk. Moreover, it would simultaneously expose the mother first to a labor and a vaginal delivery for the leading twin, and then to a cesarean delivery for the second. It follows logically that cesarean delivery is acceptable for twin pregnancies in which the second twin is in malpresentation, regardless of the presentation of the first twin. The alternative of allowing the first twin to deliver vaginally is only appropriate if skilled personnel are available to manage the anticipated malpresentation of the second twin and the gravida is fully informed about the risks, understands them, and accepts them.

This sequence of combined vaginal and cesarean delivery may not always be avoidable. It might occur, for example, when the second twin is in cephalic presentation early in labor, but then changes its presentation to breech or transverse lie when its co-twin delivers. This happens in about 10% of such cases. That frequency is high enough to question the wisdom of allowing any first twin to deliver vaginally, even if it and its co-twin are in a favorable cephalic presentation. Indeed, some have suggested that the only safe option is to undertake cesarean delivery for all twins, just as it is essentially the de facto standard of practice to do so for all higher-order multiple pregnancies (triplets and higher) these days. While this approach to twins is becoming more widespread, the cogent argument against it focuses on the good outcome results reported with series of such cases allowed to labor and deliver vaginally. We contend that the choice rests with the individual healthcare provider, evaluating her own skills and experience, and with the well-informed patient who must decide what is in the best interests of her fetus and herself.

## Growth restriction

In addition to the prematurity that so often affects twin fetuses, they are also often growth restricted. Fetal growth restriction in twins not only occurs more frequently than in singletons, but it tends to be more severe when it occurs and to carry a greater risk of untoward outcome. With higher order of multiple fetuses, the incidence of growth restriction is greatly increased and its impact is even worse. Growth restriction in which both twins are about equally affected—i.e., without discernible weight discordance—is encountered in association with a range of maternal conditions that adversely affect placental function, but is found in multiple pregnancy even in the absence of evident maternal or fetal disease.

## Weight discordance

A more threatening finding than either prematurity or equivalent growth restriction in multiple pregnancy is disparate fetal weights (Table 12.7). This can occur if one fetus has a major anomaly or infection, if twin-twin transfusion occurs, or sometimes for no discernible reason. Diagnosis of a lethal fetal anomaly as the cause of growth discordance is essential because intervening aggressively to try to salvage that fetus, often a fruitless effort, may jeopardize the well-being of its normal co-twin. Your choice of delivery route may also be affected.

A clinically important cause of growth discrepancy, results from *twin-twin transfusion syndrome*, a condition in which there is a vascular anastomosis between the two fetal circulations. These anastomoses are found almost exclusively in the shared placenta in monochorionic fetuses.

**Table 12.7** Neonatal outcome for twins by degree of growth discordance

| Degree of discordance, % | Neonatal mortality, per 1000 |
| --- | --- |
| None | 3.8 |
| 15–19 | 5.6 |
| 20–24 | 8.5 |
| 25–29 | 18.4 |
| 30+ | 43.4 |

*From Leduc L, Takser L, Rinfret D. Persistence of adverse obstetric and neonatal outcomes in monochorionic twins after exclusion of disorders unique to monochorionic placentation. Am J Obstet Gynecol 2005;193:1670–5.

Where they occur, placental vascular connections can be artery to artery, vein to vein, or artery to vein. It is important to diagnose chorionicity early in pregnancy to flag those twin cases that have to be followed especially carefully. Serial imaging for estimating the weight of both fetuses will permit you to detect weight discordance as early as possible.

At first, growth discrepancy is the only manifestation that can be detected by imaging. As the condition progresses in severity, oligohydramnios becomes apparent in the amniotic sac of the smaller or donor fetus (if there are two sacs). Eventually, if the process is allowed to progress without correction or interruption, anhydramnios in the donor twin makes it appear on imaging to be tightly apposed to the uterine wall, giving rise to the term *stuck twin*.

## Chorionicity

Twins develop either from two ova (*dizygotic*), each of which is fertilized separately, or from a single ovum (*monozygotic*) that divides after fertilization. About two-thirds of twins are dizygotic. Each dizygotic twin has its own placenta (although they may fuse) and its own amniotic sac. Each amniotic sac is surrounded by an outer chorion, and the gestation is designated *diamniotic dichorionic* (DADC). Monozygotic twins, by contrast, can have a number of different configurations, depending on when the ovum divides after fertilization. If the single fertilized egg divides within 3 days of fertilization, both fetuses will occupy separate sacs in the same DADC arrangement as dizygotic twins, and will be clinically indistinguishable from them. If the split occurs between 4 and 8 days, the twins will occupy separate amniotic sacs, with one chorion around both sacs, and no chorion in the septum between them, called *diamniotic monochorionic* (DAMC). After 8 days, both twins will occupy the same amniotic sac with chorion enveloping it, forming a *monoamniotic monochorionic* pattern (MAMC). On rare occasions and for unknown reasons, the division will be delayed more than 13 days; if this occurs, the embryo will not divide completely, resulting in conjoined twins.

This important information is relevant to your management of twin delivery. MAMC gestations stand at the high-risk end of the fetal risk spectrum. At the other end, DADC twins do best, regardless of whether they are monozygotic or dizygotic, although not quite as well as singletons of equivalent gestational age. We have already alluded to the twin-twin transfusion syndrome, which develops almost exclusively in monochorionic twins by virtue of their shared placenta and frequent vascular anastomoses. In addition, monoamniotic twins are at markedly increased risk from cord entanglement because they occupy the same sac. One-quarter of them suffer intrauterine death, usually without forewarning. The frequency of congenital anomalies is also increased among monozygotic twins, as is preterm delivery. Diagnosis of chorionicity is ideally made by ultrasonographic imaging early in gestation.

When you need to make decisions about delivery, the process is easier if the twins have been kept under close serial surveillance during pregnancy. You will thus be aware of the chorionicity and be certain of the gestational age. You will know about the presence of fetal structural anomalies as well as growth restriction of both twins and discordance of relative growth between them.

### Death of one twin

As noted earlier, it is not unusual for one twin to "vanish" over the course of pregnancy, particularly early on. When this occurs in the first half of pregnancy, it is almost always clinically silent, i.e., with no discernible impact on either the mother or the surviving co-twin.

Death of a twin in late pregnancy, however, may constitute a hazard not only for the mother, but for the surviving fetus as well. Death of one twin is especially perilous in monochorionic gestations, when the surviving fetus may be at severe and immediate risk. The mortality risk for the surviving twin is considerably elevated, and this fact will influence decisions about when it should be delivered.

### Conjoined twins

Rarely, in monoamniotic twins, there is failure of the fertilized ovum to split completely. This phenomenon causes conjoined twins in one of several forms. It is beyond our scope in this book to delve into this subject in depth, but suffice to say the most critical aspect relating to delivery is the need to diagnose the condition in a timely manner. You need to determine the type of conjoining that exists, assess for other structural abnormalities, and advise the patient of her options for the management of the pregnancy and the newborns. No one has a great deal of experience with these rare disorders, but consulting with other healthcare providers who are knowledgeable about these matters is essential.

In almost all instances of conjoined twins, cesarean delivery will be needed. It can be done on a scheduled basis after the twins are sufficiently mature to do reasonably well on their own. The delivery should be carried out at a specially-equipped facility where expert personnel are at hand. That team is needed to ensure the twins are optimally prepared and managed after they are delivered in preparation for the complex neonatal care and surgery that may be contemplated.

### Higher-order multifetal pregnancy

We noted earlier that the frequency of twins has increased over time. In the same period, higher-order multifetal pregnancies (triplets, quadruplets, etc.) have also increased, but at an even more accelerated rate. The impetus seems to be largely the result of assisted reproductive technology applied to aiding conception. Despite the newsworthy reports of survivals among such rarities as septuplets and octuplets, the reality is that high-order multiple pregnancy puts mother and fetuses at very serious risk of prenatal, intrapartum, neonatal, and life-long problems.

Your primary objective with regard to high-order multifetal pregnancy is to diagnose it early and then serially evaluate for the development of adverse features. These pregnancies almost always begin labor prematurely, and their labor is often complicated by disordered progression patterns, fetal malpresentations and cord or placental accidents. Therefore, if gestational duration reaches 34–36 weeks or so, cesarean delivery is generally considered acceptable as a safer option. If labor begins sooner, and is not amenable to suspension with tocolytics, cesarean is also indicated. These pregnancies should be delivered in a facility that can readily mobilize the full panoply of facilities and staff that will be needed to deal with the mother's needs and those of several preterm neonates.

## Managing the labor and delivery

Three important aspects of decision making as it pertains to the delivery of multiple pregnancy have to be tailored for each case. First is to designate where a gravida with twins will deliver. Second, you have to decide when to undertake delivery. Third, you have to ascertain how to deliver the fetuses. Needless to say, the latter two issues are not completely independent of each other. Choosing the route of delivery, for example, rests in large measure on the timing because preterm intervention is almost always constrained by conditions that are unfavorable for successful labor and vaginal delivery. We have tried to provide a helpful guide in the form of a decision-making algorithm to reduce the complexity of the problem by addressing each of the issues in turn (Fig. 12.1). The process encompasses decisions you have to make during the prenatal course as well as those relating to timing and route of delivery.

### Where to deliver

As to choosing where to deliver, let us consider the alternatives. In general, twin pregnancies should be delivered in a well-equipped and staffed hospital setting. Serious complications can arise with lightning speed, so the delivery unit should have the advantages of skilled personnel for detecting and responding rapidly to complications of labor and delivery. Obstetricians, anesthesiologists, neonatologists, and nurses should be in constant attendance, and an available team for emergency operative intervention available around the clock. A sophisticated neonatal intensive care unit is important as well. Further, given the high risk of postpartum hemorrhage, the full-time services of a blood bank are essential. It is even more important to have this extensive staffing and these facilities available for monochorionic twins (and still more so for higher-order multifetal pregnancy) because they are afflicted with more frequent and more severe complications. Obviously, the more premature the gestation, the greater the need will be for an array of sophisticated services.

## When to deliver

As to the second consideration, choosing the time to intervene (if at all), you may not have any option if the patient begins labor spontaneously. This happens often in these cases. If the pregnancy is very preterm and the status of mother and fetuses does not yet warrant delivery, the use of a tocolytic agent to attempt to stop the labor is certainly acceptable. Although seldom actually successful in stopping the labor for any great length of time in twin gestation, and even less so in higher-order multiple pregnancy, it may provide a short window of opportunity for treating with corticosteroids to enhance fetal lung maturity. Bear in mind, however, that the combination of enhanced blood volume in twin pregnancy and the administration of both a tocolytic agent and a corticosteroid is not without risk because it may precipitate pulmonary edema in the mother. You must be watchful for early signs of this serious complication and be ready to manage it.

If labor does not begin on its own, then timing the intervention for induction or cesarean delivery will depend on prevailing conditions. For high-order multiples, we have already addressed the preference for proceeding with cesarean delivery when the fetuses are approaching maturity. Because the labor in these cases is almost always complicated, operative intervention without waiting for the onset of labor is warranted. Sometimes, amniotic fluid evaluation to assess pulmonary maturation of one or more fetuses is performed. As we have emphasized a number of times before, from the fetal perspective, your guiding principle should be to choose a time when the fetal risks of remaining in utero exceed the risks of being born prematurely.

For twins, choosing when to intervene is a bit more nuanced than for higher-order multiples. Dizygotic twins tend to do rather well in the course of gestation unless some complicating feature develops, such as maternal pregnancy-induced hypertension or acute hydramnios. There is some controversy over the best time to deliver dizygotic twins if labor does not begin prior to term. There are those who advocate allowing them to enter spontaneous labor, even at term or beyond, and others who recommend elective intervention after 38 completed weeks of gestation. The argument

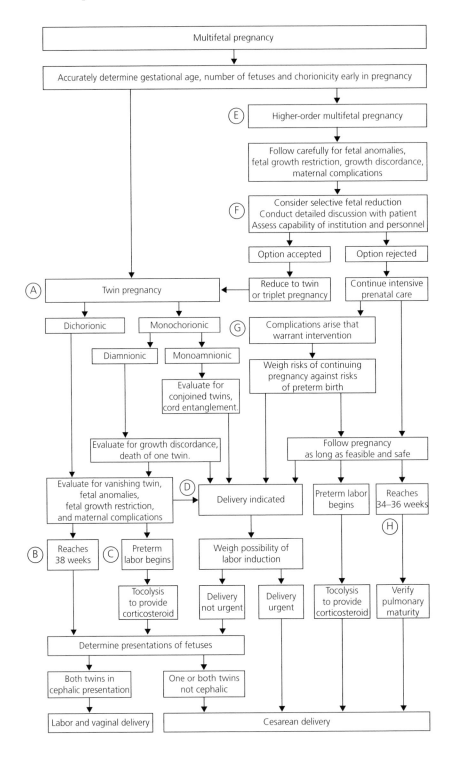

for allowing labor to begin on its own is that it ensures maximum fetal maturation; the counterarguments are that delay exposes the fetuses to risks the longer they remain in utero and to whatever risks may accrue as the consequence of the gravida being admitted for labor care at night or on the weekend when staffing and services may not be adequately prepared for emergencies that could arise. The argument for intervening electively is that it avoids those hazards; but that concern is countered by the

**Figure 12.1** Algorithm for managing multiple pregnancy.

**A**. Having diagnosed twin pregnancy early in gestation, determine accurate gestational age and chorionicity to help guide management. Twins with low-risk dichorionic placentation can be managed expectantly as for singleton pregnancies, unless adverse maternal or fetal conditions arise. Because monochorionic twins are at considerable risk for a number of potentially serious conditions, they have to be much more closely monitored.

**B**. If a gravida with uncomplicated dichorionic twins reaches 38 completed weeks of gestation, delivery can be considered. If both fetuses are cephalic, labor can either be allowed to begin spontaneously or induced if cervical conditions are favorable. If either presentation is not cephalic, consider cesarean delivery instead, particularly if you practice elective cesarean delivery for the singleton fetus in breech presentation.

**C**. If labor begins spontaneously before term in a twin pregnancy and no complication warrants urgent delivery, administer a tocolytic agent to provide time for corticosteroids to help accelerate fetal maturity. If the tocolytic agent fails to stop the labor, which is likely in twins, choose vaginal delivery if the fetuses are both cephalic or cesarean delivery if either is not.

**D**. When the risks of a developing complication threaten the well-being of the mother or the fetuses, and those risks exceed the risks of continuing the pregnancy, delivery is indicated. If the situation is truly urgent, proceed with cesarean; if not, consider labor induction.

**E**. A high-order multifetal pregnancy, including triplets or more, exposes mother and fetuses to great risk. They need specialized antepartum, intrapartum and postnatal care with back-up of knowledgeable, experienced personnel in fully-equipped facilities. Careful, detailed periodic assessments for developing complications are essential.

**F**. Selective reduction of the number of fetuses to twins (or less preferably, triplets) should be considered to help improve outcome for the mother and the remaining fetuses. If reduction is acceptable and can be safely achieved, further care will be the same as for a twin pregnancy.

**G**. Complications are quite likely to develop in the antepartum course of high-order multifetal pregnancy before fetal maturity can be guaranteed. Those complications often require delivery with varying degrees of urgency. It is sometimes possible to delay delivery until the fetuses are more mature. If delay is possible, it is worthwhile in the interest of fetal well-being, until such time as the risks of remaining in utero exceed those of premature birth.

**H**. Given the great likelihood of complications during labor in high-order multifetal pregnancy, such as unanticipated fetal malpresentation, cesarean delivery is almost always appropriate for them. If they reach 34–36 weeks of gestation without a complication demanding intervention and labor has not yet begun, assess pulmonary maturity periodically. Undertake cesarean delivery as soon as fetal maturity is verified.

possibility that the fetuses will be immature because of dating errors. We recommend the latter approach in the interest of providing orderly planning and care by the people who know the patient and her problems best, are most able to detect problems as they arise and deal with them expeditiously, and do it at a time when all needed facilities will be at hand.

We suggest the following approach for timing the delivery of dizygotic twins if the dating of the pregnancy duration is reasonably certain (or, if dates are unsure, pulmonary maturation can be assured by amniotic fluid evaluation) and labor does not begin spontaneously: Intervene at 38 completed weeks of gestational age, but no later than 40 weeks. This assumes that the pregnancy has been uneventful and fetal growth and oxygenation are deemed normal. Undertaking measures to induce labor or proceed with cesarean delivery prior to 38 weeks risks delivering twins who are not sufficiently mature to do well after they are born. Contrary to older beliefs that delivery as early as 34 weeks was acceptable in such cases, recent objective studies have shown that even singleton fetuses delivered near term, but not yet at term, experience increased morbidity and mortality. Given the greater vulnerability of twins by virtue of their smaller size and greater immaturity relative to singletons of the same gestational age, the results of these investigations provide strong support for waiting at least until 38 weeks, if possible, before intervening electively to deliver otherwise healthy dizygotic twins with no complications. Obviously, if complications develop before 38 weeks, they may require earlier delivery, depending on their severity and on how immature the fetuses are at the time.

Because monozygotic twins usually enter labor earlier and are more likely to be threatened by complicating factors requiring early intervention, there is seldom any need for you to have to decide about elective intervention to deliver or when to intervene. If monozygotic twins are in separate sacs (DAMC and DADC) and develop well and remain healthy in utero, you can manage them in the very same way as dizygotic twins, specifically by elective delivery at or after 38 completed weeks. Monoamniotic twins, however, deserve special consideration because they remain at high risk of cord entanglement and intrauterine death without forewarning until they deliver. Therefore, they may benefit from earlier elective intervention, especially if cord entanglement has been demonstrated by Doppler flow studies. For those few without complications, a reasonable compromise between delivering them too soon and waiting too long is to aim for delivery at about 34–36 weeks of gestation.

## How to deliver

Once you have made a thoughtful decision about when to deliver based on logical considerations of the best interests of your patient and her fetuses, your options for delivery should be transparent. They flow logically from a consideration of factors such as the gestational age, the number of fetuses, their presentations, the cervical characteristics, and how urgent it is to effect delivery. Urgency to deliver, if truly based on an immediate and serious threat to maternal or fetal life or well-being, surely trumps all other considerations. Yet even that overarching concern needs some modification insofar as choosing the delivery method, especially with respect to gestational age (e.g., if the fetuses are previable) and the condition of maternal soft tissues (e.g., if unfavorable for induction).

Gestational age dictates delivery mode when the fetuses are either previable or viable but very preterm. For example, if labor begins before the fetuses are viable with almost no chance of surviving, say prior to 23 weeks' gestational age, and you cannot stop the labor by tocolytic agents, cesarean delivery would certainly be inappropriate. To deliver fetuses by major surgery without any hope of salvaging them just exposes the mother to surgical and anesthetic risks without gain, unless there is a maternal indication to justify it. For fetuses that are very small, but considered viable, say between 24 and 28 weeks of gestation, it has long been felt that cesarean delivery is warranted to counter the risk of intracranial hemorrhage from the ostensibly traumatic forces of vaginal delivery. While this risk seems intuitively reasonable, there is little objective evidence to support it. Whether it is true or not, however, is immaterial given the need to effect cesarean delivery in this group for a better reason, namely, to avoid the common risk of fetal malpresentation. Since the condition of the cervix is usually unfavorable for induction, that constitutes yet another reason for proceeding with cesarean.

In high-order multifetal pregnancies, regardless of gestational age, fetal malpresentation is a commonly encountered risk, as noted above. To compound the problem, these malpresentations may not exist before labor, but often develop unpredictably during labor. The rapidly changing spatial relationships that can occur among multiple fetuses at any time means that malpresentations are thus likely to arise suddenly, often as an antecedent fetus is being delivered vaginally, perhaps in association with cord prolapse or placental abruption. These complications, alone or in combination, will necessitate emergency cesarean delivery, often under suboptimal conditions. Since it is clear from this that labor in these cases is an unsafe option, you should not consider allowing gravidas with high-order multifetal pregnancy to labor. Proceed instead directly to cesarean delivery when it is clear they must be delivered.

Vaginal delivery is usually an acceptable option in twin pregnancies at or near term, particularly when both fetuses are in cephalic presentation.

Some contend the time has come to adopt a policy of cesarean delivery for all multiple pregnancies. They base their argument on the greater risk accruing to second twins in the course of labor than first twins (from cord prolapse, abruptio placentae, and malpresentation), a fact not in dispute, and that those risks can be avoided by cesarean delivery before labor near term. Clinical evidence, however, does not support this view. We recommend vaginal delivery, therefore, when conditions permit and the delivery can be done safely.

Another contentious issue for twin delivery is how to proceed when the first twin is in breech presentation. Here, if the second twin is in cephalic or breech presentation, and you practice breech vaginal delivery for singleton pregnancies, then vaginal delivery is an appropriate consideration. If you would not consider a vaginal delivery for a singleton fetus in breech presentation, it follows that cesarean delivery for this condition in twins is in order.

When delivery of twins is urgent and vaginal delivery is being considered, choosing between vaginal and cesarean delivery will depend on the degree of urgency and the status of maternal soft tissues. We have already discussed the criteria for determining when induction of labor for singleton pregnancy is likely to be successful, in the form of the Bishop score (Chapter 10). These criteria also apply for twins. Similarly, if there are contraindications against vaginal delivery, it would be inappropriate to contemplate that route for any delivery, let alone an urgent one. In cases in which safe vaginal delivery is feasible, several alternative scenarios are possible. At one extreme, if there is great urgency and the cervix is unfavorable (Bishop score 4 or less), prudency dictates a cesarean delivery. At the other, if urgency is less pressing and the cervix is favorable for induction (Bishop score 9 or more), a trial of labor is called for, and is likely to lead to a short labor and safe, successful vaginal delivery. In between, you have the option of attempting to make the cervix more favorable by priming it pharmacologically (Chapter 10) to induce labor or to facilitate a subsequent labor induction. Once labor is under way, you can expect vaginal delivery to occur in due time. If cervical ripening fails, do not persist, but proceed forthwith to cesarean delivery lest the condition for which the induction was first undertaken gets out of hand, i.e., becomes serious enough to constitute a hazard to mother and fetuses.

The conduct of labor for gravidas with twins is somewhat different from the routine activities in singleton labors. Simultaneous electronic monitoring is necessary for both fetuses, and ultrasonographic imaging is needed to verify the fetal presentations initially, and again after the first twin is delivered. Imaging should supplement prompt vaginal examination at that time to help determine what has to be done to effect safe delivery of the second twin. One has to ascertain at this point which of the several alternatives is best: cephalic delivery, version, breech extraction, or cesarean delivery. In monochorionic twins, watch for a nuchal cord at the delivery of the first twin. If present, do not cut it because it may actually be the umbilical cord of the second twin. Slip it gently over the first twin's head instead and proceed to deal with the delivery of the second twin.

Preparations for delivery of twins expand considerably upon those preparations generally undertaken for singleton deliveries. Since postpartum hemorrhage is so common after twin delivery, two large-bore intravenous lines should be established in advance and blood cross-matched in the event transfusions become necessary. Blood bank facilities should thus be at the ready. Anesthesia services must also be mobilized to be available for the delivery. Since as many as one-third of cases in which a trial of labor is undertaken for twins ultimately need cesarean delivery, plan to do the delivery in an operating room. That will ensure against any delay in undertaking the cesarean delivery if it were to become necessary on an acute emergency basis. The operating room has to be fully-equipped and staffed to deal immediately with urgent cesarean delivery and uterine hemorrhage. Two neonatal teams also have to be present at the delivery to handle resuscitation of the twins.

## Vaginal delivery of the second twin

Once the first twin delivers, there is often a temporary cessation of intense uterine contractions. Use this interval to examine the second fetus. Determine its presentation, station, position, and whether its membranes are intact. (If you are uncertain of the presentation from your vaginal examination, sonography may be necessary, because it is very difficult to feel fetal poles through the contracted uterus at this point.) Assure its well-being by monitoring its heart rate pattern, and note any potential hazards such as excessive uterine bleeding or umbilical cord prolapse.

If the second twin is in a cephalic presentation, you can await the recurrence of strong regular contractions or, if they do not soon develop, initiate an oxytocin infusion. Observe fetal descent as you would for a singleton, and await spontaneous delivery. This usually occurs within about 20 minutes, but in exceptional cases may be delayed considerably longer. Note the fetal position frequently. Brow and face presentations are not unusual in second twins, especially when premature. There is no need to rush the delivery by applying forceps or the vacuum extractor as long as the fetal heart rate pattern is normal. If concerns about fetal well-being develop, instrumental vaginal delivery or prompt cesarean delivery is appropriate.

When the second twin is in breech presentation, proceed as you would for a singleton breech, with the goal of a spontaneous or assisted breech delivery (Chapter 8). Use complete breech extraction only if delivery is urgent and prompt cesarean delivery is not feasible.

When the second twin is a transverse lie the situation is challenging. If labor is allowed to proceed, the fetus will often convert to a longitudinal lie, and descend as a breech or cephalic presentation, which you can deal with as described above. Internal podalic version and breech extraction is possible, but requires considerable skill and carries substantial risk. Attempting external cephalic version to convert the transverse lie to a cephalic presentation is a useful option. Once you turn the fetus, hold it in position through several contractions while the uterus accommodates itself to the new fetal orientation, lest it turn right back to transverse. Once the cephalic presentation is secured, await spontaneous delivery. During all of these maneuvers, make every effort to maintain the membranes intact. Once the membranes rupture, external version is more difficult, and the risk of cord prolapse is magnified.

## Key points

- Because multiple pregnancy can be expected to be complicated, optimal care requires the attention of experienced, skillful personnel.
- Plan ahead carefully to ensure the gravida is fully informed and that all staff and facilities necessary for the delivery are mobilized.
- The greater the number of fetuses in a multifetal pregnancy, the higher the risks for mother and babies.
- Evaluate gravidas with multiple pregnancy early on for accurate gestational age, the presence of fetal anomalies, and differentiation of chorionicity.
- During the antepartum course, watch for early manifestations of chronic hypertension, pregnancy-induced hypertension, congestive heart failure, anemia, thrombophlebitis, and hydramnios.
- Fetal morbidity and mortality are increased among twins and greater still in higher-order multifetal pregnancy (triplets and more), related to premature birth, congenital anomalies, fetal malpresentations, growth restriction (reflecting uteroplacental insufficiency), and twin-twin transfusion syndrome (manifested primarily by growth discordance).
- Chorionicity is an important indicator of fetal risk, with best outcomes for dizygotic twins and worst for monoamniotic monochorionic twins.
- The death of one fetus in a twin monozygotic pregnancy in the second half of pregnancy puts the other fetus at great risk.
- High-order multifetal pregnancies are best managed by cesarean delivery.

# Further Reading

## Books and reviews

American College of Obstetricians and Gynecologists. Special problems of multiple gestation. ACOG Educational Bulletin No. 253, 1998.

American College of Obstetricians and Gynecologists. Multiple gestation: complicated twin, triplet and high-order multifetal pregnancy. Practice Bulletin No. 56, 2004.

Machin GA, Keith LG. Can twin-to-twin transfusion syndrome be explained, and how is it treated? Clin Obstet Gynecol 1998;41:104–13.

Martin JA, Hamilton BE, Sutton PD, Ventura SJ, et al. Births: final data for 2005. Nat Vital Stat Reports 2007;56:24–5.

Oleszczuk JJ, Oleszczuk AK, Keith LG. Twin and triplet birth: facts, figures, and costs. Female Patient 2003;28:11–16.

Ong SS, Zamora J, Khan KS, Kilby MD. Prognosis for the co-twin following single-twin death: a systematic review. Br J Obstet Gynaecol 2006;113:992–8.

Taylor MJ. The management of multiple pregnancy. Early Hum Dev 2006;82:365–70.

## Primary sources

Blondel B, Kaminski M. Trends in the occurrence, determinants, and consequences of multiple births. Semin Perinatol 2002;26:239–49.

Branum AM, Schoendorf KC. The effect of birth weight discordance on twin neonatal mortality. Obstet Gynecol 2003;101:570–4.

Divon MY, Martin MJ, Pollack RN, Katz NT, Henderson C, Aboulafia Y, et al. Twin gestation: fetal presentation as a function of gestational age. Am J Obstet Gynecol 1993;168:1500–2.

Kahn B, Lumey LH, Zybert PA, Lorenz JM, Cleary-Goldman J, D'Alton ME et al. Prospective risk of fetal death in singleton, twin and triplet gestations: implications for practice. Obstet Gynecol 2003;102:685–92.

Kingdom JC, Nevo O, Murphy KE. Discordant growth in twins. Prenat Diagn 2005;25:759–65.

Leduc L, Takser L, Rinfret D. Persistence of adverse obstetric and neonatal outcomes in monochorionic twins after exclusion of disorders unique to monochorionic placentation. Am J Obstet Gynecol 2005;193:1670–5.

Russell RB, Petrini JR, Damus K, Mattison DR, Schwarz RH. The changing epidemiology of multiple births in the United States. Obstet Gynecol 2003;101:129–35.

# CHAPTER 13

# Managing Shoulder Dystocia

*Shoulder dystocia* is a complication in which the fetal shoulders fail to deliver spontaneously after delivery of the head. It occurs because of impaction of one or both shoulders against the bony pelvis. Most often the anterior shoulder is trapped behind the pubic symphysis; exceptionally, descent of the posterior shoulder is also obstructed at the sacral promontory. Proper management on your part requires sangfroid and grit in greater measure than for most obstetric emergencies. You, and your obstetric team, should always be prepared to deal expeditiously with shoulder dystocia when it occurs. Anticipation of the problem and preparedness—coupled with early diagnosis and calm, knowledgeable and skilled intervention—are key to successful resolution of this serious event without fetal harm.

## Etiology

Shoulder dystocia complicates 2% or less of deliveries, but is of considerable importance because of its association with brachial plexus injury in 3–15% of cases and, less commonly, with fetal asphyxia, fracture of long bones, and even spinal cord injury. Moreover, the problem of shoulder dystocia and its accompanying complications is increasing in frequency. This may be attributable to the increase in birth weight and in the prevalence of fetal macrosomia over recent decades, a consequence of the rapidly spreading epidemic of maternal obesity.

Traction injury to the brachial plexus nerve roots during delivery has traditionally been assumed to cause brachial plexus palsy, and this undoubtedly is so in the great majority of cases. Whether sufficient traction to injure the plexus is always the consequence of excessive force applied by the obstetrician is less certain. Some cases of neonatal brachial plexus injury are alleged to occur prior to delivery, or are produced during delivery

*Labor and Delivery Care: A Practical Guide*, First Edition. Wayne R. Cohen and Emanuel A. Friedman. © 2011 John Wiley & Sons, Ltd. Published 2011 by John Wiley & Sons, Ltd.

despite what is reported to be minimal or absent interference by the attendant. Moreover, some nerve injuries occur despite the most skillful efforts to extract impacted shoulders. Brachial plexus injury occurs in the absence of documented shoulder dystocia in a substantial number of cases.

It is evident that some cases of shoulder dystocia and resulting nerve damage are neither foreseeable nor reasonably preventable despite expert obstetric care; but it is equally clear that poor management of labor or delivery can cause or contribute to brachial plexus injury. Optimal outcome in an individual case is possible only if you anticipate the problem when it is reasonable to do so, understand the nature of the disorder, and have a system of management in place to employ without delay. This should involve a detailed protocol that the team has practiced and is ready to launch at once when called upon to act. Although you have primary responsibility for managing shoulder dystocia, optimal outcome requires the concerted efforts of a team, with you—or someone else with more skill and experience—as its leader. To this end, establishment of hospital-specific guidelines that ensure an efficient and coordinated response to this emergency is very important, as are periodic drills to practice the response.

## Normal shoulder mechanism

During normal labor in the gravida with a gynecoid pelvis, the fetal head generally engages and descends to the midpelvis in a transverse position (Chapter 3). As internal rotation and delivery of the head occur, the shoulders engage in the pelvic inlet, usually in an oblique diameter (although this is quite variable).

During the second stage of labor, the shoulders and the trunk gradually accommodate passively to the architecture of the birth canal during descent. This serves to ensure proper engagement of the shoulders. The posterior shoulder passes over the sacral promontory and, with the shoulder girdle in an oblique orientation, the anterior shoulder then stems beneath the pubic symphysis and emerges beneath the subpubic arch. Several factors may, individually or in combination, confound the normal accommodation and descent of the shoulder girdle. These may relate to the fetus, to the pelvis, or to the rate of descent.

## Predisposing factors

Certain conditions are associated with increased risk of shoulder dystocia and brachial plexus injury. Some of them derive from the patient's history, some from prenatal events, and some from the labor process itself. Principal among them are fetal macrosomia, maternal diabetes mellitus, history of previous shoulder dystocia, instrumental delivery (especially midforceps), postterm pregnancy, and dysfunctional labor. Shoulder dystocia is itself the strongest risk factor for brachial plexus injury. We focus below especially on the risk indicators that you can identify while caring for your patient during labor to help you flag patients at risk, anticipate the problem, and prepare for it well in advance.

## Fetal risk factors

There is a direct relation between birth weight and the likelihood of shoulder dystocia. Risks increase exponentially as birth weight surpasses 4000 g. It is, therefore, not surprising that various factors associated with high birth weight—such as maternal diabetes, obesity, excessive weight gain during pregnancy, and a history of large babies—are also associated with shoulder dystocia.

When the fetus is very large, the shoulders may be too broad to engage normally, and both of them may remain trapped at the inlet as the head delivers. More commonly, the posterior shoulder advances beyond the promontory, while the anterior shoulder becomes impacted above or behind the symphysis pubis. Many macrosomic fetuses (especially those who develop in a mother with poor glycemic control) have a disproportionately large trunk, and especially upper torso, in relation to their head size. This helps explain the propensity for difficult shoulder delivery in large fetuses. Disproportionate growth sometimes occurs even in those with normal weights. Unfortunately, such disparate growth is not easily quantifiable prior to labor.

While large fetal size and disproportionate growth of the trunk predispose to shoulder dystocia and, in turn, to brachial plexus damage, remember that 20–50% of such neuropathies occur in average-weight babies. Also, other cases are related to obstetric factors (e.g., compound presentations) that are not associated with macrosomia.

## Pelvic risk factors

Thorough and systematic clinical pelvimetry to determine the capacity and architecture of the pelvis is helpful in interpreting or predicting the mechanism of labor (Chapters 3 and 4). Pelvimetry can also alert you to the possibility that shoulder dystocia will occur. Difficult shoulder delivery can occur even in a pure gynecoid pelvis, particularly if the pelvis is of small capacity or the fetus is large. However, certain distinctive characteristics of the pelvis increase the risk. For example, if you find foreshortening of the anteroposterior diameter of the inlet (which you will encounter primarily in a pelvis with android or platypelloid features), you should be concerned that normal engagement of the shoulders may be impeded.

A steeply inclined or unusually long pubic symphysis (common in a pelvis with anthropoid features) favors impaction of the anterior shoulder, particularly if associated with a relatively foreshortened anteroposterior pelvic dimension. A transversely narrowed midpelvis may impede rotation of the upper trunk, and an unusually flattened sacrum may inhibit descent of the posterior shoulder. A narrow subpubic arch (often associated with other abnormalities higher in the pelvis) could encumber or prevent delivery of the shoulders unless there is room for the posterior shoulder to shift deeply into the posterior portion of the pelvis. If the lower sacrum and the coccyx are also directed anteriorly, delivery of the shoulders will be difficult.

### Labor risk factors

As many of three-fourths of brachial plexus injuries are preceded by abnormal labor. This is not unexpected because fetal macrosomia is a risk factor for dysfunctional labor as well as for shoulder dystocia. Those labor dysfunctions most commonly associated with difficult shoulder delivery are characterized by either sluggish dilatation or descent or (paradoxically) by exceptionally rapid descent.

One type of abnormal labor, the prolonged deceleration phase, is a strong independent predictor of neonatal brachial plexus palsy. It is a harbinger of second stage labor abnormalities and difficulty with shoulder delivery. In this context, you can consider a prolonged deceleration phase to reflect a problem of descent as well as of dilatation. As the last portion of dilatation occurs in the active phase of labor, the cervix retracts around the fetal presenting part. For cervical retraction to occur, some descent of the presenting part is generally required. If descent cannot be readily initiated because the fetal head or shoulders are large, retraction of the cervix is delayed or prevented. When a prolonged deceleration phase occurs in the context of suspected fetal macrosomia, other first stage labor abnormalities, a long second stage, or other risk factors for brachial plexus injury, consider cesarean delivery as a safe and appropriate option to avoid shoulder dystocia and resulting fetal harm.

Many cases of shoulder dystocia follow precipitate descent. In these situations, we presume that inadequate time for normal shoulder accommodation results in the bisacromial diameter remaining in the anteroposterior diameter of the inlet when the head has delivered. The same process may explain the frequent association of operative vaginal delivery and shoulder impaction. By accelerating the rate of descent artificially, insufficient time for the shoulders to conform to the pelvis leaves them in an abnormal position at the time of their expected engagement.

Delivery by vacuum extractor or forceps confers substantial risk for shoulder dystocia and brachial plexus injury. This is particularly so when the instrumental delivery is undertaken from the midpelvic cavity, but excess risk accrues in low and outlet operative deliveries as well. It is unclear whether this is a direct consequence of the imposed traction or reflects the fact that instruments are more likely to be used in dysfunctional labors that are associated with a large fetus. We generally advise against instrumental delivery when there has been a preceding active phase or second stage labor dysfunction. This is an especially important admonition when other risk factors for brachial plexus injury are also present.

## Prediction

The ability to predict shoulder dystocia is quite limited despite the fact that several risk factors are clearly associated with it and with its adverse consequences. Unfortunately, none of these factors individually is a sufficiently sensitive or specific predictor of shoulder dystocia for you to use as a means to determine the best route of delivery. Remember, risk factors are not necessarily good predictors of an event, particularly when the risk factor is quite prevalent in the population. For example, maternal obesity is a very strong risk factor for shoulder dystocia and brachial plexus injury; but because obesity is so common, and is not usually associated with difficult shoulder delivery, you cannot reliably predict dystocia solely from the presence of obesity.

Moreover, some of the most important risk factors cannot be known prior to delivery. High birth weight, for instance, has a very strong association with shoulder dystocia and brachial plexus injury; but our ability to predict birth weight in large fetuses, even using ultrasonographic imaging, is quite limited. Similarly, precipitate descent, to the extent it is a contributing risk, is one that is not reasonably foreseeable and, once recognized, allows no time to alter management.

To make matters of prediction more complicated, the effects of many risk factors for shoulder dystocia interact, and their independent role is not easy to assess. For example, fetal macrosomia, maternal diabetes, and obesity are all risk factors. Macrosomia tends to occur in diabetic women and in obese women. Moreover, obesity and diabetes are themselves strongly related to each other. The consequence of these overlapping effects is that it is difficult to determine whether the multiple risk factors you encounter in an individual patient are additive, or if they confer the same likelihood of difficult shoulder delivery as if only one were present. There are statistical methods to help sort this out, and we are beginning to learn more about the predictive value of various factors.

Complex risk scoring systems for brachial plexus injury requiring computer analysis have been recently developed, but they are not yet validated for clinical application. Applying such prediction models could allow you to estimate the likelihood of brachial plexus injury for each individual clinical circumstance. Decision making using such models is, in essence, based on how many additional (in retrospect, unnecessary) cesarean deliveries would be required to prevent each case of neonatal brachial plexus injury. Prediction systems, which would consider only information available to you before delivery, could be programmed into electronic obstetric records. Using such techniques would eliminate a portion of brachial plexus injuries by prompting timely delivery in cases at high risk and by discouraging cesarean delivery in cases unlikely to have a complication.

Almost all cases of brachial plexus injury and other complications of shoulder dystocia could be prevented by avoiding vaginal delivery. How then do you identify patients who will probably benefit from preventive cesarean delivery without subjecting too many women unnecessarily to its risks? Most serious injury can probably be avoided if you are a sapient observer of the labor process. Using the approaches we have recommended to recognize and treat dysfunctional labor will help (Chapter 5). They allow early identification of problems and encourage proper timing of cesarean delivery. In the absence of a statistically validated electronic risk assessment system for your particular population, how should you deal with the presence of predisposing conditions? There is, unfortunately, no easy formula for this purpose.

One approach is to consider risk factors in three categories: those derived from your patient's history; those recognized during prenatal care; and those that arise during labor (Box 13.1). The influence of these hazards will, of course, be modified by their severity. Poorly controlled diabetes, for example, is of more concern than if it is well controlled. Among macrosomic fetuses, one with an estimated weight of 5500 g is at greater peril than one of 4000 g. A prior shoulder dystocia that resulted in a child with a permanent Erb palsy is more worrisome than a history of a macrosomic baby without injury.

In general, the presence of serious risk factors in two or more categories should prompt strong consideration of cesarean delivery. Thus, if you have a patient with poorly controlled diabetes and a prior delivery complicated by shoulder dystocia, she is a potential candidate for cesarean delivery, depending on her wishes and other extant medical factors. Should that patient choose to labor, the development of a documented dysfunction, especially a prolonged deceleration phase, magnifies the risks, and you should inform the patient of that. Remember, the clinical assessment of risk is not a static undertaking. You must serially reassess the likelihood of a safe vaginal delivery throughout the labor, and change your strategy and recommendations accordingly.

> **Box 13.1 Risk factors for shoulder dystocia and neonatal brachial plexus palsy**
>
> - History
>   - ○ Prior delivery with shoulder dystocia or brachial plexus palsy
>   - ○ Prior macrosomic baby
>   - ○ Diabetes mellitus (especially with poor glycemic control)
> - Prenatal care
>   - ○ Gestational diabetes mellitus (especially with poor glycemic control)
>   - ○ Maternal obesity
>   - ○ Excessive weight gain
> - Intrapartum care
>   - ○ Estimated fetal weight > 90th percentile for gestational age
>   - ○ Arrest or protraction disorders of active phase
>   - ○ Abnormal fetal descent (failed, arrested or protracted descent)
>   - ○ Long deceleration phase
>   - ○ Precipitate descent
>   - ○ Compound presentation
>   - ○ Unfavorable pelvic architecture
>   - ○ Forceps or vacuum assisted delivery
>   - ○ Induced labor

## Clinical management

You should have in mind a logical strategy to confront shoulder dystocia, recognizing that each circumstance may require modification. Every obstetric service should have a protocol that ensures all staff members understand their roles when a shoulder dystocia occurs. Simulation drills using a mannequin are helpful in developing a coordinated team approach to the problem.

There exist no data clearly demonstrating the superiority of any particular maneuver or series of maneuvers. Astute clinical judgment (i.e., taking into account all the information that is available and making a reasonable plan) and familiarity with the necessary techniques for resolving the dystocia are vital if you are to achieve a successful atraumatic delivery. Management requires keen and accurate physical examination, rapid and insightful analysis, and physical dexterity and skill. We recommend the sequence presented in Fig. 13.1. It is important that whatever efforts you make to effect delivery be done with slow, steady application of force applied as gently as consistent with accomplishing the objective. Persistence over time is less likely to result in injury than the same forces applied over a short time. Maneuvers applied prophylactically to prevent shoulder dystocia do not appear to be beneficial.

You should be alerted to the possibility of shoulder dystocia when the head delivers (often with disquieting slowness) and retracts back against the perineum. This phenomenon has been descriptively called the "turtle sign," reflecting the turtle that retracts its head beneath its carapace. Less commonly, the head emerges without reluctance, but the shoulders do not follow as swiftly as you would expect. Whenever you suspect shoulder dystocia, it is important that you make no effort to exert downward traction on the head, even the gentle traction you ordinarily use with most normal deliveries. At this point, there may already be considerable tension on the brachial plexus because it is stretched between the impacted anterior shoulder high in the pelvis and the base of the head fixed at the outlet. The nerve roots may not be able to tolerate further stretching without injury.

In these situations, a sense of urgency and dread is understandable, especially for the inexperienced. While it is obviously important that you address the problem with appropriate dispatch, you can do more damage in shoulder dystocia cases by mindless floundering or imprudent pulling on the fetus than could ever accrue from delaying intervention for a minute to allow thoughtful analysis, followed by a logical series of skillful maneuvers. While the amount of available time to rescue the fetus varies according to its state of oxygenation prior to emergence of the head, and to other factors, under most circumstances a delay of 5 minutes between delivery of the fetal head and body will cause no asphyxial harm.

When you face a probable shoulder dystocia, do not panic, do not rush, and do not place any traction on the fetal head and neck. It is usually a good idea to await the next uterine contraction before attempting to release the impacted shoulders. The extra time sometimes allows gradual accommodation of the shoulder girdle to the birth canal. If that occurs, you will see the shoulders spontaneously assume an oblique position. The anterior shoulder is then readily delivered. Even if this does not occur, the extra time allows for the team of personnel to be assembled, and for you to organize your thoughts and direct the team.

When you suspect shoulder dystocia, ask the mother to stop pushing. Call for assistance and initiate your delivery unit's protocol. Carry out a vaginal examination to assess the position of the shoulders, the location of the fetal back, and the degree of descent of the posterior shoulder. In addition, look for a compound presentation (see below).

When shoulder dystocia occurs, it is prudent for you to make a generous episiotomy. It can provide the room necessary to carry out manipulations within the vagina to help resolve the problem. Descriptions of various maneuvers cannot convey the fact that, especially with a macrosomic fetus filling the birth canal, there is very little room to insert your hand, no less perform delicate maneuvers with it. Episiotomy can facilitate that work.

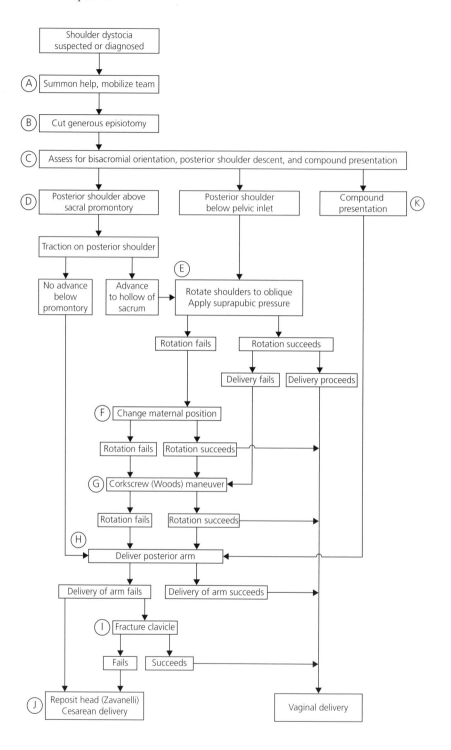

When you examine the patient with shoulder dystocia, most of the time you will find the posterior shoulder below the sacral promontory, in the hollow of the sacrum at the level of the ischial spines. The bisacromial diameter of the fetus will be in the direct anteroposterior diameter of the pelvis. If you find these conditions, your first step should be to attempt to rotate the shoulders into an oblique diameter of the pelvis.

Use of the *McRoberts maneuver* at this stage is commonplace, but it is not the panacea many believe it to be. The McRoberts maneuver involves flexing the mother's thighs against her abdomen in an effort to make the pelvic geometry more favorable for delivery. It often works, and is widely recommended as the first step in relieving shoulder dystocia. Use of this maneuver, however, may not be wise because it places more stretching force on the brachial plexus than do attempts to rotate the shoulders directly.

**Figure 13.1** Algorithm for managing shoulder dystocia.

**A.** As soon as shoulder dystocia is diagnosed or suspected, summon help. Another obstetrician and another nurse are vital; an anesthesiologist will sometimes be required for the mother, and a pediatrician is essential for managing the newborn.

**B.** An episiotomy can markedly increase the available room for intravaginal or intrauterine manipulations.

**C.** Determine the orientation of the shoulders (usually anteroposterior) and the fetal back. Look for a compound presentation and determine whether the posterior shoulder has descended below the sacral promontory. At this stage of diagnosis and assessment, avoid fundal pressure, strong maternal bearing down efforts, or *any* traction on the head. Explain the situation to the patient, and prepare her for the manipulations to follow.

**D.** If the posterior shoulder is fixed above the pelvis, attempt to pull it into the sacral hollow.

**E.** If there is a compound presentation and the posterior arm is prolapsed, attempt to deliver it. If the anterior arm is presenting, rotate the fetus 180 degrees using the posterior arm for traction and rotation. If a leg is presenting, try to reposit it.

**F.** Rotate the fetal shoulder into an oblique diameter of the outlet. Have your assistant use suprapubic pressure directed posterolaterally in the same direction you are attempting rotation. Once the shoulders have been rotated, have the mother bear down.

**G.** If 45 degrees of rotation is successful, but the anterior shoulder does not deliver, continue rotation to 180 degrees, if possible. Have the mother bear down during this maneuver.

**H.** If shoulder rotation is not effective, consider alternative positions if time permits. The lateral position is most readily attained. The hands and knees position may also useful, as may squatting if conditions permit.

**I.** If the change in maternal position is unsuccessful, or if you choose not to do it, attempt to deliver the posterior arm.

**J.** If delivery of the posterior arm is not availing, repeat the previous maneuvers. If delivery is still unsuccessful, consider extreme measures, including replacement of the head back into the vagina and cesarean delivery or clavicle fracture.

Moreover, when the McRoberts maneuver does not work, it may have the potential to worsen the situation or cause maternal complications. With the brachial plexus roots already under stretch when the fetal head is restrained at the introitus and the anterior shoulder is fixed behind the pubic symphysis, forcefully flexing the mother's thighs may increase the tension on the nerve plexus. If the shoulder delivers promptly, there may be no harm; but if the anterior shoulder does not slide under the pubic arch, the McRoberts position worsens tension on the nerve roots and potentially results in (or enhances) their injury. Reports of pathologic separation of maternal pelvic joints and maternal nerve injury have also appeared. As a consequence of these concerns and the absence of documentable benefit, we recommend against using the McRoberts maneuver as a means for dealing with shoulder dystocia.

To accomplish rotation of the anterior shoulder from its anteroposterior orientation, insert at least two fingers of one hand into the vagina against the dorsal aspect of the anterior shoulder. Start by applying firm pressure to the anterior shoulder (i.e., counterclockwise if the fetal back is on the mother's left) with your fingers behind the scapula. This may have the added benefit of flexing the shoulder girdle and reducing the bisacromial diameter. At the same time, apply force in the opposite direction with fingers of your other hand against the ventral surface of the posterior shoulder. If the fetal trunk does not turn readily, reassess the fetal position, focusing on the location of the fetal back. If your original assessment was correct, move on to another maneuver; if incorrect, you should attempt to rotate the shoulders in the opposite direction.

When you are trying to move the shoulders from the anteroposterior pelvic axis to an oblique one, an assistant should provide suprapubic pressure. (Note that this should not be fundal pressure.) This pressure should be directed posterolaterally on the mother's lower abdomen in the same direction as the direction you are using to move the shoulder with your intravaginal fingers. The suprapubic pressure is designed to help you push the anterior shoulder in the desired direction by supplementing the forces being applied intravaginally. Communicate clearly with your assistant to be sure your efforts are coordinated. Often these maneuvers alone are sufficient to effect vaginal delivery.

If rotation of the shoulders into an oblique position is successful but the anterior shoulder does not stem beneath the symphysis, you should next attempt to rotate the posterior shoulder through a full 180 degrees. For best results, use simultaneous downward traction to bring the posterior shoulder around anteriorly and outward below or beyond the symphysis pubis. This corkscrew maneuver (also called the *Woods maneuver*) will often result in emergence of the anterior shoulder (previously posterior) beneath the pubic arch. The remainder of the delivery can be expected to proceed uneventfully if this succeeds.

If attempts to rotate the shoulders into an oblique orientation are not successful, consider changing your patient's position. Various positions may promote resolution of shoulder dystocia, although objective data to support the practice are wanting. Squatting may be helpful, but is not always practical, especially if your patient has epidural anesthesia. Simply turning the patient onto her side is sometimes beneficial, and in many cases encourages the posterior shoulder to descend and deliver. If that does not work, and the mother is able to do so, have her move to her hands and knees (that is, up on "all fours").

If alternative positioning is of no avail, return the patient to her back with her knees and hips moderately flexed, and try to deliver the posterior arm. Insert your hand (use your left hand if the fetal back is on the mother's left) into the posterior vagina along the ventral surface of the fetus and locate the posterior arm, which is often extended. While this sounds straightforward, there may be surprisingly little room in which to maneuver your hand, especially if the fetus is very large. A generous amount of lubricant on your glove will help, as will the aforementioned generous episiotomy. Once your hand reaches the fetal arm, flex it gently at the elbow. Grasp the forearm or hand, and draw it across the fetal chest, taking care not to force the arm into an unphysiologic position. Continue traction until the arm out of the vagina. Fracture of the humerus frequently results, especially if the arm is extracted by traction without first flexing the elbow. Once you extract the arm, the other shoulder usually delivers easily. If it does not, rotation of the trunk (the Woods maneuver) is almost always effective. To facilitate truncal rotation, you can apply rotational traction on the extracted arm.

When one or more of the above-described maneuvers fails, do not hesitate to try them again. Sometimes incremental progress with one maneuver will facilitate good results from another. Be mindful, however, of the amount of time that is passing, and do not squander it on efforts that seem clearly to be fruitless.

When none of the above maneuvers is effective, more radical approaches to shoulder dystocia have been advocated. *Symphysiotomy* has been utilized effectively in some parts of the world, but it has never achieved acceptance in the United States or Europe. It can have serious complications and its success rate is unknown. The *Zavanelli maneuver* involves pushing the head back into the vagina by reversing the prior mechanism of labor, and then proceeding with cesarean delivery. A number of reports of success with this maneuver have appeared, but so have accounts of serious complications, including fetal death, cervical dislocation, and hypoxic-ischemic encephalopathy. The ratio of its benefits and risks is uncertain, but the Zavanelli maneuver is a reasonable alternative when all else fails.

Intentional fracture of the clavicle is often mentioned as a technique for managing arrested shoulders. Indeed, once the clavicle breaks, the shoulder girdle can more readily collapse and the obstruction to delivery is thereby relieved. Although no doubt it may be helpful, intentional clavicle fracture is seldom practiced and rarely achieved. It may be categorized as more easily said than done. Injury to the subclavian vessels or lung and entry into the pleural space may occur if the bone splinters posteriorly. To fracture the clavicle, place four fingers of your dominant hand behind the fetal back. Position your thumb on the superior surface of the middle of the clavicle and exert force inferiorly. Restrict the use of large cleidotomy scissors, which can cause considerable harm, as a last resort for managing shoulder dystocia in the dead fetus who is undeliverable by other means, taking special care not to injure the mother.

Whatever maneuvers you use to treat this disorder, several principles should be paramount. Remain calm and give clear instructions to your assistants; do not rush; use a logical sequence of maneuvers to resolve the dystocia. Be sure that any suprapubic pressure used is directed properly, that is, not posteriorly, but posterolaterally. The primary purpose of the suprapubic force is to assist in rotation and perhaps secondarily to narrow the shoulder girdle. Once the anterior shoulder begins to stem beneath the symphysis pubis, some experts sanction the use of fundal pressure, but this is controversial and probably inappropriate under most circumstances (see below). Forsake attempts to deliver the anterior shoulder by traction on the neck and head. Doing so is both ineffective and potentially quite harmful. Manipulate the shoulders or the arms only. It is remarkable how little force is sometimes necessary to produce brachial plexus injury, even if it is applied in the correct direction. You will not be able to prevent every case of brachial plexus injury, but if injury occurs, you and your patient will take comfort in the knowledge that you did everything reasonable and appropriate to prevent it.

## Special situations

### Compound presentations

Compound presentations complicate 2–5% of cases of shoulder dystocia. While compound presentation classically refers to the combination of limb and head (or breech) presenting together, a partially prolapsed limb reaching only down to the shoulder needs to be included here because the problems produced in cases of shoulder dystocia are essentially the same. Presumably, the fetal arm or leg lying alongside the head or shoulders alters the ability of the shoulder girdle to accommodate to the pelvis and enlarges the combined fetal dimensions at that level to make delivery even more difficult. Whether prolapse of the arm can indicate preexisting *in utero* malfunction of the brachial plexus is not known.

When your initial examination after shoulder dystocia diagnosis reveals a compound presentation, identify the limb to determine if it is an arm or a leg. This important differentiation is not always easy; it requires special attention to ensure your assessment is correct (see Chapter 8 for details). If it is a prolapsed leg, try to reposit it. If that is not possible, proceed with cesarean delivery. With a prolapsed posterior arm, attempt to extract the arm first, as described above. If the anterior arm presents, rotate the shoulders 180 degrees and then deliver the presenting arm, now located posteriorly. Use the more accessible posterior arm for this purpose, as in the Woods maneuver described above. The direction for optimal rotation should be the one that allows the anterior arm to cross the ventral surface of the fetus spontaneously (clockwise if the right arm is anterior and the fetal back is on the mother's left). While delivery of the presenting arm in a compound presentation generally requires little force, its extraction can be exceptionally difficult when the fetus is quite large. This affords little space for manipulation and flexion of the elbow. Moreover, fractures are not uncommon, despite the best efforts of the operator.

### Unengaged posterior shoulder

As noted previously, when you examine the patient with suspected shoulder dystocia, you will generally find that the posterior shoulder has entered the true pelvis and can be felt easily in the sacral hollow. If it is higher and has not negotiated the sacral promontory, the standard maneuvers described above cannot be expected to succeed unless you are able to draw the posterior shoulder into the midpelvis. To do so, insert two fingers behind the pubis along the fetal back to gain a purchase on the scapula. By gentle suprapubic pressure and slight traction on the shoulder, push the anterior shoulder to one side in the direction of the fetal chest so as to reduce the shoulder width. Then try to dislodge the posterior shoulder from the sacral promontory by passing your hand high into the posterior vagina over the fetal back. Aided by gentle but firm external suprapubic pressure on the anterior shoulder (Fig 13.2), grasp the posterior shoulder and turn the shoulder girdle into an oblique diameter as you simultaneously draw the shoulder down into the hollow of the sacrum.

### Alternative positions

Most of the maneuvers described above are designed to be performed with your patient in the traditional, modified lithotomy position. Be aware that other maternal positions are believed by some to help you to alleviate shoulder impaction. Although controlled data are lacking, votaries of alternative positions for delivery say that shoulder dystocia is rare when women deliver in upright postures. Squatting for delivery has several potential advantages in this regard. Delivery with the mother in the lateral position may also be

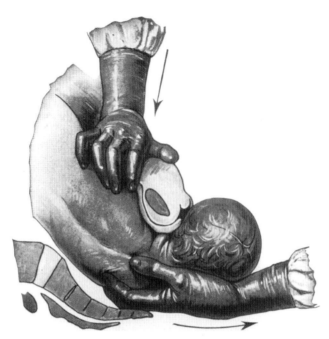

**Figure 13.2** A method for dislodging the posterior shoulder into the sacral excavation in a case of impacted shoulders. Have an assistant exert light suprapubic pressure against the anterior shoulder, pressing it into the right anterior quadrant, while you pull the posterior shoulder downward and into the left posterior quadrant of the pelvis.

beneficial, and good clinical success has been reported with the "all fours" position (i.e., with the patient on her hands and knees). Do not hesitate to try one or more of these approaches. If you try an alternative delivery position, do not introduce undue delay into the process of resolving the dystocia.

### Unusual causes

Rarely, the arrest of delivery after emergence of the head is not due to shoulder dystocia per se, although it will appear that way at first. Always keep in mind the possibility of a fetal malformation or other pathologic condition that alters the fetal anatomy so much that delivery is impossible. Examples include large sacrococcygeal teratomas, conjoined twins, and massive fetal ascites or anasarca.

## Documentation

It is vital that you detail the events associated with a shoulder dystocia case in the medical record. Such documentation allows unambiguous interpretation of the delivery by those evaluating it in retrospect. This

**Box 13.2 Elements of documentation in shoulder dystocia cases**

- Time of delivery of the head
- Time delivery completed
- Personnel present at time of delivery
- Description of the antecedent course of labor (with specific description of disorders of dilation and descent)
- Use of anesthesia
- Use of episiotomy
- Identification of which shoulder was anterior and what the position of the shoulders was when you recognized the problem
- Presence of a compound presentation
- A list of the maneuvers done to relieve the dystocia in the order in which they were done
- An indication that throughout the maneuvers you maintained the fetal spine in the axial plane of the fetus
- Maternal birth canal injury
- Difficulties with patient compliance or behavior that could affect outcome
- Examination of the newborn in the delivery room
- When appropriate, make a recommendation regarding a subsequent delivery. If you feel that cesarean delivery should be done, record that opinion in the record, and say it directly to the mother.

may be important from the points of view of risk management, education, and research. While a detailed annotation of the delivery is obviously important, so too is evidence that you considered any risk factors and other pertinent findings in your clinical decision making prior to delivery.

You should scrupulously record the existence of any historical, prenatal, and intrapartum factors that are associated with an increased risk of shoulder dystocia, beginning at the first prenatal visit and continuing through delivery. If risks arise, include an assessment of them and how they influence your plans for managing labor and delivery. The record should demonstrate that consideration was given to the probability of difficulties at delivery, and the thoughtful preparation for them. Document that any perceived risks were discussed with the mother. In fact, it is wise to include a discussion of shoulder dystocia with all prenatal patients, and to document the content of this discussion in the medical record.

Always create a detailed delivery note shortly after the delivery. This note should contain, at a minimum, the information listed in Box 13.2. To the extent that all of the above can be recorded through menus in an electronic medical record, this may suffice. We recommend, however, that any pertinent details be placed in a narrative description of the events of delivery as well.

The neonatal record, in addition to a physical examination pertinent to identifying possible injuries, should include birth weight, head circumference, thoracic circumference, and abdominal circumference measurements of the newborn.

## Shared responsibilities

Every obstetric unit should have a protocol for the anticipation and management of shoulder dystocia. Because it is often an unexpected event, you must call upon all the necessary interdisciplinary resources and have them available promptly. Each member of the team (obstetricians, midwives, nurses, anesthesiologists, neonatologists, etc.) should be familiar with her role in the event a shoulder dystocia occurs. Practice drills to ensure smooth operation of the protocol should be done periodically. Some obstetric units now require satisfactory participation in these drills for reappointment to the hospital staff. While each obstetric unit should assign responsibilities appropriate to its particular staffing and organization, a general approach is outlined in Box 13.3.

The major pitfalls in care relate to the failure to be prepared for and to optimally manage shoulder dystocia. Preparation is obviously important when risk factors exist, although you must bear in mind that this complication occurs frequently in the absence of any demonstrable risk factors. Therefore, assume that the potential for shoulder dystocia exists in any delivery. The likelihood of a good outcome is enhanced if appropriate anticipatory action has been taken to address it. This anticipation specifically involves being sure that timely observations are made before and during labor, that emerging risk factors are identified, and that adequate help is promptly available in the delivery room from all the required team personnel.

If shoulder dystocia occurs, retrospective analysis of the record should reveal that the obstetrician exercised reasonable care in anticipating it, advised the patient appropriately, and took all reasonable measures to manage it. This would include the following documentation:
- A discussion of shoulder dystocia during prenatal care
- Estimated fetal weight prior to labor and during labor
- Results of the prenatal glucose challenge test and oral glucose tolerance test
- Maternal obesity or excessive weight gain
- Prior birth weights if the patient is a multipara
- Prior shoulder dystocia if the patient is a multipara
- A history of instrumental vaginal delivery

**Box 13.3 Roles and responsibilities during shoulder dystocia management**

- Obstetrician or Midwife
  - Diagnoses probable shoulder dystocia
  - Assumes leadership role unless more experienced person is present
  - Informs delivery room nurse to initiate shoulder dystocia protocol
  - Explains situation to patient and reassures her
  - Determines position of the shoulders
  - Assesses level of descent of posterior shoulder
  - Assesses need for episiotomy or bladder catheterization
  - Initiates maneuvers to resolve the dystocia
- Delivery Room Nurse
  - Records time of delivery of head
  - Notifies Head Nurse of shoulder dystocia
  - Assists with catheterization, position change, reassurance of patient
  - Applies posterolateral suprapubic pressure at the direction of the obstetrician or midwife
- Head Nurse
  - Summons another staff nurse to assist in room
  - Summons anesthesiologist, neonatologist, and senior obstetrician
  - Prepares operating room for possible emergency cesarean delivery
- Staff Nurse
  - Takes over documentation from Delivery Room Nurse
  - Announces elapsed time at intervals
  - Records sequence of maneuvers used
- Senior obstetrician
  - Assists primary obstetrician or midwife in management
  - Assumes leadership role if most experienced
- Anesthesiologist
  - Provides intravenous access if needed
  - Provides sedation or anesthesia as appropriate after consultation with obstetrician
  - Assists with resuscitation of newborn, as necessary
- Neonatologist
  - Prepares resuscitation equipment
  - Examines newborn in delivery room
  - Performs neonatal resuscitation as necessary
  - Communicates with patient and family and provides emotional support

- Clinical cephalopelvimetry done during labor
- Recognition of labor abnormalities
- Fetal position and the mechanism of labor
- A specific tabulation of those factors influencing the decision to proceed with a trial of labor and vaginal delivery, i.e., a serial reevaluation of the probability of safe vaginal delivery when appropriate
- Details of a frank, detailed discussion with the parents after the incident, including appropriate expressions of sorrow if there was an injury

## Key points

- Assume that the potential for shoulder dystocia exists in any delivery.
- All obstetric units should have a protocol for the anticipation and management of shoulder dystocia.
- Record the existence of any historical, prenatal, and intrapartum factors associated with an increased risk of shoulder dystocia beginning at the first prenatal visit and continuing through labor and delivery. There is a direct relation between birth weight and the likelihood of shoulder dystocia, but 20–50% of cases of brachial plexus injury occur in average-weight babies.
- As many of three-fourths of brachial plexus injuries are preceded by abnormal labor. Prolonged deceleration phase is a particularly strong independent predictor of brachial plexus injury.
- A steeply inclined or unusually long pubic symphysis, a transversely narrowed midpelvis, a flattened sacrum, and a narrow subpubic arch can encumber shoulder delivery.
- If shoulder dystocia occurs, remain calm and give clear instructions to assistants; do not rush; use a logical sequence of maneuvers to resolve the problem.
- Changing the maternal position may help alleviate shoulder impaction.
- Always create a detailed narrative note shortly after the delivery.

## Further Reading

### Books and reviews

Gherman RB, Chauhan S, Ouzounian JG, Lerner H, Gonik B, Goodwin TM. Shoulder dystocia: the unpreventable obstetric emergency with empiric management guidelines. Am J Obstet Gynecol 2006;195:657–72.

Goffinet F, Cabrol D. Shoulder dystocia. In: Kuryak A, Chervenak FA (eds) *Textbook of Perinatal Medicine, second edition*. Informa UK Ltd, London, 2006: 1928–35.

Morrison JC, Sanders JR, Magann EF, Wiser WL. The diagnosis and management of dystocia of the shoulder. Surg Gynecol Obstet 1992;175:515–22.

Naef RW III, Morrison JC. Guidelines for management of shoulder dystocia. J Perinatol 1994;14:435–41.

Schifrin BS, Cohen WR. The maternal fetal medicine viewpoint: causation and litigation. In: O'Leary JA (ed) *Shoulder Dystocia and Birth Injury*, 3rd edition. Humana Press, New York, 2008: 227–47.

### Primary sources

Acker DB, Gregory KD, Sachs BP, Friedman EA. Risk factors for Erb-Duchenne palsy. Obstet Gynecol 1988;71:389–92.

Acker DB, Sachs BP, Friedman EA. Risk factors for shoulder dystocia in the average-weight infant. Obstet Gynecol 1986;67:614–18.

Benedetti TJ, Gabbe SG. Shoulder dystocia: a complication of fetal macrosomia and prolonged second stage of labor with midpelvic delivery. Obstet Gynecol 1978;52:526–9.

Bruner JP, Drummond SB, Meenan AL, Gaskin IM. All-fours maneuver for reducing shoulder dystocia during labor. J Reprod Med 1998;43:439–43.

Deaver JE, Cohen WR: A prediction model for brachial plexus injury. J Perinat Med 2009;37:150–5.

Dyachenko A, Ciampi A, Fahey J, Mighty H, Oppenheimer L, Hamilton EF. Prediction of risk for shoulder dystocia with neonatal injury. Am J Obstet Gynecol 2006;195:1544–9.

Gonen R, Bader D, Maha A. Effects of a policy of elective cesarean delivery in cases of suspected fetal macrosomia on the incidence of brachial plexus injury and the rate of cesarean delivery. Am J Obstet Gynecol 2000;183:1296–300.

Gross TL, Sokol RJ, Williams T, Thompson K. Shoulder dystocia: a fetal-physician risk. Am J Obstet Gynecol 1987;156:1408–18.

Gurewitsch ED, Johnson E, Hamzehzadeh S, Allen RH. Risk factors for brachial plexus injury with and without shoulder dystocia. Am J Obstet Gynecol 2006;194:486–92.

Gurewitsch ED, Kim EJ, Yang JH, Outland KE, McDonald MK, Allen RH. Comparing McRoberts' and Rubin's maneuvers for initial management of shoulder dystocia: an objective evaluation. Am J Obstet Gynecol 2005;192:153–60.

Hopwood HG. Shoulder dystocia: fifteen years' experience in a community hospital. Am J Obstet Gynecol 1982;144:162–6.

McFarland LV, Raskin M, Daling JR, Benedetti TJ. Erb/Duchenne's palsy: a consequence of fetal macrosomia and method of delivery. Obstet Gynecol 1986;68:784–8.

Rouse DJ, Owen J, Goldenberg RL, Cliver SP. The effectiveness and costs of elective cesarean delivery for fetal macrosomia diagnosed by ultrasound. JAMA 1996;276:1480–6.

Rubin A. Management of shoulder dystocia. JAMA 1964;189:835–7.

Weizsaecker K, Deaver JR, Cohen WR: Labour characteristics and neonatal Erb's palsy. BJOG 2007;114:1003–9.

Woods CE. A principle of physics as applicable to shoulder delivery. Am J Obstet Gynecol 1943;45:796–804.

# CHAPTER 14

# Using Forceps and the Vacuum Extractor

The ability to use instruments to facilitate vaginal delivery is an important obstetric skill, albeit one used with diminishing frequency today. Obstetric forceps and the vacuum extractor are designed to expedite delivery of the fetus during the second stage of labor. Use them when it is important for you to hasten delivery. The decision to use instruments for vaginal delivery depends on whether you judge them to be preferable, from the standpoint of fetal or maternal safety, to the alternatives of proceeding with immediate cesarean section or delaying to allow further time in labor.

The vacuum extractor, first introduced in the 1950s, has become increasingly popular in the United States over the last 20 years, and now accounts for the majority of operative vaginal deliveries in most units. The use of forceps has diminished correspondingly. Both types of instruments have their virtues, limitations, and passionate advocates. Less important than the choice of instrument is that you have complete familiarity with its use in the circumstance to which you intend to apply it. Both vacuum extractor and forceps delivery do have the potential to reduce the risks of labor, but they can also cause serious harm to fetus and mother. You can minimize that harm by using them gently and skillfully, by recognizing their prerequisites, indications, and limitations, and even more important, by choosing only appropriate situations in which to employ them.

Forceps and vacuum extractor operations are classified according to the level in the pelvis from which the fetus is extracted and the degree of rotation they impart to the head. In general, the higher the station at which you apply the instrument and the greater the degree of rotation necessary for delivery, the more likely it is to cause injury. In every case you must weigh the risks and benefits of instrumental delivery against those of the alternatives. Before you begin an operative vaginal delivery, write down details of this analysis and the conclusions that flow from it, in the patient's record.

*Labor and Delivery Care: A Practical Guide*, First Edition. Wayne R. Cohen and Emanuel A. Friedman. © 2011 John Wiley & Sons, Ltd. Published 2011 by John Wiley & Sons, Ltd.

## Obstetric forceps

### Types of forceps operations

Aside from application to the aftercoming head in breech deliveries, forceps operations as applied to the fetal head in cephalic presentation are classified as *outlet forceps*, *low forceps*, *midforceps*, and *high forceps* (Box 14.1). They are defined on the basis of the fetal station and the position of the head at the time the instrument is applied. These definitions can be considered to apply as well to vacuum extractor-assisted deliveries.

An outlet forceps operation is the application of the instrument to the fetal head when the skull has reached the pelvic floor and the sagittal suture is no more than 45 degrees off the anteroposterior diameter of the pelvic outlet. A low forceps operation is one done with the fetal head at or below station +2 but above the pelvic floor. A midforceps operation is one done when the fetal head is engaged but the conditions for low forceps have not been met. In the context of this term, any procedure requiring artificial rotation of more than 45 degrees would be designated midforceps.

A high forceps operation is the application of the instrument at any time prior to the engagement of the fetal head. High forceps delivery carries such great risks to mother and fetus that it is never justified.

In this chapter we focus primarily on the performance of outlet and low instrumental delivery. Midcavity procedures have become so uncommon in most American obstetric facilities that it is difficult for any obstetrician to develop the necessary skills to perform them safely.

---

### Box 14.1 Criteria for classification of forceps and vacuum extraction deliveries

- Outlet
  - Scalp is visible at introitus without separating the labia
  - Fetal skull has reached pelvic floor
  - Position is OA, OP, LOA, ROA, LOP or ROP
  - Rotation is 45 degrees or less
- Low
  - Leading edge of fetal skull is at or below station +2 but has not reached the pelvic floor
  - Rotation is 45 degrees or less
- Mid
  - Fetal head is engaged
  - Station of head is between 0 and +2
  - Any procedure requiring rotation of more than 45 degrees (regardless of fetal station)
- High
  - Fetal head is not engaged

## Forceps instruments

Distinguish the two major categories of obstetric forceps by the configuration of their shanks. Simpson-type forceps have separated shanks, whereas Elliot-type forceps have overlapping shanks (Fig. 14.1). The significance of this difference lies in the shape of the arc that results from the excursion of the blade out from its heel to the maximum point of separation (the cephalic curvature). A flatter, shallower arc results when the blade starts further out from the midline of the instrument with separated shanks; a fuller, rounder arc is produced by overlapping shanks. Thus, Simpson-type forceps have a tapered cephalic curve whereas that curve is more rounded in Elliot-type forceps.

Based on these differences in the cephalic curve, you should use the Simpson-type forceps for elongated molded heads and the Elliot-type for rounded, relatively unmolded heads. There are dozens of variants of each of these basic types, all with minor differences in length, curvature, fenestration, thickness of the blades, lengths of the shanks, the kinds of locking or articulating devices, design of the handles, and mechanisms for traction. Safe use of any forceps requires adherence to the same principles.

You can use obstetric forceps to provide traction, rotation, and flexion or extension of the head. Forceps designed for special situations exist, but are used uncommonly today. Examples include Kielland forceps for rotation of the head from an OT or OP position to an OA position in an anthropoid pelvis; or Barton forceps for effecting descent or delivery in an OT position in a platypelloid (flat) pelvis.

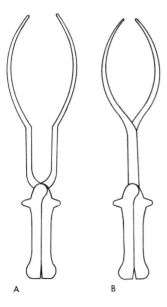

A          B

**Figure 14.1** Comparison of Simpson type of forceps (**A**) and Elliot type (**B**). Note parallel versus overlapping shanks, which create a tapering or rounded cephalic curve, respectively.

Although not generally appreciated, compression of the head by forceps is inevitable. Bear in mind that the widest dimension between the two articulated blades is no greater than 7.5 cm in all contemporary obstetric forceps. Since the biparietal diameter of a term fetus is about 9.5 cm, some head compression has to take place whenever a forceps procedure is done on a term fetus. To minimize this, we recommend preventing the forceps handles from closing completely during traction or rotation by inserting your finger or a doubly folded 4 × 4 inch surgical sponge between them.

Compression of the fetal head has a potentially harmful effect on the brain, especially if prolonged. Circulation may be hindered, causing ischemia and hemorrhages in addition to direct injury to the cranial bones. Internally, the tentorium, the falx, the vessels, and even the brain itself can be injured. Most such serious injuries occur during midcavity procedures, especially those involving rotation of the fetal head. Nevertheless, improperly done or unduly forceful outlet or low forceps operations can also result in significant fetal trauma, particularly when undertaken in the presence of cephalopelvic disproportion. More rarely, technically adequate operations can also cause harm. Neither forceps nor the vacuum extractor should be used except under optimal circumstances and in the hands of skilled, knowledgeable, experienced personnel.

While traction is the dominant function of forceps, if you are skillful, you can use them also as a rotator to correct the position of the fetal head without injury to mother or fetus. Unless you have acquired considerable experience, you should not be doing forceps deliveries that require rotation through more than about 45 degrees. Remember, however, that even smaller degrees of rotation require proper technique. Rotation with forceps must take into account the angle between the blades and the handle, a relation that forms the pelvic curve of the forceps. In order to make the head rotate around its own axis, you must gently sweep the handles through a large circle outside the pelvis (Fig. 14.2). Describing this large arc with the handles will impart the necessary rotary motion to the head within the pelvis.

The objective of forceps traction is to mimic nature in the amount of force, the direction in which it is applied, and its intermittent characteristic. Only by employing great care and gentleness will you protect the fetus and the mother from injury.

## Indications

Most forceps operations in the past were done ostensibly as prophylactic measures, a concept introduced by DeLee in the United States in the 1920s. The purported benefits of an elective forceps procedure are that it will reduce the effort and discomfort of the second stage of labor, save the pelvic floor from overstretching, reduce blood loss, and protect the fetal

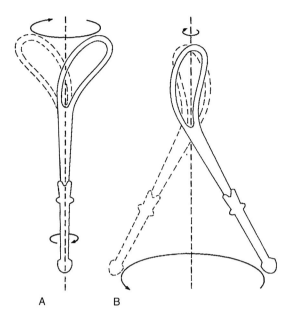

A          B

**Figure 14.2** Principle of forceps rotation. If handles of classic forceps were to be rotated as shown in (**A**), the blades would describe an arc in the pelvis, risking damage to the vagina and fetus. Rotating the handles correctly through a wide arc (**B**) imparts a smooth confined rotary movement to the blades in the pelvis.

brain from prolonged compression. Whether these claims are true has never been convincingly verified. Intelligent expectancy should be your guide and you should intervene with forceps or the vacuum extractor only when its risks can be justified in the presence of evident or potential danger to mother or fetus. Because even small risks cannot be justified without a balancing benefit, do not do prophylactic or purely elective forceps or vacuum extraction (i.e., instrumental procedures with no demonstrable medical indication or benefit).

Most clinically indicated forceps procedures (Box 14.2) are done to rescue a fetus from an acute hypoxemic situation or to overcome an arrest of progress with the fetal head on or near the pelvic floor. The latter situation occurs in association with insufficient uterine and expulsive force, excessively resistant or inelastic perineal tissues, or large fetal head diameters relative to the pelvic capacity to accommodate the fetal head safely. Combinations of these factors are common. While the risks of properly executed outlet forceps procedures are minimal, delivery from higher in the pelvis can be fraught with hazard. The very factors that can result in delayed descent or rotation are the ones that make instrumental vaginal delivery particularly dangerous. While each case must be judged individually, cesarean delivery is usually a safer alternative unless you find that

**Box 14.2 Indications and contraindications for instrumental vaginal delivery**

- Indications*
  - Maternal condition precluding pushing efforts (e.g., certain cardiopulmonary or cerebrovascular diseases)
  - Maternal condition requiring shortening labor (e.g., sepsis, acute critical illness)
  - Fetal hypoxemia requiring urgent delivery
  - Arrest of descent without evidence of cephalopelvic disproportion
- Contraindications
  - Clinical suspicion of cephalopelvic disproportion
  - Known fetal skull or brain malformation
  - Known fetal bleeding diathesis
  - Known fetal bone demineralization or connective tissue disorder
  - Prior scalp blood sampling (applicable to vacuum extraction)
  - Gestational age < 34 weeks (applicable to vacuum extraction)

*Indications require your considered judgment that instrumental delivery in a particular situation will carry less risk than the alternatives, namely, either urgent cesarean delivery or allowing further labor with or without oxytocin stimulation.

disproportion is very unlikely to be present. If you choose forceps or vacuum extractor in those situations, be especially sure that you have made an accurate determination of the true degree of descent of the head and of both the architecture and the capacity of the pelvis. Do not allow yourself to be deceived by extensive cranial molding into thinking the head is deeply engaged and descending; and never attempt to force delivery through a pelvis not anatomically suited to it. The result in either case can be disastrous.

Acute fetal hypoxia warrants a forceps operation if conditions are safe and appropriate for vaginal delivery. You must always weigh the relative risks of this procedure against the alternatives of cesarean section, or further delay to allow more optimal conditions to evolve for spontaneous delivery or for a less hazardous instrumental procedure.

Complications that affect the mother or fetus may also justify using forceps or vacuum extraction when the alternatives are judged less likely to result in a satisfactory outcome. Such situations include massive placental abruption (with severe blood loss or fetal compromise), prolapse of the umbilical cord, or maternal cardiopulmonary collapse (e.g., from amniotic fluid embolism). In certain medical conditions (e.g., cerebral arteriovenous malformation or aneurysm, severe cardiac or pulmonary disease), the physical effort and the Valsalva maneuver required for bearing-down efforts may be dangerous, and thus contraindicated. In some of these cases, instrumental delivery may be necessary for vaginal delivery to occur. These situations can sometimes even justify midforceps or mid-cavity vacuum extractions.

Maternal exhaustion is often given as a reason to perform instrumental delivery. Sympathy for a patient who is physically and emotionally spent after having been in labor for a long time is appropriate, and the impulse to terminate the labor is decent and understandable. Your patient may even request (or demand) that you use forceps or vacuum extractor. Outlet extractions are justifiable for this purpose, given their minimal morbidity, provided conditions are optimal. But think twice before embarking on a procedure with more risk in this situation. Also, long, exhausting labors may render you fatigued as well. Do not let your own need for rest cloud your judgment. In addition to fetal risks, the vaginal and vulvar venous engorgement and edema that accompany a long second stage make these tissues especially vulnerable to severe laceration. There are alternatives that might help your patient endure further labor. Allow her to rest, and encourage her not to push with every contraction. Bearing down with every other contraction or every third contraction may suffice for a while as she recoups her strength. Epidural anesthesia is very helpful in this regard. In these situations, do not feel strictly bound by second stage duration in making a decision to use instruments. While a long second stage demands evaluation and close surveillance, it does not itself constitute an indication for undertaking a potentially harmful delivery procedure.

In every situation in which you intend to use forceps or vacuum extractor, write a thorough preoperative note in the patient's record. At a minimum, this note should describe the indication for the procedure, the fetal position and station, the fact that you have considered (and discussed with the patient) the risks, benefits, and alternatives to the operation, and that she understands and has consented. After the delivery, document the details of the procedure (Box 14.3).

## Conditions for forceps delivery

Before you undertake instrumental delivery, certain conditions must be fulfilled in order to minimize maternal and fetal hazards.

1. Never apply instruments if you are uninitiated or unskilled in their use. The requisite skills are gained by mannequin practice and closely supervised extensive experience under various clinical circumstances.
2. The pelvis must be large enough to permit safe delivery of an undamaged fetus. A procedure in which the instrument is applied when this fact is unknown or in doubt is considered a *trial forceps,* and is rarely performed in modern obstetrics.
3. The cervix must be completely effaced and dilated.
4. The bladder and rectum must be empty.

---

**Box 14.3 Medical record documentation of instrumental vaginal delivery**

- Prior to procedure
  - Rationale and indication
  - Estimated fetal weight
  - Fetal position, station, attitude, asynclitism, molding, and caput succedaneum
  - Findings of cephalopelvimetry with assessment of pelvic architecture and capacity and especially of adequacy of cephalopelvic relationship
  - Details of informed consent discussion
- After delivery
  - Position and station at application
  - Position and station at delivery
  - Type of anesthesia
  - Estimated blood loss
  - Number of pulls
  - Number of dislodgements (applicable to vacuum extraction)
  - Use of episiotomy
  - Maternal lacerations and repairs done
  - Newborn condition

---

5. Anesthesia is required.
6. The fetus must be in cephalic presentation. The only exception is the application of Piper forceps to the aftercoming head in a vaginal breech birth (Chapter 8).
7. The fetal presentation and position must be known precisely.
8. The head must be engaged.
9. The membranes must be ruptured.

## Technique

The ideal or normal application of forceps (Fig. 14.3) occurs with the sagittal suture of the fetal head in the anteroposterior diameter of the pelvis. The forceps is applied to the head so that the axis of the shanks is perpendicular to the sagittal suture, with the toes or apices of the blades anchored around the zygomatic processes of the maxilla bilaterally. The superior edge of each blade (i.e., the shorter arc of the concavity) should lie just in front of the fetal ear. The proximal portions of the superior edges of the blades are close to and equidistant from the lambdoidal sutures on either side. The heels of the blades override the parietal bones. If these conditions are met, the head will be grasped in the most favorable manner and delivery will be attended with the least difficulty and the least risk of harm.

A forceps procedure consists of five separate sequential maneuvers: (1) applying the blades to the fetal head; (2) checking the application;

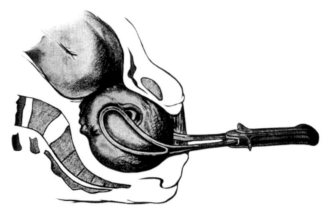

**Figure 14.3** The forceps applied in its most favorable position to a head in a direct OA position. Note position of blades in front of the fetus's ear, with the blades' toes anchored below the zygoma.

(3) adapting, adjusting, and locking the forceps; (4) extracting the fetal head; (5) removing the instrument.

## Application to the fetal head

The patient's bladder should be empty. Catheterize it if necessary. Pass two fingers into the vagina to ascertain that all conditions are met for instrumental delivery. Determine the fetal station and position precisely. Do not begin any kind of instrumental application until you are certain about these. Some form of anesthesia, usually epidural, is necessary, although an outlet forceps delivery can be performed under pudendal nerve block when necessary.

Your choice of the type of forceps will depend on the degree of fetal head molding anticipated, the shape of the pelvis, the type of operation planned, and any special problems encountered or anticipated. Generally, for the well-molded head resulting from a long labor, especially in a nullipara, a Simpson-type forceps can be used to advantage. For a relatively unmolded head in a multipara after a short labor, choose one of the Elliot forceps types.

The blade you insert first depends on the position of the fetal head. For OA and LOA positions, apply the left blade first (Fig. 14.4); for a ROA position you should insert the right blade first. When you apply the more posterior blade initially, you prevent the head from rotating to the posterior during the wandering maneuver that must take place while you adjust the other (anterior) blade.

Sometimes, the occiput will rotate anteriorly during the insertion of the posterior blade. In fact, it is a common practice to make a deliberate effort to effect anterior rotation by applying slight internal pressure (clockwise

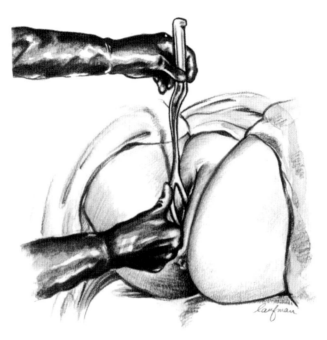

**Figure 14.4** The left blade of the forceps, which is held loosely in the left hand, is inserted into the left side of the pelvis along the left side of the fetal head in an OA position.

in a ROA position). When a single blade of a forceps is used alone in this manner it is called a *vectis*; it is occasionally quite useful in this regard.

Extra care is required when the right blade is introduced first. The construction of all forceps necessitates laying the right blade on top of the left, where the lock is located, to articulate the forceps properly. Contrastingly, when you place the right blade first, you will have to recross the handles outside the vulva after the application. While this is not a difficult manipulation, be sure to perform it gently and with minimal excursions of the blades; otherwise, it can cause injury.

If the left blade is chosen, hold its handle lightly in your left hand and introduce your right hand into the vagina along the left side of the maternal pelvis. The toe of the forceps blade is introduced along the palm of the hand in the vagina (Fig. 14.4). Poise the handle vertically over the introitus at first so that the blade can be passed along the pelvic curvature with utmost gentleness and delicacy. As you slip the blade along your fingers into the vagina, hold the toe of the blade close to the head. Use the thumb of your right hand to guide and press the blade into place. Lower the handle progressively as the blade advances inside the pelvis. Never force the blade into position or apply pressure to the handle to advance the blade; to do so may cause great damage. Properly positioned and maneuvered, the forceps blade should slide smoothly into place, falling into the correct position almost by its own weight.

Then pass the right blade in a like manner into the right side of the maternal pelvis along the right side of the fetal skull, inserting four fingers of your left hand to act as a guide. If the fetal position is directly OA, introduce the right blade precisely as you did the left one. If the position is LOA, however, the left blade will lie in the left posterolateral aspect of the pelvis; the right blade must be wandered by the left hand in the vagina using gentle pressure in a clockwise direction until it is seated properly alongside the head in the right anterolateral pelvis. The same technique is used if the position is ROA, except you would introduce the right blade first into the right posterolateral pelvis. Then insert the left blade and wander it to the left anterolateral location. Following this, you can cross the shanks and handles to lock the instrument in place.

### Checking the application

After both blades are in place, articulate them and carefully check to be sure the placement is correct. The points to be remembered are as follows: (1) the shanks should be exactly perpendicular to the sagittal suture; (2) the lambdoidal sutures should each be about 1 cm anterior to the front edge of the forceps blades and equidistant from them; (3) you should be able to insinuate no more than one fingertip under the heel of each blade over the parietal bones.

If the shanks are not perpendicular to the sagittal suture, the instrument is not aligned properly with the head. This error is confirmed if you find that the lambdoidal sutures are not equidistant from the front of the blades. In that case, unlock and adjust the blades one at a time so that they are moved clockwise or counterclockwise to fit the head more correctly.

If you find the lambdoidal sutures are equidistant but more than 1 cm from the blades, this usually means that you have applied the forceps to a deflexed head; this, too, will have to be adjusted, by first unlocking the forceps and then individually moving each arm anteriorly until they are properly positioned on the fetal head, where they can again be locked in position. If there is more than one fingertip of space between the heels of the blades and the skull, it is likely that the forceps you chose is too long or too tapered for the head. This usually results when a forceps designed for use on a molded head (that is, a Simpson type) is being incorrectly used on an unmolded head. Alternatively, the toes of the blades are anchored above the zygomas; this results when a short Elliot-type forceps is used on an elongated, molded head. Both possibilities are very serious errors because of the danger of trauma from slippage of the blades, a complication that is likely to result when traction is applied.

### Adapting, adjusting, and locking

Further necessary modifications of the forceps application to the fetal head will depend on its presentation and position. To ensure minimal exposure of the fetus to harm from forceps delivery, it is imperative that you apply the blades to fit the head in the best way. If the head is low in the maternal pelvis and the occiput is directly anterior, the blades will fit naturally to the sides of the head. Often, however, they need a little adjusting before it is possible to close the lock smoothly with no force at all. The easiest way to bring the blades into position is to press the unlocked handles gently downward onto the perineum. Forced locking considerably enhances the risk of injury to mother or fetus.

If the blades do not lock easily you have most likely diagnosed fetal position incorrectly. To correct this, remove the forceps and reassess the sutures and fontanels in detail so you are sure of the fetal position. Then reapply the forceps to correct the direction and the degree of error according to the guidelines just described. If the error is rotational (the fetal head is in LOA position but the forceps is applied as if it were direct OA, for example), adjust the blades smoothly to the sides of the head by wandering one blade a little anteriorly and the other a little posteriorly. The wandering maneuver involves unlocking the blades and, with the appropriate hand in the vagina (the right hand for the left blade), lifting or lowering the blade gently into place. The external hand applies no pressure whatsoever and merely supports the handle.

If the error is one of deflexion, correct this by disarticulating the blades and raising them toward the occiput one at a time before rearticulating and locking them. The error of poor fit (toes anchored behind the zygomas, for example) connotes a poor choice of instrument or a badly misapplied forceps. In either instance, remove the forceps entirely. If a new application or more appropriate instrument does not correct the problem, abandon the attempt at forceps delivery.

### Extracting the fetal head

The principles of traction are the following:

1. Imitate a uterine contraction with each pull. Use gradually increasing force while pulling to slowly reach an acme. Hold for a moment and then slowly relax the pull.
2. Use as little force as possible, regulating the amount by the advance of the fetal head. Keep your elbows at your sides and your arms flexed to ensure against using excessive traction. Do not rush. Open the handles somewhat between each pull, allowing cerebral blood flow to reestablish itself in the fetus.
3. If rotation is complete, the traction should be simple and directed in the proper pelvic axis. Never use pendulum, corkscrew or twisting motions. All are dangerous and not productive.

4. Traction should not be directed straight out, but forward and downward, following the curve of the pelvic canal. You can achieve the proper direction by gripping the handles with one hand and simultaneously placing the other hand over the shanks. Pull directly toward yourself with the handles, while using an equivalent force to press directly downwards with the hand on the shanks. The vector force that results from this combined approach (the Saxtorph-Pajot maneuver) will be directed in the pelvic axis.

5. Insinuate a finger or folded gauze pad between the handles to reduce head compression, as previously emphasized.

Apply traction as indicated above in terms of intensity, timing, and direction (Fig. 14.5). Carefully determine the progress of descent achieved while

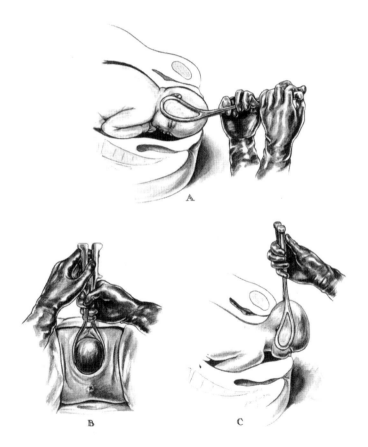

**Figure 14.5** Outlet forceps delivery. **A.** The forceps is in place; the handles are separated with the left index finger and thumb; the pull is directed downward (i.e., posteriorly) and toward you with combined forces. **B.** Traction is continued, but with gradual extension of the head; the handles are separated to avoid excess head compression. **C.** The head is delivered by further extension over the perineum.

traction is being applied and allow the fetal head to recede very slowly. Loosen the forceps after each traction effort, but do not separate the handles too far. After a minute, make another and slightly stronger traction, if necessary. Pull during uterine contractions, and have the mother bear down to take advantage of the combined forces of her expulsive efforts, uterine contractility, and forceps traction.

As the head begins to distend the perineum, pull in a more upward trajectory, along the external projection of the pelvic axis. To complete the delivery of the fetal head, grasp the forceps at the shank with one hand and gently and slowly draw the head out and over the perineum, mimicking the spontaneous delivery mechanism. Allow the perineum to stretch slowly, taking at least as much time as natural delivery would require. Be especially careful to avoid sudden decompression of the fetal head as it delivers, thereby preventing injury from rapid changes in intracranial pressure.

### Removing the forceps

When the widest diameter of the fetal head is about to pass the vulvar ring, you can remove the forceps, although you can also await completion of head delivery to do so. The slight lessening in the presenting circumference (by 5–8 mm) from removing the instrument may help avert tissue injury. Remove the forceps by reversing the process of application, taking care not to injure the fetal scalp or ear or the maternal soft tissues. Disarticulate the blades, and remove them one at a time, holding them by the handles and pulling gently in an upward direction toward the opposite side, maintaining the cephalic curve and toe closely applied the head. As the blade comes off the head, the handles come to lie over the mother's abdomen (the handle of the left blade goes to the right lower abdominal quadrant).

### Rotation in outlet and low forceps operations

To perform an outlet or low forceps delivery, you may need to rotate the fetal head as much as 45 degrees. This small degree of rotation, if you do it properly, adds minimal risk to the procedure. As noted previously, if you keep the handles horizontal and rotate the handles of classic obstetric forceps, the toes of the blades describe a large arc, and severe vaginal lacerations or fetal trauma can result. To rotate the head from an anterior oblique position to a direct OA position, verify that the forceps is applied correctly. Then depress the handles (thus ensuring flexion of the head), and rotate them in a wide arc to accomplish the rotation (Fig. 14.2). Recheck the application before applying traction.

## Forceps in occiput posterior positions

When you need to deliver a fetus in an OP position by forceps, it is usually prudent to deliver the fetus in the direct OP orientation. Rotation to an anterior position can be done with forceps (or, sometimes, manually), but the risk of trauma is considerable, unless you are certain that the pelvic architecture would better accommodate the head as an OA. In most persistent OP presentations the pelvis is android or anthropoid. Prominent ischial spines and a narrow forepelvis in such cases would likely prevent you from rotating the head past the transverse position without damaging it.

As noted, to qualify as an outlet or low forceps procedure, the sagittal suture of the fetal skull must be in (or within 45 degrees of) the anteroposterior diameter of the outlet. This belies the potentially more difficult and dangerous features of the procedure done with the head in an OP position, as compared to an OA position.

Excess risks accrue to OP deliveries for several reasons. The head is more likely to be markedly molded, making correct application of the blades difficult. The leading edge of the molded head may have reached the pelvic floor, but the biparietal diameter may still be quite high in the pelvis. This is so because the head is extended and elongated by much molding. The perineum and the pelvic floor are more likely to be injured. Moreover, the vectors for traction are different and more difficult to master than those for OA positions.

The technique of forceps delivery for the fetal head in an OP position is very similar to that for OA presentations. Apply the forceps as if the head actually were in the anterior position. Note, however, that since the instrument must fit the pelvis, it is actually applied in inverted fashion to the head so that the posterior fontanel is located toward the back of the blades rather than to the front (Fig. 14.6). Moreover, flex-

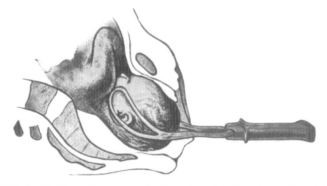

**Figure 14.6** Application of forceps to a head on the pelvic floor in an OP position. The large presenting diameters (compared to OA positions) require more distention of the perineum and delivery by flexion of the head through the pelvic curve.

ion of the head tends to be rather poor in this position, and you will need to correct this before applying traction for the delivery. In addition, since the presenting fetal diameters are larger and the actual plane of the biparietal diameter tends to be higher than in anterior positions, the axis of traction must be lower, i.e., directed more posteriorly than ordinarily. This kind of delivery puts great stress on the perineum and pelvic floor. A large episiotomy is advisable but injury is, nevertheless, common.

## Vacuum extractor

The vacuum extractor, long popular in other parts of the world, has now become the predominant instrument for assisted vaginal delivery in the United States. The technique makes use of a traction cup that is attached to the fetal scalp by applying negative pressure to create a "chignon" of artificial caput succedaneum within the cup. Once the cup is firmly affixed to the scalp in this way, traction can be applied. Sequential traction should be synchronized with uterine contractions and applied in the appropriate pelvic axis to accomplish delivery. During descent, the head undergoes any rotation necessary to accommodate itself optimally to the pelvic dimensions. The direction of traction should, therefore, be changed as appropriate along the pelvic axis.

Vacuum cups in common use today are either soft or rigid, and are 5–7 cm in diameter. The soft cups are bell-shaped and made of a pliable material such as silicone or polyethylene. Rigid cups are also made of disposable plastic material. Both types of cup are suitable for any delivery, but you will find the rigid cups, which do not have a long stem for attachment of the vacuum pump, are easier to apply to the OP-presenting head.

The vacuum can be produced using an electric or a hand pump. Many devices have a hand pump that is integral to the apparatus and easy to use. Often a gauge is included that allows you to know when the correct negative pressure has been applied. A wide variety of instruments is available, and you should familiarize yourself with one or two that you can use regularly.

Vacuum extraction is generally associated with a lower risk of severe perineal and vaginal lacerations than forceps, but the vacuum extractor is more likely to produce fetal scalp injury. Both instruments have the capacity to cause skull and brain trauma if not used properly or if used without appropriate indications.

Indications and contraindications for vacuum extractor delivery are the same as for forceps (Box 14.2), but the vacuum extractor should never be used before 34 weeks' gestation because of the greater risk of injury to the small head. Trauma to the scalp is common, and can take the form of minor abrasions or more serious scalp lacerations, cephalhematomas, and even life-threatening subgaleal hemorrhage. Although even with correct use, instrumental delivery can result in trauma, often (as is the case with forceps) serious fetal or maternal injury from vacuum extraction procedures is caused by improper technique. Persistent attempts at delivery with inappropriately extended periods of traction, improper cup placement, and failure to recognize probable cephalopelvic disproportion all too commonly result in maternal and fetal injury.

Paradoxically, the ease with which this device can be used by the unskilled is perhaps its greatest disadvantage. Forceful traction is too easily substituted for critical study of cephalopelvic relationships, good clinical judgment, and understanding of pathologic labor mechanisms. Thus, some of the trauma reported to result from the use of the vacuum extractor may reflect its use under unfavorable circumstances, perhaps even when operative vaginal delivery should not have been undertaken.

## Application of the vacuum extractor

Before applying the vacuum extractor, perform a thorough examination to verify the position and the station of the head, as well as the presence and degree of molding, caput succedaneum, or asynclitism. Knowledge of all these factors is essential to ensure that you will apply the cup properly, and to help you decide if instrumental delivery is even appropriate. If you do not make a correct assessment, you might apply the vacuum cup at the wrong place on the head. This will make delivery more difficult and increase the risk of fetal trauma.

The mother should be in dorsal lithotomy position. Anesthesia, as for forceps delivery, is required. After ascertaining the position and other characteristics of the head as described above, identify the *flexion point*. This is where you will attach the vacuum cup. The flexion point is about 3 cm anterior to the center of the posterior fontanel in the midline. With the cup centered here, traction will encourage flexion and bring the vertex easily through the curve of the birth canal. Once the cup is in place, verify its position before exerting any traction. The edge should be about 3 cm from the center of the anterior fontanel.

Be careful that no maternal soft tissues, such as cervix or fold of vagina, are included in the cup. Once you are satisfied with placement, create the vacuum gradually over 1–3 minutes. Read the manufacturer's instructions to determine the appropriate vacuum pressure for the device you are using. Generally, this is about 0.6–0.8 kg/cm$^2$ (about 500–600 mmHg).

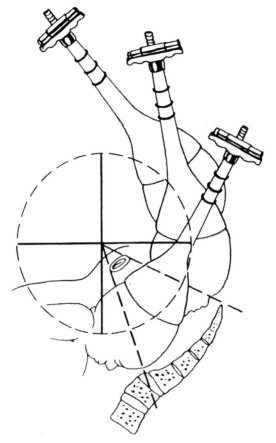

**Figure 14.7** Changes in the required direction of traction as the fetal head descends through the curve of the birth canal. This is demonstrated for the vacuum extractor; the same directional changes are used with forceps. (O'Grady JP, Gimovsky ML, McIlhargie CJ (eds) *Vacuum Extraction in Modern Obstetric Practice*. The Parthenon Publishing Group, New York, 1995: p. 66, fig. III.7.)

Use your dominant hand for traction. Place the other hand on the fetal scalp adjacent to the edge of the cup. This helps to steady the instrument and to identify cup dislodgement early. In addition, it is a useful way to judge progress in descent. Never use rocking motions, and do not attempt to rotate the head by twisting the cup. This can cause serious scalp injury. In any case, if rotation is required for delivery to occur, it will usually develop passively as you pull the head through the pelvis. Be sure you pull in the midline of the pelvis; oblique traction makes the cup more likely to dislodge, and can provoke head injury.

Build the force of your traction in concert with the crescendo of the uterine contraction and relax the force as the contraction subsides. Have

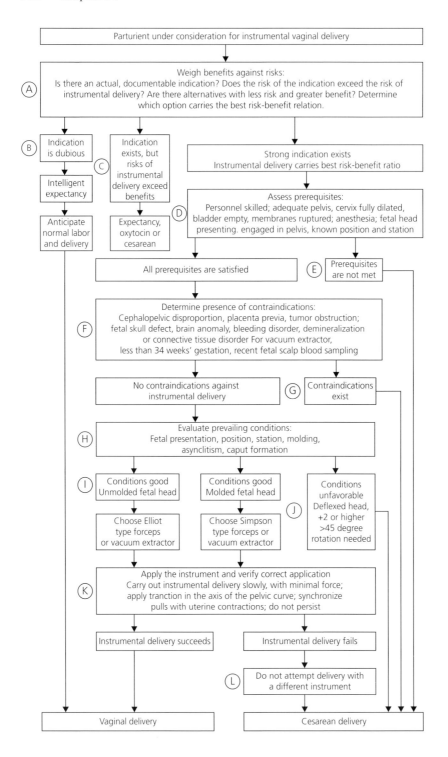

(A) Parturient under consideration for instrumental vaginal delivery

Weigh benefits against risks:
Is there an actual, documentable indication? Does the risk of the indication exceed the risk of instrumental delivery? Are there alternatives with less risk and greater benefit? Determine which option carries the best risk-benefit relation.

(B) Indication is dubious

(C) Indication exists, but risks of instrumental delivery exceed benefits

Strong indication exists
Instrumental delivery carries best risk-benefit ratio

Intelligent expectancy

(D) Assess prerequisites:
Personnel skilled; adequate pelvis, cervix fully dilated, bladder empty, membranes ruptured; anesthesia; fetal head presenting. engaged in pelvis, known position and station

Anticipate normal labor and delivery

Expectancy, oxytocin or cesarean

All prerequisites are satisfied

(E) Prerequisites are not met

(F) Determine presence of contraindications:
Cephalopelvic disproportion, placenta previa, tumor obstruction; fetal skull defect, brain anomaly, bleeding disorder, demineralization or connective tissue disorder For vacuum extractor, less than 34 weeks' gestation, recent fetal scalp blood sampling

No contraindications against instrumental delivery

(G) Contraindications exist

(H) Evaluate prevailing conditions:
Fetal presentation, position, station, molding, asynclitism, caput formation

(I) Conditions good
Unmolded fetal head

Conditions good
Molded fetal head

(J) Conditions unfavorable
Deflexed head, +2 or higher >45 degree rotation needed

Choose Elliot type forceps or vacuum extractor

Choose Simpson type forceps or vacuum extractor

(K) Apply the instrument and verify correct application
Carry out instrumental delivery slowly, with minimal force; apply tranction in the axis of the pelvic curve; synchronize pulls with uterine contractions; do not persist

Instrumental delivery succeeds

Instrumental delivery fails

(L) Do not attempt delivery with a different instrument

Vaginal delivery

Cesarean delivery

**Figure 14.8** Algorithm for using forceps and the vacuum extractor.

**A**. Given the risks inherent in forceps or vacuum extractor delivery, no matter how skilled the operator or how well the procedure is done, ensure that the hazard of the indication for its use outweighs those risks. Evaluate the risk–benefit ratio of alternatives, including expectancy, oxytocin stimulation, or cesarean delivery. Choose the one that carries the least risk and greatest benefit. Document this analysis, share your conclusions with the patient, and obtain her written consent.

**B**. Elective or prophylactic instrumental delivery, i.e., without a medical indication, is not justified because the risks of the procedure, even if small, are greater than the nonexistent risks of not doing it.

**C**. If the risks of instrumental delivery exceed those of the indication, an alternative approach is desirable. If time permits allowing the labor to continue or, if needed, stimulating it with oxytocin is preferable. If there is not enough time to try these conservative measures, cesarean delivery is appropriate.

**D**. If it is clear that instrumental delivery carries the best risk–benefit ratio of available options, next ensure all prerequisites are met. Foremost is the availability of someone with the technical skills to conduct the procedure safely and the knowledge necessary to understand when to proceed—and, when to desist. Other prerequisites include pelvic adequacy, anesthesia, and definitive information about cervical dilatation, fetal station, fetal position, and membrane status.

**E**. If prerequisites are not met, an urgent indication for delivery usually merits cesarean delivery.

**F**. Before embarking on an instrumental delivery, consider any contraindications. Aside from birth canal obstructions, such as overt or suspected disproportion, or cervical fibroids, be alert to fetal skull or brain anomalies, coagulopathies, and genetic demineralization disorders. Prematurity (<34 weeks) and recent fetal scalp blood sampling interdict use of the vacuum extractor.

**G**. If contraindications against the use of instruments for delivery exist, vaginal delivery by any means may also be contraindicated. If so, proceed with cesarean delivery. Alternatively, if unaided vaginal delivery is acceptable and time permits, consider either expectancy or uterotonic stimulation with oxytocin.

**H**. Having satisfied the need to ensure a favorable risk–benefit ratio, compliance with all prerequisites, and the absence of contraindications, do a final check to ensure conditions are optimal for proceeding with delivery. If you plan to use forceps and the fetal head is molded, it requires a forceps blade with a tapered cephalic curve (Simpson-type) if unmolded, the rounded head is best served by forceps with a rounded cephalic curve (Elliot-type).

**I**. If conditions are favorable for instrumental delivery—i.e., the head is well flexed and below station +2 and the occiput is within 45 degrees of the direct anterior position, apply the instrument.

**J**. If these conditions are unmet, difficult and potentially traumatic, reconsider other options. Unless you have the requisite skills and experience, and there are overriding, pressing reasons to proceed, prudence dictates cesarean as a safer choice.

**K**. Apply the instrument. Apply traction gently, pulling synchronously with uterine contractions. In the absence of contractions, apply traction to simulate their timing. Pull in the axis of the birth canal, i.e., directed more posteriorly with a relatively high head, changing the direction as the head advances. For vacuum extractor delivery, do not angulate the direction of your traction or rotate the cup; limit the number and duration of pulls. For any instrument, if no advance is perceived, do not increase the force you apply and do not persist. Proceed instead with cesarean delivery.

**L**. If the instrument you have chosen does not effect descent and delivery, do not think that a different instrument will be more successful. Using it exposes mother and fetus to trauma without benefit.

the mother bear down during these efforts. Increase traction smoothly and gradually; jerking the cup may displace or dislodge it. The direction of your pulls should mimic the expected progress of the head along the curve of the pelvic axis. As with forceps, higher stations require the direction of pull to be more steeply posterior (Fig. 14.7).

In general, if the cup dislodges three times, or if more than four or five pulling efforts are required, you should abandon further attempts at vacuum extractor delivery. Do not assume that dislodgement of the cup from the head is a built-in safety mechanism. Injury can occur prior to the cup separating from the scalp.

## Trial of instrumental delivery

In a sense, you should consider every attempt at instrumental delivery to be a trial of forceps or vacuum extractor. Low and outlet instrumental deliveries are generally safe if you have chosen appropriate candidates and you use the instruments gently and skillfully. Unfortunately, it is difficult to judge when you are applying excessive force, and that force may vary considerably according to circumstances. Never allow your pride and earnest desire to effect vaginal delivery to cloud your good sense. If a procedure does not progress smoothly and without incident, abandon it and move to an alternative course of action. A suggested approach to instrumental delivery is described in Fig. 14.8.

Sequential use of vacuum extractor and forceps is generally to be decried. It is specious to assume that if one type of instrument proved inadequate for delivery, subsequent use of the other will be effective. Under most circumstances, your inability to deliver suggests that a degree of cephalopelvic disproportion exists that would make further attempts at instrumental delivery hazardous. In fact, the sequential use of vacuum extractor and forceps increases the chances of fetal injury substantially. Combining the two procedures can be justified only in rare circumstances. Cesarean delivery with the head at a very low station can be difficult, and is not without its own risks and complications, but it is almost always a better option from the perspective of safety after cautious efforts to effect vaginal delivery by forceps or vacuum extractor have failed.

## Key points

- Use of instruments to aid vaginal delivery requires knowledge about indications, contraindications, and prerequisites as well as technical skills acquired by training and experience.

- Before undertaking an instrumental vaginal delivery, analyze the risks and the benefits of using them in a given case. Compare those with the risks and the benefits of alternative approaches; these may include allowing the labor to continue as is, stimulating the labor with oxytocin or proceeding with cesarean delivery.
- Document the details of this analysis and add critical information pertaining to the conditions prevailing at the time the instrument is applied, such as indication, fetal position, station, molding, asynclitism, and caput formation.
- Include a statement to verify that the gravida understands the conclusions of the risk–benefit assessment and consents to the procedure.
- Recognize that two major variants of classic forceps are designed for different applications: Simpson types are intended for molded fetal heads by virtue of their tapered cephalic curve, while Elliot types are meant for unmolded heads because of their rounded cephalic curve. Choose accordingly in any given case.
- Understand the important differences in the type of instrumental procedure you are contemplating (i.e., outlet, low, and midpelvic applications) and the risks associated with each. Be particularly aware that the higher the fetal station and the more rotation required to achieve an optimal occiput anterior position, the greater the risk of fetal and maternal trauma will be.
- There is no place in safe obstetric practice today for purely elective or prophylactic instrumental delivery. Intelligent expectancy is preferable in the absence of an objectively justifiable indication to counterbalance known risks.
- Limit the use of forceps and vacuum extractor to conditions in which the benefits clearly outweigh the risks. Such indications include an acute fetal hypoxic event or a maternal problem that mandates prompt delivery, provided the vaginal delivery is likely to be accomplished safely.
- Prerequisites for applying instruments to effect vaginal delivery include personnel with the necessary knowledge and skills; a gravida with an adequate pelvis, cervix fully dilated, ruptured membranes, an empty bladder; anesthesia; and a fetus in cephalic presentation with engaged head and precisely known position and station.
- Always use minimal force when performing an instrumental delivery, extracting the fetal head by slow, gentle traction and rotation, pulling synchronously with uterine contractions (or mimicking them when they are not present). Direct your traction along the trajectory of the pelvic curve.
- While the risks of the vacuum extractor are somewhat less than those of forceps, it is not harm-free. Its use, therefore, requires the same knowledge and skills as the use of forceps for vaginal delivery.
- The risks of vaginal delivery by vacuum extractor can be reduced, but not entirely eliminated, by avoiding excessive force, pulling for long periods, applying traction that is not directed along the pelvic curve,

rotating the instrument, and placing it improperly. Be especially careful not to use the vacuum extractor if vaginal delivery is contraindicated, such as when there is evidence of disproportion.

• If one instrument fails to achieve vaginal delivery, do not consider using another because it is unlikely to succeed. Doing so exposes mother and fetus to substantial risk with no discernible benefit.

## Further Reading

### Books and reviews

American College of Obstetricians and Gynecologists. Operative vaginal delivery. ACOG Practice Bulletin 17. Washington, DC, ACOG, 2000.

Danforth DN , Ellis AH. Midforceps delivery – a vanishing art? Am J Obstet Gynecol 1963;86:29–37.

Hopp H, Husslein P. Instrumental Delivery. In: Kurjak A, Chervenak FA (eds) *Textbook of Perinatology, Second Edition*. Informa, London, 2006:1888–98.

Johanson RB, Menon BKV. Vacuum extraction versus forceps for assisted vaginal delivery. Cochrane Library 2000;2:1–7.

Miksovsky P, Watson WJ. Obstetric vacuum extraction: state of the art in the new millennium. Obstet Gynecol Surv 2001;56:736–51.

O'Grady JP. Instrumental delivery. In: O'Grady JP, Gimovsky ML (eds) *Operative Obstetrics*, 2nd edition. Cambridge University Press, New York, 2008:455–508.

Yeomans ER. Operative vaginal delivery. Obstet Gynecol 2010;115:645–53.

### Primary sources

Bofill JA, Rust OA, Schorr SJ, Brown RC, Martin RW, Martin JN, et al. A randomized prospective trial of the obstetric forceps versus the M-cup vacuum extractor. Am J Obstet Gynecol 1996;175:1325–30.

Castillo M, Fordham LA. MR of neurologically symptomatic newborns after vacuum extractor delivery. Am J Neuroradiol 1995;16(Suppl):816–8.

Demissie K, Rhoads GG, Smulian JC, Balasubramanian BA, Gandhi K, Joseph KS, Kramer M. Operative vaginal delivery and neonatal and infant adverse outcomes: population based retrospective analysis. BMJ 2004;329:24–9.

Friedman EA, Sachtleben MR, Bresky PA. Dysfunctional labor XII: long-term effects on infant. Am J Obstet Gynecol 1977;127:779–83.

Friedman EA. Patterns of labor as indicators of risk. Clin Obstet Gynecol;1973;16: 172–83.

Huang LT, Lui CC. Tentorial hemorrhage associated with vacuum extraction in a newborn. Pediatr Radiol 1995;25(Suppl 1):S230–2.

Ngan HY, Min P, Ko L, Ma HK. Long-term neurological sequelae following vacuum extractor delivery. Aust NZ J Obstet Gynaecol 1990;30:111–14.

Towner D, Castro MA, Eby-Wilkens E, Gilbert WM. Effect of mode of delivery in nulliparous women on neonatal intracranial injury. N Engl J Med 1999;341:1709–14.

Yancey MK, Herpolsheimer A, Jordan GD, Benson WL, Brady K. Maternal and neonatal effects of outlet forceps delivery compared with spontaneous vaginal delivery in term pregnancies Obstet Gynecol 1991;78:646–50.

# CHAPTER 15

# Obstetric Case Studies

This chapter contains 30 case studies. Each is presented to emphasize aspects of clinical management of labor that we have addressed in this book. Each case is followed by one or more questions. Choose what you feel would be the best response or responses in the circumstances provided.

You can verify your answers on pages 338–53. The answers reference the chapter in which relevant information can be found in the text.

In each case, make the following assumptions, unless otherwise stated: (1) the pregnancy is at term; (2) fetal oxygenation, as measured by fetal heart rate monitoring or other techniques, is normal; (3) the parturient has no medical problems that would alter management of labor or delivery other than those described in the presentation; (4) no medications have been administered, except as stated; (5) cesarean delivery can be accomplished within less than 30 minutes.

## Case 1

A woman who had three previous vaginal deliveries at term begins labor at 15:00 (hour 0). Her contractions are moderately strong, and are occurring every 3–5 minutes when you examine her at 18:00 (3rd hour of labor). You find the cervix to be thick and nearly closed. Spontaneous rupture of membranes occurred two days previously. She reports no fever, but her temperature on admission is 100.2 °F. The uterus is not tender. Her general physical examination and history reveal no source for the fever. At 23:00 (hour 8), the cervix is 2 cm dilated, soft, and 0.5 cm long (80–90% effaced). Maternal temperature is unchanged. At 05:00

*Labor and Delivery Care: A Practical Guide*, First Edition. Wayne R. Cohen and Emanuel A. Friedman. © 2011 John Wiley & Sons, Ltd. Published 2011 by John Wiley & Sons, Ltd

(hour 14), the cervix is 3 cm dilated, and prolonged latent phase is diagnosed. The patient is exhausted and frustrated after many hours of labor and little change in cervical dilatation. You prescribe therapeutic rest, and give a dose of meperidine, 150 mg intramuscularly.

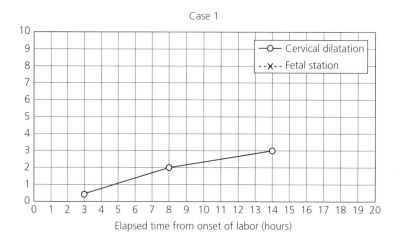

Case 1

## Question
Your treatment for prolonged latent phase:

**A** Is appropriate, especially given the patient's physical and emotional strain
**B** Should not have been instituted until 20 hours had elapsed in the latent phase
**C** Is likely to result in neonatal respiratory depression
**D** Should have instead been oxytocin administration

## Case 2

A 40-year-old primigravida begins to have regular uterine contractions at 08:00 (hour 0). You examine her at 12:00 (hour 4) and find a longitudinal lie with a cephalic presentation. The cervix is 4 cm dilated and very thin. The fetal head is at station –1. You estimate the fetal weight to be 3900 g. The ischial spines are not prominent, the sacral curve is deep, the sacrosciatic notch is wide, and the pelvic sidewalls are parallel. At 14:00 (hour 6), you find the cervix to be fully dilated. The head is at station 0, well flexed in an ROA position. You encourage her to begin bearing-down efforts. Two hours later, at 16:00 (hour 8), the vertex has reached station +3. There is moderate caput succedaneum formation and molding.

Case 2

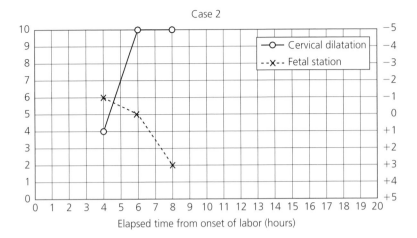

Elapsed time from onset of labor (hours)

## Question

What would be the best option at this time?

**A** Recommend cesarean delivery for protracted descent with cephalo-pelvic disproportion

**B** Allow the second stage to continue, because progress thus far is normal

**C** Recommend vacuum-assisted delivery because spontaneous delivery is not imminent after 2 hours in the second stage

**D** Recommend cesarean delivery because spontaneous delivery is not imminent after 2 hours in the second stage, and instrumental delivery would be too risky

## Case 3

You initiate induction of labor in a multipara at 39 weeks of gestation because she presented with a history of having ruptured her membranes spontaneously 36 hours previously. She had three prior vaginal deliveries. The most recent was done by vacuum extraction 3 years ago. A shoulder dystocia occurred in a 4250 g fetus, but there was no neurologic injury. During the last 3 years your patient has gained considerable weight, and her body mass index now is 34.6 kg/m$^2$. On abdominal examination you find a cephalic presentation with half of the fetal head palpable suprapubically. You estimate the fetal weight to be 4000 g. Vaginal examination when oxytocin infusion is begun at 08:00 (hour 0) reveals a cervix 2–3 cm dilated with the vertex palpable at station –1. She is afebrile and has a normal white blood cell count. At 13:00 (hour 5), the cervix is 8–9 cm dilated. The fetal head is at station –1 in a LOT position. At 15:00 (hour 7), only a thin rim of cervix remains. Firm contractions recur every 2–3 minutes. Station and position are –1 and LOT. At 16:30 (hour 8.5), the cervix becomes fully dilated, and at 18:30 (hour 10.5), the fetal head is crowning.

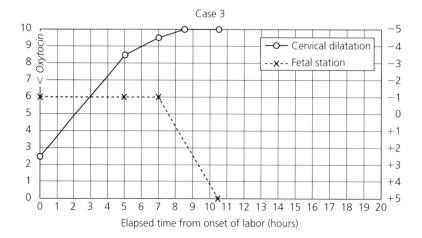

Case 3

Elapsed time from onset of labor (hours)

## Questions

1  How would you characterize labor progress at the time of your 15:00 (hour 7) examination?
   **A** Normal
   **B** Protracted active phase
   **C** Failure of descent
   **D** Prolonged deceleration phase

2  What should you do therapeutically at 15:00 (hour 7)?
   **A** Continue to observe for the development of dysfunctional labor
   **B** Push the rim of cervix over the fetal head and have the patient begin bearing down
   **C** Increase the oxytocin infusion rate
   **D** Recommend cesarean delivery

## Case 4

The vaginal delivery in Case 3 (see above) was complicated by shoulder dystocia. The head emerges very slowly at 19:10 (hour 11.2) in the OA position and, after it delivered spontaneously, it seems to be fixed at the perineum in that position.

### Question

What should you have done next?
   **A** Apply gentle downward traction to the head to bring the anterior shoulder beneath the pubic symphysis
   **B** Call for help

**C** Acutely flex the mother's hips against her abdomen and exhort her to bear down forcefully

**D** Assess the orientation of the shoulders and the degree of descent of the posterior shoulder

## Case 5

You have been providing prenatal care to a 21-year-old primipara (secundigravida) whose first pregnancy was terminated by cesarean delivery in a rural area of the developing world. You have not been able to obtain the records of that procedure from the hospital where it was done. The patient recalls that her midwife had to call a surgeon for assistance when delivery had not occurred after 24 hours of labor. Your patient has a vertical skin incision. She would like to deliver this baby vaginally.

### Question
What should you recommend?

**A** A trial of labor is always advisable, even though the type of the uterine scar is unknown

**B** A trial of labor is never allowable when the type of uterine scar is unknown

**C** Because her cesarean may have been done by a general surgeon in a remote region, there is a substantial likelihood it was a classical cesarean. Inform her of the associated risks and benefits of a trial of labor in this circumstance and arrive at a joint decision

**D** Induction of labor at 36–37 weeks

## Case 6

A multipara who had three previous uncomplicated term vaginal deliveries begins to have regular uterine contractions at 21:00 (hour 0) on her estimated date of delivery. She arrives at the hospital at 02:00 (hour 5). Your evaluation reveals a lean woman. You can barely palpate part of the fetal head above the symphysis pubis on the same side as the fetal back, which is on the mother's left. Fetal small parts are felt on the right. Estimated fetal weight is 2900 g. On vaginal examination, you find the cervix 9 cm dilated and completely effaced. The presenting part feels firm, but lumpy. During your examination, a contraction occurs and the cervix retracts around the presenting part to attain full dilatation. You now can feel the fetal orbits and chin, confirming your suspicion of a face presentation. It is in a left mentum anterior position at station +2.

## Question

What should you do next?

  **A**  Prepare for immediate cesarean delivery
  **B**  Anticipate spontaneous vaginal delivery
  **C**  Manually flex the head to convert to a vertex presentation
  **D**  Summon a pediatrician to be present at delivery

## Case 7

A 38-year-old multipara (Gravida 3 Para 2002) presents in labor at 06:00
(hour 6), about 6 hours after onset of strong uterine contractions. Her children had birth weights of 3000 g and 3400 g and were born after uncomplicated labors. Your evaluation reveals a body mass index of 45 kg/m².
The pelvis has a diagonal conjugate measurement of 14 cm. The ischial
spines are prominent, and the sacrum is long and deeply curved. Your
estimated fetal weight is 3500 g. The fetal head is at station –2. The cervix
is 3 cm dilated and about 1 cm long (70% effaced). At noon (hour 12),
it is unchanged. Uterine contractions are occurring every 3–4 minutes. At
14:00 (hour 14), the cervix is 7 cm dilated and 0.5 cm in length (80–90%
effaced). You find the head to be in direct OP position, at station –2.
At 16:00 (hour 16), cervical dilatation and fetal station are unchanged.

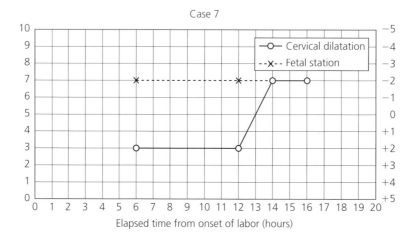

## Question

At this time, the labor pattern is most consistent with the diagnosis of:

  **A**  Arrest of dilatation
  **B**  Arrest of dilatation and arrest of descent
  **C**  Failure of descent
  **D**  Normal labor

## Case 8

A 19-year-old nullipara begins to have regular uterine contractions at 22:00 (hour 0). She is admitted to the hospital 6 hours (hour 6) later with strong contractions occurring every 2–3 minutes. You find a cephalic presentation with less than half of the fetal head palpable above the symphysis. The cervix is 2 cm dilated and very thin. The fetal head is at station 0. The patient is having severe pain with her contractions and is having trouble coping with her discomfort. You confer with an anesthesiologist, and your patient is given an epidural block using dilute bupivacaine beginning at 05:00 (hour 7). Within 30 minutes she is feeling only mild pressure during her contractions. Testing shows a level of anesthesia at the eighth thoracic dermatome level. At 12:00 (hour 14), there is no change in cervical dilatation or fetal station. Contractions are occurring every 4–5 minutes.

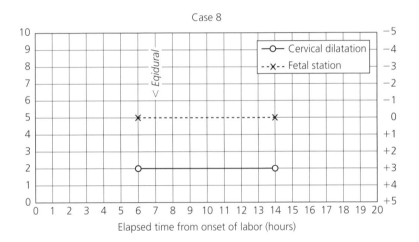

Case 8

Elapsed time from onset of labor (hours)

### Questions

1 How would you characterize her labor progress at 12:00?
   **A** Normal
   **B** Prolonged latent phase
   **C** Protracted active phase
   **D** Failure of descent
2 What should be done?
   **A** Recommend cesarean delivery
   **B** Continue to observe and maintain the epidural level
   **C** Administer an oxytocin infusion
   **D** Allow the epidural block to partially abate

# Case 9

A very thin, 34-year-old nulliparous woman is admitted in early labor at 16:00 (hour 8). Regular contractions began 8 hours previously, and are now quite strong, recurring every 2–3 minutes. The fetus is in cephalic presentation. You can feel most of the head above the pelvis, and you think you can identify the forehead or chin through the abdominal wall. You find the fetal shoulder quite lateral to the mother's midline. Estimated fetal weight is 4100 g. The cervix is 5 cm dilated, and is not well applied to the fetal head, which is at station −3. With some difficulty you can reach the fetal head with your intravaginal fingers and you are able to feel both fontanels. The position is ROP.

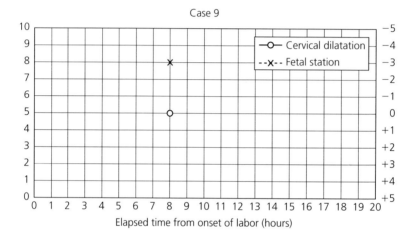

Case 9

## Questions

**1** How would you characterize the labor at this initial evaluation?
   **A** Normal
   **B** Failure of descent
   **C** It is indeterminate
   **D** Arrest of dilatation

**2** What is the significance of feeling both fontanels?
   **A** It confirms the head position is OP
   **B** It demonstrates the head is deflexed
   **C** It suggests a cranial malformation is present
   **D** It indicates that atraumatic vaginal delivery is unlikely

**3** What should be done?
   **A** Observe and reexamine in 1–2 hours
   **B** Cesarean delivery for arrest of dilatation
   **C** Administer oxytocin
   **D** Undertake clinical pelvimetry

## Case 10

A patient comes to you for a second opinion regarding vaginal birth after cesarean (VBAC). Her obstetrician has informed her that she is not an appropriate candidate for an attempt at VBAC. Her first pregnancy was terminated by low transverse cesarean section at 37 weeks in active phase labor because a breech presentation was diagnosed. Her second pregnancy was uncomplicated and she underwent repeat cesarean delivery prior to labor at 39 weeks of gestation. Her current (third) pregnancy has reached 20 weeks and has been uncomplicated.

### Question
You should advise her that:
  **A** You agree with her physician. Attempting VBAC with two previous cesarean deliveries is too risky. She should have another repeat cesarean at term
  **B** The success rate for attempts at VBAC after two prior cesarean deliveries is similar to that of women with one prior cesarean, and that she should attempt VBAC if she wishes
  **C** It would be in the best interests of all concerned (her, the fetus, the obstetrician, and the hospital) if she had a repeat cesarean at 39 weeks
  **D** A trial of labor is reasonable, but only if it is conducted in a tertiary care center

## Case 11

A 37-year-old Gravida 3 Para 2002 arrives for evaluation at 41 weeks of gestation, early in the latent phase of labor. Her obstetric history included two spontaneous vaginal deliveries. Records are not available, but she says that both pregnancies were uncomplicated. Birth weights were 4100 g and 4240 g. Both children are currently healthy. From the mother's description, you infer that both previous babies may have had a transient brachial plexus neuropraxis that lasted for about 1 week after delivery and resolved completely.

During the current pregnancy the 50 g glucose challenge test result was 145 mg/dL. The oral glucose tolerance test was normal. The mother's body mass index is 45 kg/m². She has gained 25 kg during this pregnancy.

Contractions are mild and occur every 10 minutes. You find the fetus in cephalic presentation with the head at station −1. The cervix is 4 cm dilated and 1 cm long (70% effaced). The fetal position is OP. You feel the pelvis is capacious, but the symphysis is quite long, and the sacrum is flattened and somewhat anterior. Physical examination reveals an estimated fetal weight of 4000 g.

## Question

What should you do?

**A** Offer the patient cesarean delivery now to avoid the risk of brachial plexus injury

**B** Stimulate with oxytocin to shorten the latent phase and expedite delivery

**C** Allow spontaneous labor to evolve

**D** Get a more accurate estimated fetal weight by ultrasonography before making a management decision

## Case 12

The patient from Case 11 does not want a cesarean. She prefers to undergo labor and "see what happens." The evolution of labor progress is depicted in the figure. The cervix became fully dilated 1 hour ago (hour 12). The fetal skull has reached station +2. The position is LOP. She has had no anesthesia or analgesia and is coping well with the pain from her contractions.

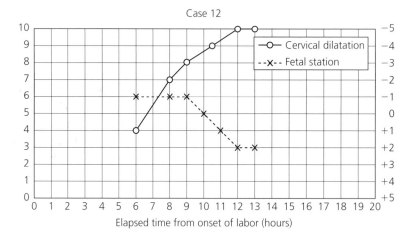

Case 12

## Question

What would be the best management at this time?

**A** Continue to observe the labor, as progress has been normal thus far

**B** Administer oxytocin to treat dysfunctional labor

**C** Urge your patient to undergo cesarean delivery now

**D** Proceed with low forceps delivery to prevent further risks during labor

## Case 13

A 40-year-old Gravida 1 Para 0 is admitted for induction of labor because the gestational age is 41.5 weeks. Her prenatal care was uncomplicated. She has a body mass index of 26.2 kg/m². Estimated fetal weight is 3500 g. Presentation is cephalic. Your abdominal examination suggests a posterior position of the occiput. The cervix is 2 cm dilated and uneffaced. The fetal head is at station −1. The pelvis has a large anteroposterior dimension relative to its transverse diameter, and the pubic symphysis is long and steeply inclined. The sacral excavation is flat.

Oxytocin is begun at 08:00 (hour 0). Examination at 12:00 (hour 4) shows no change in dilatation or station. At 16:00 (hour 8),the cervix is 3 cm dilated. At 20:00 (hour 12), dilatation is 4 cm, cervical length 1 cm (70% effaced), and the station still −1. At 20:00, a decision for cesarean delivery is made. The indications are failed induction of labor and failure of descent.

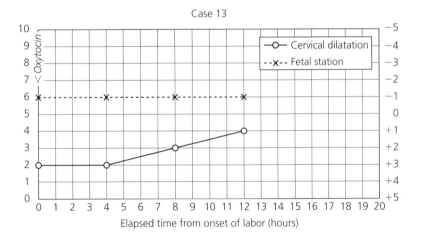

Case 13

Elapsed time from onset of labor (hours)

**Question**

How would you characterize the progress of labor at 20:00?

**A** Abnormal dilatation and descent

**B** Abnormal dilatation, normal descent

**C** Normal dilatation, abnormal descent

**D** Normal dilatation and descent

## Case 14

A multipara with four previous vaginal deliveries arrives at 03:00 (hour 3) in labor. She has been having regular uterine contractions every 4–5 minutes since midnight (hour 0). The cervix is 2–3 cm dilated, 1 cm long (70% effaced), and the fetal head is at station −2. At 09:00 (hour 9), the cervix is 3 cm dilated. At 10:30 (hour 10.5), its dilatation is unchanged, and it is about 3 mm long (90–95% effaced). The head remains at station −2. Membranes are intact. Contractions continue to be moderate in intensity and recur every 4 minutes. Oxytocin infusion is ordered.

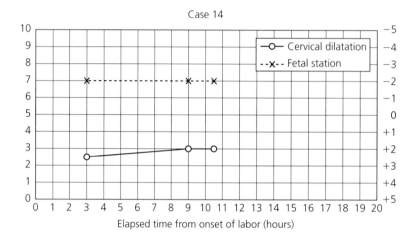

Case 14

Elapsed time from onset of labor (hours)

### Question
Which is correct?
  **A** Oxytocin is indicated to treat prolonged latent phase
  **B** There is an arrest of descent
  **C** The labor is normal
  **D** There is an arrest of dilatation

## Case 15

A healthy 32-year-old is in labor at 39 weeks in her first pregnancy. The estimated fetal weight is 3900 g. The first stage of labor was normal. She has had no analgesia or anesthesia. Full dilatation occurred at 17:00

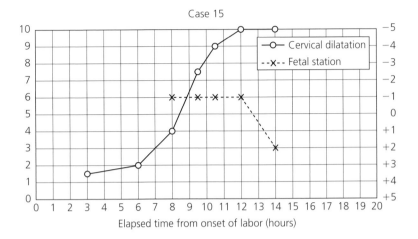

Case 15

(hour 12) with the fetal head at station −1. At 19:00 (hour 14), the station is +2; fetal position is ROP.

### Question
What should you do?
  **A** Recommend cesarean delivery because the second stage is 2 hours long and delivery is not imminent
  **B** Administer oxytocin because there is a malposition and the progress of descent is protracted
  **C** Allow the labor to continue its spontaneous evolution because it is normal
  **D** Offer the option of vacuum delivery

## Case 16

A primigravida at 41 weeks of gestation arrives in the labor and delivery unit at 00:15 (hour 6), having been in labor for about 6 hours. The cervix is 8–9 cm dilated. The head is direct OP position, station 0. Another person provided prenatal care, and she indicated in the chart that the pelvis is "adequate for a 3600 g baby." Your estimated fetal weight is 3500 g. At 02:00 (hour 7.8) there is just a rim of cervix, and at 03:30 (hour 9.2) just a thin anterior lip of cervix remains. The leading edge of the skull is at station 0. There is a large amount of caput formation and moderate molding. The pelvis has prominent ischial spines and an anteriorly inclined flat sacral surface. A Müller-Hillis maneuver creates no descent or rotation of the head.

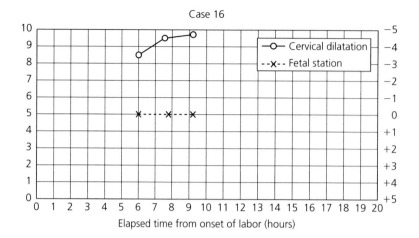

Case 16

Elapsed time from onset of labor (hours)

## Question
Which is a reasonable management option?
  **A** Push the remaining lip of cervix over the head and continue observation
  **B** Recommend a cesarean for failure of descent
  **C** Rotate the head manually to OA
  **D** Administer oxytocin

## Case 17

A multipara with two previous uncomplicated cesarean deliveries presents in advanced labor in her third pregnancy, during which she has had no prenatal care. Within 20 minutes of arrival she has a normal spontaneous delivery of a healthy neonate. Fifteen minutes after delivery there is only a small amount of vaginal bleeding. The placenta has not delivered despite oxytocin administration and uterine massage. You gingerly insert two fingers into the uterus and palpate the edge of the placenta on the lower anterior uterine wall.

## Question
What should you do?
  **A** Type and cross-match blood
  **B** Attempt a Brandt maneuver to deliver the placenta
  **C** Wait another 15 minutes and, if the placenta has not delivered, do a manual removal
  **D** Inject 10 units of oxytocin diluted in 10 mL of saline into the umbilical vein

## Case 18

A 25-year-old primipara arrives in labor at 01:00 (hour 5), 5 hours after the onset of regular uterine contractions. Two years previously she uneventfully delivered a 4520 g baby after a short labor. The current pregnancy has been unremarkable, and testing for diabetes mellitus was negative. Maternal weight gain was 12 kg, and her body mass index is 28.5 kg/m². Your estimated fetal weight is 4500 g. The pelvis seems capacious, with gynecoid features. The cervix is 2–3 cm dilated and the presenting vertex at station −1. At 02:30 (hour 6.5), she complains of severe pelvic pressure. Examination reveals the cervix to be 8 cm dilated, with the vertex at station 0. The fetal position is ROT. The patient is very uncomfortable and requests epidural anesthesia. This is provided, and a good sensory block is in place by 03:30. At that time (hour 7.5), the cervix is 9 cm dilated, and the head has descended to station +1. Throughout the labor, her contractions have been strong and regular at 2- to 3-minute intervals. At 04:30 (hour 8.5), the cervix is still 9 cm dilated, and is becoming edematous. At 06:30 (hour 10.5), the cervix is fully dilated and the vertex at station +3. Despite strong expulsive efforts by the mother, there is no descent after 3 hours of second stage (hour 13.5). There is so much caput and molding that fetal position can no longer be determined from the orientation of the cranial sutures. The vacuum extractor is applied, and delivery of the head accomplished after 15 minutes (hour 13.8) of steady traction. A shoulder dystocia occurs, and is resolved after 4 minutes by delivering the posterior arm of the fetus after other maneuvers failed. The baby had an Erb palsy and a fractured humerus. Birth weight is 5489 g.

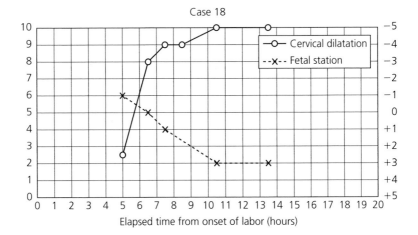

Case 18

## Questions

1 What labor abnormalities were present in this case?
 **A** Prolonged deceleration phase
 **B** Protracted descent
 **C** Arrest of descent
 **D** Failure of descent

2 What features of the instrumental delivery were inappropriate?
 **A** The vacuum was applied without knowledge of the fetal position
 **B** Sustained traction over 15 minutes was potentially hazardous
 **C** Instrumental delivery in the wake of several antecedent labor dysfunctions is contraindicated because of the high risk of associated trauma and of shoulder dystocia
 **D** Forceps would have been a better choice of instrument

## Case 19

A 24-year-old nullipara just delivered a 3750 g fetus and suffered a midline perineal laceration that traversed the anal sphincters and created a 3 cm longitudinal tear in the wall of the anal canal beginning at the anal verge.

## Question

Which is true of the repair?
 **A** The internal and external anal sphincters should each be reapproximated
 **B** A tear in this location cannot involve the internal sphincter
 **C** This laceration will not affect the patient's future continence
 **D** Nonabsorbable suture should be used to repair the laceration

## Case 20

You admit a 31-year-old nullipara in the latent phase of labor at 09:00 (hour 9). Regular uterine contractions had awakened her at midnight (hour 0). She is obese (body mass index 40 kg/m²) and has gestational diabetes mellitus, controlled with insulin. Your estimate of fetal weight is 3800 g. The cervix is 3 cm dilated and the fetal head is at station −1. At 12:30 (hour 12.5), the cervix has advanced to 7 cm dilatation, and 2 hours later (hour 14.5) is unchanged. A diagnosis of arrest of dilatation is made. Clinical cephalopelvimetry reveals the head to be in direct OP position with minimal molding. The sacrum is flat and directed more anteriorly than normal. Oxytocin infusion is begun at 14:45 (hour 14.8). Within 20 minutes, strong contractions are occurring every 2 minutes. At 18:30 (hour 18.5), the cervix is found to be still 7 cm dilated and the fetal head at station −1.

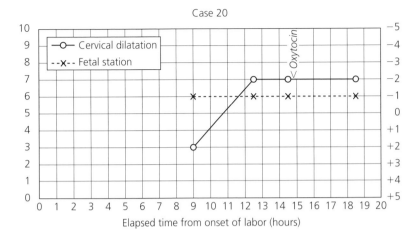

Case 20

Elapsed time from onset of labor (hours)

## Question

What should you do?

  **A** Continue oxytocin infusion

  **B** Recommend cesarean delivery

  **C** Perform artificial rupture of the membranes

  **D** Administer narcotics for therapeutic rest

## Case 21

You first examine a lean, 42-year-old nullipara at 03:00 (hour 8) after she has been in labor for 8 hours. Contractions are moderate in strength and occur every 5 minutes. The cervix is 3 cm dilated and 1 cm long (70% effaced). At 05:00 (hour 10), the cervix has reached 4 cm in dilatation. At 07:00 (hour 12), dilatation is 5 cm, and the cervix is 0.5 cm (80–90% effaced) in length. The fetal head is at station −1. An epidural catheter is placed, and a dose of bupivacaine and sufentanil is administered through it. Good pain relief follows, with a tenth thoracic dermatome level of analgesia. At 09:00 (hour 14), the cervix is 6 cm dilated and completely effaced; at 10:00 (hour 15), full cervical dilatation is reached, with the fetal head at station 0 and in LOA position. At 11:00 (hour 16) and at 12:00 (hour 17), the station is +3. The fetal head has a mild degree of caput and moderate molding of the cranial plates. The position remains LOA. Contractions are firm, and occur every 3 minutes. The pelvis has prominent ischial spines, parallel sidewalls, and a somewhat narrow sub-pubic arch. You perform a Müller-Hillis maneuver at the peak of a contraction. During the maneuver the head rotates to OA, and descends about a centimeter.

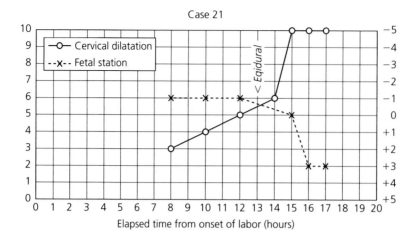

Case 21

Elapsed time from onset of labor (hours)

## Questions

**1** How would you characterize the labor progression?

   **A** Normal

   **B** Protracted active phase

   **C** Arrest of descent

   **D** Prolonged latent phase

**2** What would you do at this point?

   **A** Recommend cesarean delivery

   **B** Apply the vacuum extractor and deliver the fetus

   **C** Administer oxytocin

   **D** Manually rotate the head to OA.

# Case 22

You admit a 39-year-old nullipara at 22:00 (hour 4), 4 hours after the onset of regular uterine contractions. On admission the cervix is a fingertip dilated and very thin. The fetus is in a cephalic presentation at station +1. Contractions occur every 4–5 minutes. During the next 4 hours (hour 8), contractions gradually increase in frequency and intensity. The cervix is now 1 cm dilated and the fetal head is at station 0. The position is ROT, based on your abdominal examination. At 03:30 (hour 9.5), the cervix is 3 cm dilated, and the head at station 0. You administer 50 mg meperidine intravenously because she is quite uncomfortable and requests pain relief. Subsequent examinations done at 04:30, 05:30 and 07:00 (hours 10.5, 11.5 and 13) found the cervix to be 4, 5, and 7 cm dilated, respectively. At 06:30, you per- form amniotomy in the hope that it will speed cervical dilatation. At 08:00 (hour 14), the cervix is 8–9 cm dilated, and the head is between +1 and +2 station. You give another dose of meperidine. At 08:30 (hour 14.5), the station is +2, and the head remains ROT. At 09:30 (hour 15.5, the head has reached +3 when the cervix attains full dilatation. A third dose of meperidine is given. At 11:45 (hour 17.8), the head has reached station +4, is in ROP position, and has marked cranial molding and caput formation. Because the second stage has lasted 2 hours, and your patient is exhausted from a long labor, you decide to apply the vacuum extractor. You deliver a 3900 g baby with Apgar scores of 6 and 7 at 1 and 5 minutes, respectively. The baby has a large subgaleal hemorrhage that resulted in hyperbilirubinemia and the need for transfusion. The mother has a deep vaginal sulcus laceration that requires repair. Her estimated blood loss for the delivery was 800 mL.

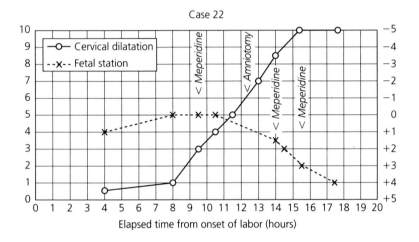

Case 22

### Questions
1 How would you characterize the patient's labor progress?
  A Normal
  B Failure to progress
  C Arrest of dilatation and arrest of descent
  D Protracted active phase and protracted descent
2 How should the patient's labor have been managed differently?
  A It required no different management
  B She should have received oxytocin to enhance dilatational progress
  C Epidural anesthesia should have been given for pain relief
  D The second stage should have been allowed to continue

## Case 23

A 33-year-old primipara's previous delivery was done by outlet forceps after a long labor. Her current pregnancy has been uncomplicated, and she is awakened with the onset of regular uterine contractions at 04:00 (hour 0). Spontaneous rupture of membranes occurred 1 hour later. You examine her at noon (hour 8). Her body mass index is 28 kg/m². On abdominal examination, you feel the fetus in a cephalic presentation with the head floating over the inlet. The cervix is 3 cm dilated, soft, and about 0.5 cm long (70% effaced). The head is at station −3. The pelvis has a light bony structure, with flat ischial spines, an average size sacrosciatic notch, and parallel sidewalls. The subpubic arch is wide. At 14:00 (hour 10), the cervix has dilated to 6 cm and is completely effaced. The head is at station −2, and you determine it is in a direct OP position. There is minimal molding and caput formation. At 16:00 (hour 12), the cervical examination is unchanged.

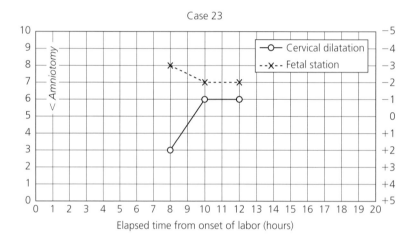

Case 23

## Questions

1 How would you categorize labor progress at 16:00?
   **A** Normal
   **B** Prolonged latent phase
   **C** Protracted descent
   **D** Arrest of dilatation

2 What action would you recommend?
   **A** Continued observation and support
   **B** Oxytocin stimulation
   **C** Epidural anesthesia
   **D** Cesarean delivery

## Case 24

A nullipara is first examined at 15:00 (hour 8), 8 hours after the onset of regular uterine contractions. Membranes are intact. The estimated fetal weight is 3800 g. You find the fetus in a cephalic presentation, and about half of the head is palpable over the pelvic inlet. Pelvic examination finds the vertex presenting at station –1. The cervix is 2 cm thick (30–40% effaced), firm, and 1 cm dilated. The subpubic arch is wide, the diagonal conjugate about 13 cm, and the sacrospinous ligament long and thin. Contractions are moderate in intensity and recur every 3–4 minutes. At midnight (hour 17), the cervical examination is unchanged, and at 03:30 (hour 20.5), the cervix is 1 cm long (70% effaced) and 2 cm dilated. The fetal head is at station –1. Contractions are regularly spaced every 3 minutes.

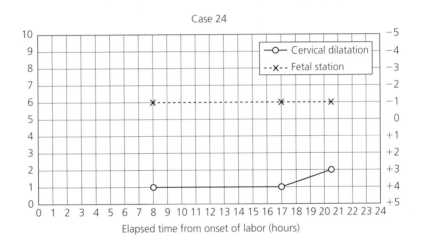

Case 24

Elapsed time from onset of labor (hours)

### Questions

1  How would you characterize labor progress?

   **A** Normal

   **B** Prolonged latent phase

   **C** Protracted active phase

   **D** The patient is not in labor

2  What would be the best treatment?

   **A** No intervention is necessary

   **B** Stimulate labor with oxytocin

   **C** Recommend cesarean delivery for failure to progress

   **D** Administer meperidine, 150 mg intramuscularly

## Case 25

A nulliparous patient with a known dichorionic diamniotic twin gestation enters spontaneous labor at 37 weeks of gestation. On admission, you note the first twin to be in vertex presentation at station +2. The cervix is 3 cm dilated and fully effaced. The first stage of labor proceeds normally, and a spontaneous delivery of a healthy first twin occurs at 10:00. After the delivery, the uterus ceases contracting.

### Questions

1 Your next step should be to:

   **A** Do an internal podalic version and total breech extraction of the second twin

   **B** Do a vaginal examination to assess the presentation and membrane status of the second twin

   **C** Begin an oxytocin infusion

   **D** Deliver the placenta of the first twin

2 If you determine that the second twin is in a frank breech presentation, you should:

   **A** Recommend prompt cesarean delivery

   **B** Perform total breech extraction

   **C** Await further labor and descent of the second twin

   **D** Perform internal podalic version

## Case 26

You have an obese multiparous patient who gained 20 kg during an otherwise uncomplicated pregnancy. At 39 weeks of gestation, spontaneous labor began at 01:00 (hour 0). She arrives on the labor unit at 04:00 (hour 3) having regular contractions every 4–5 minutes. You examine her at 08:00 (hour 7) and find a longitudinal lie. You have difficulty palpating the fetus thoroughly because of the patient's obesity. The estimated fetal weight on an ultrasound done 10 days previously was 3800 g. Your vaginal examination finds the cervix to be 3 cm dilated and the head at station 0. At noon (hour 11), the cervix is 6 cm dilated, and at 14:00 (hour 13), it is 9 cm dilated; the head remains at station 0, and the position is ROP. The AP diameter of the pelvis seems considerably greater than the transverse diameter. The ischial spines are prominent, and the sacrum is long and flat. Two hours later, at 16:00 (hour 15), you find just a small remaining anterior lip of cervix palpable with the head at station +1. Contractions are quite strong, and recur at 1- to 2-minute intervals.

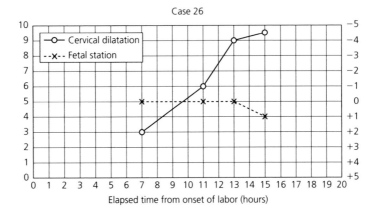

Case 26

Elapsed time from onset of labor (hours)

## Question

What should you do?

  **A** Have the patient begin pushing

  **B** Recommend cesarean delivery

  **C** Continue to observe

  **D** Administer oxytocin.

## Case 27

You admit a nulliparous patient at term; she has been in labor for about 10 hours. Contractions are strong and occur every 1–2 minutes. On abdominal examination, you find a longitudinal lie. Just to the left of the midline in the fundus is a hard firm prominence that you suspect is the fetal head. You feel the fetus suprapubically, but cannot detect the typical findings of a breech pole. On vaginal examination, you find one leg of the fetus in the vagina with the foot nearly at the introitus. You have difficulty palpating the cervix, and presume it is fully dilated. You can feel the other foot high in the vagina. Thick meconium is evident on your glove when you remove your examining hand. The mother is screaming and having difficulty remaining still.

## Question

What should you do?

  **A** Perform an immediate total breech extraction

  **B** Rush the patient to the operating room for cesarean delivery

  **C** Attempt external cephalic version

  **D** Summon help from an anesthesiologist and prepare for assisted breech delivery

## Case 28

You admit a 34-year-old nullipara for induction of labor because her otherwise uncomplicated pregnancy has reached 41 weeks' gestation. The lower uterine segment is thick, and the fetal head is floating above the inlet. The cervix is undilated and uneffaced. You administer a prostaglandin vaginal insert to ripen the cervix, and 12 hours later you find it to be 1 cm dilated, 1 cm long (70% effaced), and firm. One hour later, at 08:00 (hour 0), you begin oxytocin infusion, and you rupture the membranes shortly thereafter. At 16:00 (hour 8), you find the cervical dilatation unchanged, but the cervix is about 0.5 cm long (80–90% effaced). Contractions occur every 2–3 minutes. The mother's temperature is 100.6°F, and the amniotic fluid leaking from the vagina smells foul.

## Question
What should you do?

**A** Continue the current therapy

**B** Administer antibiotics and continue oxytocin

**C** Recommend cesarean delivery for failed induction of labor with chorioamnionitis

**D** Administer another prostaglandin insert to enhance oxytocin effects

## Case 29

A 29-year-old lean nullipara is first examined (hour 12) in active phase labor. Regular contractions began 12 hours previously and were quite strong from the outset. Your abdominal examination reveals the fetus is in an LOT position. You can easily palpate most of the fetal head above the pubic symphysis. The cervix is 8 cm dilated. You find the leading edge of the fetal head at station +2. There is considerable overlapping of the parietal bones. The pelvic sidewalls are convergent. One hour later (hour 13), the cervix is 9 cm dilated. The head is palpable between stations +2 and +3. You feel the same portion of the head above the pubic symphysis as you did previously. Membranes are intact.

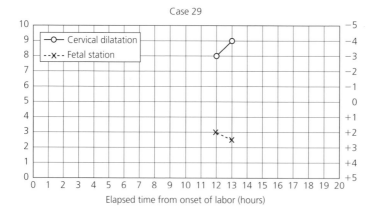

Case 29

## Question

What should you do?

  **A** Recommend cesarean delivery
  **B** Administer oxytocin
  **C** Continue observation, and be alert for signs of cephalopelvic dispro-
   portion
  **D** Rupture the membranes to encourage further dilatation.

## Case 30

A 42-year-old presents at 38 weeks of gestation in her fourth pregnancy.
Three previous uncomplicated gestations ended in normal vaginal deliveries, with birth weights between 3000 g and 3500 g. She has a body mass
index of 45 kg/m², and has been on insulin treatment for gestational
diabetes mellitus since her early second trimester. Regular contractions
began at 03:00 (hour 0), 6 hours before admission. Your initial examination (hour 6) reveals the cervix to be 4 cm dilated and very thin. The fetal
head is at station –3. The pelvis was deemed to be adequate by the obstetrician who provided prenatal care. You estimate the fetal weight to be
3500 g. You next examine her at noon (hour 9), when the cervix is 7 cm
dilated. One hour later (hour 10), it has reached 8 cm, and the fetal head
remains at station –3. No medications or anesthetic agents have been
given. Reevaluation of the pelvis reveals gynecoid features. The diagonal
conjugate exceeds 12.5 cm.

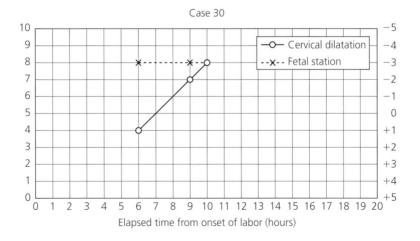

Case 30

## Questions

  **1** Which characteristics of the case known at this point are associated
   with an increased risk of dysfunctional labor?

    **A** Maternal obesity

    **B** Unengaged fetal head at term in labor

    **C** Maternal age of 40 years

    **D** Gestational diabetes mellitus

**2** How would you characterize labor progress at 13:00 (hour 10)?

    **A** Normal

    **B** Arrest of descent

    **C** Protracted active phase

    **D** Failure of descent

**3** What would be the appropriate treatment at 13:00 (hour 10)?

    **A** Close observation and emotional support

    **B** Epidural anesthesia

    **C** Oxytocin infusion

    **D** Cesarean delivery

# Answers to Obstetric Case Studies

## Case 1

D. The patient did have a prolonged latent phase, diagnosed correctly when it reached 14 hours in duration in this multipara. Prolonged latent phase is diagnosed in nulliparas after 20 hours. Under most circumstances, therapeutic rest with narcotic administration is a reasonable choice for treatment of this disorder, especially if the mother wishes some rest before having to cope with the challenges of the active phase. In this case, however, oxytocin administration would have been the required treatment because of the history of prolonged rupture of membranes and fever. Without another documentable cause, her fever should have been presumed to be from chorioamnionitis. The suspicion of intrauterine infection requires that time in labor be minimized. In this case, oxytocin treatment should in fact have been initiated soon after admission, as soon as the presumptive diagnosis of chorioamnionitis was made. The patient slept for about 3 hours and awoke with strong contractions, a temperature of 102.5 °F and a tender uterus. The cervix was still 3 cm dilated. Prompt cesarean delivery was required because of severe chorioamnionitis. The baby had evidence of sepsis. Earlier use of oxytocin stimulation would probably have prevented much of the infectious morbidity. (For more details, see Chapter 5.)

## Case 2

B. This case highlights the dilemma encountered when the second stage is judged solely by its length. Although it has been 2 hours since full cervical dilatation was attained, the rate of descent (1.5 cm/h) has been normal in this case. Considering that the fetus is not felt to be unusually large, that

*Labor and Delivery Care: A Practical Guide*, First Edition. Wayne R. Cohen and Emanuel A. Friedman. © 2011 John Wiley & Sons, Ltd.
Published 2011 by John Wiley & Sons, Ltd

the pelvis has predominantly gynecoid characteristics, and that fetal posi-tion is appropriate for the pelvis, safe vaginal delivery is likely without any operative interventions. It would probably take another hour for the pelvic floor to be distended by the descending head. Cesarean delivery is unnecessary. There is neither a protracted descent nor strong clinical evidence to raise the suspicion of disproportion. Similarly, there is no rea-son to perform a low forceps or vacuum-assisted delivery, which could be unnecessarily traumatic for mother and fetus. Note that it is not unusual for active phase dilatation to be normal (or even precipitate), followed by slow (or even abnormal) descent. The converse can occur as well.

*The patient had a normal vaginal delivery at 16:45. Mother and baby did well.* (For more details, see Chapters 4 and 5.)

## Case 3

1 C and D. The deceleration phase of the first stage of this labor does not normally exceed 1 hour in a multipara. In this case it lasted at least 3 hours, and therefore constituted a prolonged deceleration phase. This disorder is often associated with cephalopelvic dispropor-tion, and is often followed by second stage labor abnormalities and shoulder dystocia. A failure of descent is also present because fetal station has not changed between early labor and well into the decel-eration phase. Normally, descent should have begun by that time.

2 D. Doing a cesarean delivery early in labor would have been accept-able because the patient had a history of shoulder dystocia in a pre-vious pregnancy and had the additional risk factors for neonatal brachial plexus injury of maternal obesity and induction of labor. Allowing a trial of labor would also have been reasonable. However, when the labor manifested a prolonged deceleration phase and a failure of descent while on oxytocin, the probability of a safe vagi-nal delivery was quite remote. Cesarean delivery should have been recommended shortly prior to or at the time the cervix became fully dilated. See Case 4. (For more details, see Chapters 5 and 13.)

## Case 4

B and D. When shoulder dystocia is suspected there is no need to rush, and no benefit (but potential harm) to applying any traction to the fetal head or neck, no matter how gentle it seems. The first steps in manage-ment are to summon help and to assess the situation carefully. Even if you are experienced, it is important for you to get another physician to provide requisite assistance. If you are not skilled, having knowledge-able help present is critical. In addition, midwife, nurse, pediatrician, and anesthesiologist may each play helpful roles. Determine the orientation of the shoulders and whether the posterior shoulder has descended past the sacral promontory. Flexing the mother's hips (McRoberts maneuver), though widely practiced, is not the best option at this point.

*In this case, the McRoberts maneuver was unsuccessful, and was followed by upward traction on the head to attempt to deliver the posterior shoulder. This did not work, and after 5 minutes the posterior arm was delivered. The rest of the delivery followed promptly. The baby had a permanent right Erb palsy.* (For more details, see Chapter 13.)

## Case 5

C. If a classical incision were used for the previous cesarean, the risk of its scar rupturing in this pregnancy is several-fold higher than if it had been a low segment transverse incision. Because you have no way of determin-ing what kind of scar exists, it is not unreasonable to recommend repeat cesarean. However, a trial of labor can be appropriate with an unknown scar category, as long as the patient understands and accepts the asso-ciated risks. In fact, trials of labor in women with an unknown type of scar have overall outcomes quite similar to those in women with known lower segment transverse scars. This is probably because classical incisions are performed so uncommonly. You can refine your assumptions about the nature of the scar to help in decision making. If your patient has a transverse abdominal scar, and the cesarean delivery was done at or near term during labor in the developed world, it is highly likely that a lower uterine segment transverse incision was made. If the skin incision was vertical, however, and the cesarean was done well before term or in an area with limited access to trained obstetricians, it is more likely that the previous incision involved the upper uterine segment. In all cases, you should discuss your risk assessment with your patient. She should have the major role in the decision making, provided she can deliver in a hos-pital capable of managing acute uterine rupture. Induction of labor in the presence of a uterine scar is probably riskier than awaiting spontaneous labor because it increases the likelihood of uterine rupture. Induction of labor when there is even a chance the scar is a classical one is never a good idea.

*The patient had a repeat cesarean delivery that was technically challenging because of dense adhesions between the uterine corpus and the anterior abdom-inal wall. The previous cesarean scar was classical.* (For more details, see Chapter 11.)

## Case 6

B and D. Most cases of face presentation will deliver spontaneously without difficulty, although the trend is toward cesarean delivery. In this case, the patient has arrived in advanced labor, and there may be insufficient time to perform a cesarean delivery, even if that were your preference. Fortunately, this is a favorable case for vaginal delivery. The patient is a multipara, the fetal weight is not large, the head is likely engaged (or will be soon), and the mentum is anterior. Allow the labor and delivery to proceed spontaneously. A generous episiotomy may be helpful. A pediatrician should be present to evaluate the baby immediately after delivery.

*The baby delivered as a mentum anterior 30 minutes after full cervical dilatation. Its condition was excellent. Some facial edema and bruising were present and resolved within a few days of delivery.* (For more details, see Chapter 7.)

## Case 7

A. At 14:00 the labor was in its active phase, and with no further progress in dilatation over the next 2 hours, an arrest of dilatation should be diagnosed. It is too early in labor to diagnose an arrest or a failure of descent because you should not expect active descent to begin until the deceleration phase or the second stage of labor. The OP position is probably appropriate in a pelvis that has anthropoid features. An evaluation for the cause of the arrest disorder should be done. If clinical cephalopelvimetry reveals no strong evidence of disproportion, oxytocin stimulation would be appropriate. However, if disproportion is found to be likely, proceed with cesarean delivery.

*In this case oxytocin was begun. Two hours later the cervix was fully dilated. After a second stage of 90 minutes, the fetus delivered vaginally in OP position, and was in good condition.* (For more details, see Chapters 4, 5, and 7.)

## Case 8

1 A. This patient arrived in the latent phase of labor with very painful contractions. At 12:00, the latent phase had lasted for about 14 hours, which is well within the normal limit of 20 hours for a nullipara. The active phase has not begun. A failure of descent cannot be diagnosed until the deceleration phase of dilatation or the second stage.

2 C and D. Although the latent phase is not prolonged, it is longer than one would usually expect when labor begins with the cervix ripened

and the head engaged. An inhibitory effect is probably being exerted by the epidural block, which is too high. Anesthesia to the tenth thoracic dermatome is the ideal sought in the first stage of labor. Allowing the anesthesia to abate partially would be appropriate. Adding oxytocin as well is acceptable in order to overcome the inhibitory effects of the anesthesia on contractility. Continuing the excessive level of anesthesia would be inappropriate, as would discontinuing the epidural and exposing your patient to unnecessary pain.

*In this case no oxytocin was given. After 2 more hours the level of anesthesia has decreased to the T10 dermatome. Two hours after that the active phase began and progressed rapidly. Delivery was uncomplicated after a normal second stage. (For more details, see Chapters 3 and 5.)*

## Case 9

**1** C. When the first examination of a parturient in labor reveals the cervix to be this far dilated, it is impossible to determine whether the labor is still in its latent phase, is in a normal active phase, or (worst case) manifests an arrest of dilatation.

**2** B. When the head is well flexed, it is usually not possible to feel the anterior fontanel on vaginal examination. When you feel both fontanels, it indicates the head is deflexed, a common situation when the head is OP.

**3** A and D. The only way to determine what is happening with labor progress is to observe the patient and reassess the cervix. Further progress in dilatation will reveal a normal or a protracted active phase. Lack of progress will suggest that an arrest of dilatation is present or possibly that the patient is still in the latent phase of labor. In this case, given the malposition and unengaged deflexed head, it would probably be best to assume the worse case, i.e., that this is an arrest disorder, and evaluate accordingly. Part of that evaluation should involve a thorough assessment of the cephalopelvic relations to determine the likelihood that further labor would result in a safe vaginal delivery.

*Two hours later, the cervix was 6 cm dilated and completely effaced. The fetal head was still floating over the inlet. The sacral promontory was easily reached by vaginal examination. The sacrospinous ligaments were short and thick, and the subpubic arch quite narrow. The diagnosis of protracted active phase dilatation was made. Uterine contractions were occurring every 3 minutes. The combination of a large estimated fetal weight, active phase labor dysfunction, and clinical evidence of a pelvis with android characteristics made the likelihood of safe vaginal birth low. Cesarean deliv-*

*ery was indicated at that time. Unfortunately, her obstetrician viewed the continued progress in dilatation as a reassuring sign, and felt that an inadequate contractile pattern was causing slow progress. She began oxytocin infusion, and had an epidural catheter inserted for pain relief. The cervix reached full dilatation within 5 hours. After 2 hours in the second stage, the head had reached station +3 and was thought to be OA. The patient was exhausted, and a vacuum-assisted delivery was performed. Fifteen minutes of traction was required, and a 4265 g baby was delivered. The mother sustained a fourth degree laceration. The head at delivery was in OP position. Although the Apgar scores were good, the baby deteriorated. It was diagnosed with a large subgaleal hemorrhage and an underlying subdural hematoma. Permanent neurologic injury ensued.* (For more details, see Chapters 3, 4, 5, and 14.)

## Case 10

B. The patient is a reasonable candidate for a trial of labor, because most evidence supports the notion that the risk of uterine rupture during labor is about the same (0.5–0.9%) whether the patient had one or two prior lower uterine segment transverse cesarean incisions. If she has been informed objectively of all the risks and benefits pertinent to the alternatives of a trial of labor or repeat cesarean, she should have the major voice in the decision. Trials of labor in women with a prior hysterotomy scar should only be done in an institution with the personnel and resources to perform prompt cesarean delivery and to deal with the maternal and fetal complications of uterine rupture. All tertiary care centers, and many community hospitals, are well suited to those requirements.

*The patient had an uneventful labor and vaginal delivery.* (For more details, see Chapter 11.)

## Case 11

A. The best choice, given the several historical and prenatal risk factors for brachial plexus injury (probable prior brachial plexus injury, obesity, abnormal glucose challenge test, large weight gain, large estimated fetal weight, and pelvic architecture predisposing to shoulder dystocia), would be cesarean delivery. Allowing the labor to evolve would be less desirable. If chosen, be alert for the development of intrapartum risk factors for brachial plexus injury. If an active phase or second stage dysfunction occurs, cesarean is appropriate. If vaginal delivery ensues, be prepared to manage obstructed shoulder delivery. Ultrasonography is no better than clinical estimation of weight of large fetuses at term, so this option will not improve your risk assessment. (For more details, see Chapter 13.)

## Case 12

C. The labor has two manifest abnormalities: a prolonged deceleration phase and protracted descent. These are additional risk factors for
shoulder dystocia and brachial plexus injury. Further observation is
unlikely to reveal anything that would decrease that risk. It would be
unwise to use oxytocin in the context of so many risk factors for difficult shoulder delivery. Moreover, there is no evidence that oxytocin
is beneficial in resolving protracted descent. Cesarean delivery would
be the best choice. Given the many risk factors for shoulder dystocia
and brachial plexus injury (probable prior brachial plexus injury, obesity, abnormal glucose challenge test, large weight gain, large estimated
fetal weight, pelvic architecture predisposing to shoulder dystocia, prolonged deceleration phase, protracted descent), the likelihood of a safe
uncomplicated vaginal delivery is very low. Using forceps or the vacuum
extractor would not be beneficial, and are likely to be harmful under
the circumstances; it would increase further the likelihood of brachial
plexus injury.

*The patient reluctantly agreed to cesarean delivery. A healthy 5309 g baby was
born.* (For more details, see Chapters 5 and 13.)

## Case 13

D. This labor, after 12 hours of oxytocin stimulation, is still in a normal
latent phase. The latent phase in nulliparas can normally extend to 20
hours. Considering that this is an induced labor and that oxytocin was
begun with a relatively unripe cervix, a latent phase longer than 12 hours
would be common. The induction of labor has not failed. There has been
no descent of the presenting part thus far, a normal finding in the latent
phase. Failure of descent cannot be diagnosed until late in active phase or
in early second stage.

*The cesarean was complicated by lateral extension of the uterine incision into
the vessels of the left broad ligament. Three units of packed red cells were required,
and the mother was discharged with a hemoglobin of 9.5 g/dL. The 3020 g baby
did well.* (For more details, see Chapters 3, 5, and 10.)

## Case 14

C. This labor is still in a normal latent phase (<14 h in a multipara), as
evidenced by the very slow changes in cervical dilatation and gradual
effacement. An unengaged fetal head during the latent phase is not an

indicator of any problem in a multipara. Descent in such cases may not begin until late in the active phase of dilatation. There was no indication for oxytocin stimulation of this normal labor.

*Oxytocin administration resulted in the appearance of strong uterine contractions every 1–2 minutes with minimal relaxation between them. Recurrent late decelerations accompanied each contraction, and a cesarean was done because of concern about fetal oxygenation. The baby had Apgar scores or 3 and 5 at 1 and 5 minutes, respectively. He required 2 days on assisted ventilation.* (For more details, see Chapter 5.)

## Case 15

C. Fetal descent during the second stage has thus far been normal. Although the second stage has lasted 2 hours, the prognosis for a spontaneous vaginal delivery is good. The OP position is important to keep in mind. It may become a factor in your decision making; but for now, there is no reason to intervene with cesarean or instrumental delivery. Oxytocin would be contraindicated in a normally progressing labor.

*Labor continued, and at 20:00 the head, at station +3, rotated to ROA position and delivered spontaneously at 20:20. The baby appeared healthy.* (For more details, see Chapters 3, 5, and 7.)

## Case 16

B. This labor manifests two dysfunctions, both of which have a strong association with cephalopelvic disproportion: prolonged deceleration phase and failure of descent. Of the options provided, cesarean delivery or oxytocin augmentation of contractions should be considered. However, given the malposition, cranial molding, lower pelvic features that might impede descent and rotation, and the results of the Müller-Hillis maneuver, there is little to be gained by continuing this labor with its potential for fetal and maternal injury. Cesarean delivery should, therefore, be recommended. By no means should you artificially force complete dilatation by pushing the remaining cervix over the fetal head.

*In this case, full dilatation was created by pushing the cervix back over the head and oxytocin infusion was begun. Vaginal delivery occurred 80 minutes later and was complicated by a severe shoulder dystocia that was finally resolved using the Zavanelli maneuver to push the head back into the birth canal and then doing a cesarean delivery. The baby has a permanent brachial plexus palsy and asphyxial brain injury.* (For more details, see Chapters 4, 5, and 13.)

## Case 17

A. Under most circumstances, it is appropriate to wait 30 minutes before assuming the placenta is abnormally retained. Injection of oxytocin into the umbilical vein sometimes promotes placental separation, and is a reasonable procedure to try, as is the Brandt maneuver. In this particular situation, however, you should be very concerned about the possibility of a placenta accreta. The patient is at high risk for an accreta because of her previous cesarean deliveries and a placenta that is implanted over the uterine scars. Before doing anything that might provoke massive bleeding, such as attempts at manual placental delivery, be sure that blood for transfusion and adequate help are available.

*In this case, a cross-match was ordered. After waiting another 15 minutes 10 units of oxytocin diluted in 20 mL of saline was injected into the umbilical vein, with no results. Once the blood was available and the operating room team alerted, an attempt at manual removal of the placenta was made. No cleavage plane was identifiable, and severe bleeding developed. Immediate laparotomy was performed and a hysterectomy was necessary to arrest bleeding from a placenta accreta. After a day in the intensive care unit and transfusion of 5 units of red blood cells, the patient recovered well.* (For more details, see Chapter 6.)

## Case 18

1 A, B, and C. It is often erroneously assumed that the previous delivery of a large baby guarantees that subsequent deliveries will be unencumbered by disproportion. In this case, the pelvis was clearly quite ample for delivery of a 4500 g fetus; but the presence of dysfunctional labor patterns should have been a clue that this fetus may have been considerably larger than her first. The combination of three labor abnormalities made the chance of an atraumatic delivery very small.

2 A, B, and C. Choosing to do any form of instrumental delivery in this situation must be considered to have been faulty judgment because of the high associated risks, noted above. Forceps would have conferred no less fetal hazard. Using the vacuum extractor or forceps without certain knowledge of fetal position can magnify the risks of delivery. If cranial features are obscured, palpation of the fetal ear can establish position. Vacuum-assisted delivery should consist of intermittent traction coinciding with uterine contractions. Sustained traction over extended periods of time is never appropriate. As soon as the prolonged deceleration phase was identified (which was possible by 04:30) thorough cephalopelvimetry would probably have revealed evidence of disproportion and prompted cesarean delivery. (For more details, see Chapters 4, 5, and 14.)

## Case 19

A. Fourth degree lacerations must be repaired anatomically, using fine absorbable sutures. It is especially important that the internal anal sphincter be identified and reapproximated, because it plays an important role in maintaining anal continence. Even well-repaired lacerations can sometimes lead to problems with continence later in life.

*Two years after the delivery this patient has normal fecal continence. While she is still at risk for long-term problems, proper anatomic repair of her laceration should minimize this possibility.* (For more details, see Chapter 9.)

## Case 20

B. Administration of oxytocin was appropriate in this patient with an arrest of dilatation. Although there was a malposition, no strong evidence of cephalopelvic disproportion existed. However, the lack of progress in dilatation after nearly 4 hours of oxytocin stimulation bodes poorly. The probability of this labor terminating with a safe vaginal delivery is small. Further stimulation with oxytocin is likely to be unavailing, and potentially harmful to the fetus. Cesarean delivery is the best option.

*This was done. The birth weight was 4460 g. The baby was in good condition.* (For more details, see Chapters 4 and 5.)

## Case 21

1 C. The first stage of labor was normal. The latent phase was somewhat unusual in that progressive dilatation occurred, at a rate of about 0.5 cm/h. The active phase began after the cervix was about 6 cm dilated. Descent began normally, but arrested at station +3. Distinguishing a latent phase with steady cervical dilatation from a protracted active phase can be difficult. As a generalization, rates of dilatation below 0.6 cm/h are most likely not active phase. Also, it is unusual for a labor to still be in the latent phase after 6 cm of dilatation. Exceptions do occur, especially in multiparas who begin labor with the cervix already dilated to 4 or 5 cm.

2 B. An arrest of descent requires careful evaluation to identify its possible etiology. In this case there was no malposition, no evidence of infection, and an anesthetic level that was not excessive. The presence of cephalopelvic disproportion can be reasonably excluded,

at least at this level in the pelvis, by the results of the Müller-Hillis maneuver, lack of severe molding, and generally favorable pelvimetry. The patient's age may be a factor, in that arrest disorders are more common in older gravidas. The epidural block may also mute the force of the patient's bearing-down efforts. The prominent spines may be resisting full internal rotation. However, based on the rotation and descent noted when fundal pressure was applied during a contraction, this is not an insurmountable obstacle. All things considered, this is an arrest of descent in which oxytocin should be given, and in which safe vaginal delivery will probably occur. Close observation to be sure there is a good response to oxytocin is, nevertheless, important.

*Oxytocin was administered, and a normal vaginal delivery occurred 45 minutes later.* (For more details, see Chapters 3, 4, and 5.)

## Case 22

1 D. This woman experienced both protracted active phase dilatation and protracted descent. As is generally the case with these disorders, once a rate of dilatation and descent is established it rarely increases, but may be readily diminished by analgesia or anesthesia. In this case the rate of dilatation was not enhanced by amniotomy but, contrary to usual expectation, did not seem to be diminished by three doses of narcotic analgesia. In this woman the active phase had been entered by 03:30, despite the cervix being only 3 cm dilated. This emphasizes the need to distinguish active from latent phase on the basis of the achieved rate of dilatation, and not on attainment of a particular degree of dilatation.

2 D. Oxytocin would not likely have increased the rate of dilatation or descent in this case. It typically does not alter the course of a labor beset by a protraction disorder, unless that disorder has been precipitated by some inhibitory factor such as heavy dose of sedative or analgesic drugs. Epidural anesthesia would have provided more sustained pain relief without the risk of narcotic-induced neonatal respiratory depression. The decision to perform a forceps procedure was ill-advised. Although the leading edge of the head was deep in the pelvis, the considerable molding, the OP position, and the protracted descent made instrumental delivery particularly hazardous for fetus and mother. It would have been better to allow the second stage to continue beyond 2 hours and await spontaneous delivery. (For more details, see Chapters 5, 7, and 14.)

## Case 23

1 D. This labor entered the active phase and then dilatation ceased for 2 hours, an arrest of dilatation. This disorder is associated with fetal malpositions, cephalopelvic disproportion, intrauterine infection, excess analgesia, maternal obesity, and the presence of a hysterotomy scar. You should evaluate the patient for all of these potential causes.

2 B. There is no evidence of infection, and the patient has had no pain medication. She is not obese, and there is no suggestion of disproportion. There is, however, a malposition. The fetus is OP, and the pelvis has primarily gynecoid features, making it unsuitable for the mechanism of labor common to posterior positions of the occiput. You can conclude that the fetal position is not appropriate for this pelvis, and is probably the reason for the arrest of dilatation. Stimulation with oxytocin will probably correct the problem.

   *Oxytocin infusion commenced at 16:15, and within 30 minutes strong contractions occurred every 2–3 minutes. At 19:00 the cervix was 9 cm dilated and the head had descended to station +1, still in OP position. Full dilatation occurred at 20:00, and the patient began bearing-down efforts. The head continued to descend and rotated to OA after another hour. An uneventful spontaneous delivery followed.* (For more details, see Chapters 3, 4, 5, and 7.)

## Case 24

1 B. This is a straightforward case of prolonged latent phase. By 03:30 the latent phase had been ongoing for 20.5 hours. This exceeds the 20 hour limit of normal for nulliparas. The patient began labor with an unripe cervix, predisposing her to a long latent phase. The presence of painful regular uterine contractions with some cervical change indicates she is indeed in labor and the small degree and low rate of dilatation is inconsistent with the active phase. A small percentage of cases like this will stop contracting, indicating they were actually in false labor.

2 B or D. Prolonged latent phase can be treated by suspending labor temporarily with a dose of narcotic analgesic such as morphine or meperidine. Alternatively, the labor can be stimulated with oxytocin. The choice depends on whether there are any fetal or maternal conditions that would make prolonging the labor unsafe, as well as on the patient's preference. Both treatments are equally effective in making the labor transition to active phase. After narcotic rest, about 10% of patients will not be in labor, indicating in retrospect

that they had presented with false labor. About 5% will awaken with uterine contractions that require oxytocin to advance dilatation effectively.

*This patient strongly desired to continue with her labor. Oxytocin was administered, and the subsequent patterns of dilatation and descent were normal.* (For more details, see Chapters 3 and 5.)

## Case 25

1 B. The first step in deciding how to deliver the second twin is to do a careful examination to determine its presentation and position, and to establish its well-being.

2 A, B, or C. There are several options for management. Cesarean delivery is an acceptable option, especially if you do not possess the skills necessary to manage the breech presentation safely. However, vaginal delivery in this situation is also a reasonable choice. Total breech extraction is possible, but it is generally better to wait for spontaneous descent of the fetus and a spontaneous or assisted breech delivery.

*In this case, once the presentation and the well-being of the second twin were established, oxytocin infusion was begun because contractions were mild and infrequent. Once strong contractions were reestablished, the fetus began to descend. Forty-five minutes after delivery of the first twin, an uneventful assisted breech delivery was performed.* (For more details, see Chapter 12.)

## Case 26

C. The ROP position in this case is appropriate to the pelvis, which has anthropoid qualities. The deceleration phase is prolonged, not an unusual event with a persistent posterior position. The prominent ischial spines and the lack of a deep sacral hollow are of some concern, and demand close observation of progress in descent. Avoid the temptation to manually reduce the remaining lip of cervix, or to have the patient begin pushing efforts before full dilatation is attained. Oxytocin is best withheld, considering the frequent spontaneous contractions.

*At 17:00 the cervix became fully dilated, with the head at station +2. After an hour of strong contractions and intense bearing-down efforts, the head was still at station +2, and there was marked molding palpable. The Müller-Hillis maneuver revealed no descent or rotation. A cesarean delivery was carried out because of the arrest of descent and clinical evidence of disproportion.* (For more details, see Chapters 3, 5, and 7.)

## Case 27

E. Cesarean delivery would be appropriate for footling breech presentations in most circumstances. In this case, there may not be enough time to mobilize a cesarean team before vaginal delivery ensues. Judgment is necessary to decide what will likely be the safest route of delivery. Having the fetus emerge untended while preparations are being made for cesarean would be the worst scenario.

The best approach in this situation would be to control the patient's pain as promptly as possible and allow a spontaneous or assisted breech delivery to occur. Remember that a leg can prolapse into the vagina when there is a transverse lie, but this malpresentation has been ruled out by your abdominal and vaginal examinations. In a breech, the cervix can be difficult to palpate once the foot (or feet) has reached the introitus. Therefore, do not assume full dilatation is present. A total breech extraction in a footling presentation is ill-advised. The cervix may not be fully dilated. Even if it is, you may cause nuchal or extended arms to develop, or the head may be entrapped. Proceed with deliberate haste to calm, reassure, and instruct your patient about the situation, to control her pain and anxiety, to summon the necessary help, and to move her to the safest place available for delivery. However, haste is not necessary for the delivery itself. The more manipulation of a breech presentation during delivery, the greater the risk of harm.

*In this case, an uncomplicated spontaneous breech delivery occurred under the watchful care of an obstetrician experienced in the management of vaginal breech delivery and its complications.* (For more details, see Chapter 8.)

## Case 28

C. This is a case in which too many interventions created the need for prompt delivery. While induction of labor at 41 weeks is a common and acceptable approach, the alternative of awaiting spontaneous labor for another week, with the fetus under surveillance, is equally effective. It may less often lead to cesarean, especially when the cervix is very unripe at 41 weeks. Early artificial rupture of the membranes can diminish the duration of an induction, but increases the risk of ascending infection, as probably occurred here. Prompt cesarean delivery is in the best interests of the fetus in this case, because the labor is likely to be quite long, and there is a risk of fetal and neonatal sepsis.

*A cesarean was performed. The neonate was treated for sepsis, and the mother had a prolonged hospitalization for the treatment of endomyometritis.* (For more details, see Chapter 10.)

## Case 29

A. Although the lowest portion of the fetal head is felt relatively deep in the pelvis, the persistence of so much of it palpable suprapubically suggests that marked molding has occurred, and not true descent. This is confirmed by finding evidence of overlapping of the cranial bones. The convergent sidewalls make further safe progress unlikely. Cesarean delivery is the best approach. Were a careful abdominal examination and evaluation of cephalopelvic relations not done, the fetus might be subjected to further unavailing labor and risk of trauma. Oxytocin would add risk and no benefit in this situation.

*The obstetrician applied a vacuum extractor and attempted delivery, but each time she applied traction the cup popped off the head. Unable to effect delivery, and feeling the head to be OA, Simpson forceps were applied. These also failed, and a cesarean delivery was done. The baby emerged in the OP position. It had a facial nerve palsy and a depressed parietal skull fracture. Its long-term neurologic status is guarded.* (For more details, see Chapters 2, 4, 5, and 14.)

## Case 30

1 A and C. Both advanced maternal age and marked obesity are associated with dysfunctional labor. An unengaged head in an early multiparous labor is common, and not itself a poor prognostic sign. Gestational diabetes is only indirectly related to dysfunctional labor insofar as it may be associated with fetal macrosomia.

2 C. Cervical dilatation in active phase labor has been steadily progressive at about 1 cm/h, considerably slower than the minimum 1.5 cm/h expected from a multipara. Therefore, a protracted active phase exists. An arrest of descent cannot be diagnosed until the second stage of labor. Failure of descent is not diagnosable until the deceleration phase of labor (which is probably about to begin) or the onset of the second stage.

3 A. Labors with protraction disorders tend to be long, frustrating, and arduous. Epidural anesthesia will not improve labor progress; it may actually inhibit it. However, some patients will benefit from the pain abatement. If an epidural is given, be aware of the possibility it will worsen or arrest dilatational progress. Oxytocin will generally not improve the rate of dilatation in a protracted active phase, regardless of the existing pattern of uterine contractility, unless there is an inhibitory factor to overcome, such as excess anesthesia. Amniotomy is also not usually helpful, and increases the risk of intrauterine infection. Close attention to subsequent progress is necessary because

there is increased risk of further disorders and of developing evidence of disproportion. In this case, maternal age and obesity may be affecting progress in the absence of disproportion. Patience (yours and the patient's) and vigilance are the keys to a safe outcome.

*An epidural anesthetic was administered, and an infusion of oxytocin was begun. At 15:30 the cervix became fully dilated. After a 30-minute second stage an uneventful vaginal delivery occurred.* (For more details, see Chapter 5.)

# Glossary

**abruptio placentae**  Premature separation of the normally implanted placenta. An acute condition that may threaten the well-being of both fetus (from hypoxic damage, death) and mother (from coagulopathy, hemorrhage), often requiring rapid intervention either by cesarean delivery or uterotonic stimulation to try to effect prompt vaginal delivery.

**acceleration phase**  Transition period of the cervical dilatation process during which the rate of dilatation increases from the low or zero slope of the latent phase to the maximum slope of the linear midportion of the active phase.

**active phase**  The portion of labor that extends from the end of the latent phase of the first stage until complete cervical dilatation.

**aftercoming head**  The fetal head in a vaginal delivery of a fetus in breech presentation that follows after the delivery of the fetal body. (See hyperextension, fetal head; nuchal arm; Piper forceps)

**algorithm**  A schematic representation to illustrate the sequential steps in a decision tree; flow chart, paradigm or protocol.

**amniocentesis**  Procedure for inserting a needle transabdominally into the amniotic sac for obtaining a sample of amniotic fluid or for draining off excess amniotic fluid in the presence of hydramnios. (See amnioreduction)

**amnion nodosum**  Visible nodules in the amnion, often multiple, consisting of metaplastic squamous epithelium. Seen most commonly in the presence of chronically reduced amniotic fluid volume (oligohydramnios).

**amnioreduction**  Procedure for reducing amniotic fluid volume in acute hydramnios by means of amniocentesis (transabdominal needle puncture of the amniotic sac) in the interest of relieving maternal discomfort and

*Labor and Delivery Care: A Practical Guide*, First Edition. Wayne R. Cohen and Emanuel A. Friedman. © 2011 John Wiley & Sons, Ltd. Published 2011 by John Wiley & Sons, Ltd

symptoms, such as dyspnea and orthopnea. Amnioreduction provides only short-term relief.

**amniotomy**   Transcervical procedure for artificially rupturing the chorioamniotic membranes.

**android pelvis**   A heavy-boned male-type pelvis in a female, characterized by heart-shaped inlet, converging sidewalls (typical of a funnel pelvis), narrow forepelvis, prominent ischial spines and acutely-angled subpubic arch. It is often associated with an posterior oblique mechanism in labor, a high probability of cephalopelvic disproportion, and the frequent need for cesarean delivery. (See anthropoid pelvis; funnel pelvis; flat pelvis; gynecoid pelvis; platypelloid pelvis)

**anencephaly**   Severe lethal fetal anomaly in which there is absence of the bones of the cranial vault and rudimentary cerebrum, cerebellum and other parts of the brain.

**anthropoid pelvis**   Pelvic architectural type with elongated anteroposterior diameter and constricted transverse dimension, plus posteriorly-directed deeply-concave sacrum, narrow forepelvis and pubic arch, and prominent ischial spines. Usually associated with an occiput posterior mechanism in labor and an increased need for cesarean delivery. (See android pelvis; funnel pelvis; flat pelvis; gynecoid pelvis; platypelloid pelvis)

**aortocaval compression**   Complete or partial occlusion of the abdominal aorta and the inferior vena cava by the pregnant uterus, usually occurring during the third trimester when the gravida is in the supine position. (See supine hypotension syndrome)

**arrest of descent**   A labor disorder of the active portion of descent in which descent ceases for 1 hour or more.

**arrest of dilatation**   A labor disorder of the active phase of cervical dilatation in which dilatation ceases for at least 2 hours.

**assisted breech delivery**   Partial breech extraction; a vaginal delivery process in which the fetus in breech presentation is allowed to deliver spontaneously to the umbilicus and is then manipulated manually to effect the remainder of its delivery.

**asynclitism**   Absence of parallelism between the axis of the fetal presenting part and the axis of the pelvis in labor, with either the anterior parietal bone preceding the posterior parietal bone in descent (anterior or Nägele asynclitism) or vice versa (posterior or Litzmann asynclitism). It is encountered in severe form in labors associated with cephalopelvic disproportion. (See synclitism)

**atony, uterine**   Failure of the uterus to contract effectively and remain contracted after the fetus and the placenta are delivered so that profuse bleeding will occur from large maternal venous sinuses in the placental bed.

**attitude**   The relation of the various parts of the fetal body to one another. Applied most often to describe the degree of flexion of the head. Normally, the head is flexed. It may have various degrees of axial deflexion, lateroflexion, or even hyperextension. (See deflexion, fetal head; hyperextension, fetal head)

**augmentation of labor**   The process of administering a uterotonic (ecbolic) agent during the course of an already established labor to stimulate the uterus to contract more vigorously. (See hypercontractility, uterine; hyperstimulation, uterine; oxytocin; prostaglandins)

**Bandl ring**   Pathologic retraction ring; an indented band formed around the uterus during obstructed labor, located where the thinned-out lower uterine segment joins the thick upper uterine segment. It may precede uterine rupture. Bandl ring is encountered in gravidas with cephalopelvic disproportion who have been allowed to labor unduly long. (See cephalopelvic disproportion)

**Barton forceps**   Obstetric forceps designed specifically for application to a fetal head in occiput transverse position in a platypelloid pelvis. Its curved posterior blade is a fixed curve and its anterior blade is hinged. (See deep transverse arrest; flat pelvis; platypelloid pelvis)

**battledore placenta**   A placental variant in which the umbilical vessels insert at the margin of the placenta instead of eccentrically into the chorionic plate.

**birth canal**   The cavity enclosed by the maternal pelvis, uterus, vagina and perineum through which the fetus passes during the labor process.

**bisacromial diameter**   The distance between the acromial processes of the scapulae. Useful as an objective means to assess the width of the shoulder girdle. (See shoulder dystocia; suprapubic pressure)

**Bishop score**   Scoring system used to determine readiness of a gravida for induction of labor, evaluating cervical dilatation, effacement, consistency and position, plus fetal station. It is also used to predict the probability of successful induction. (See induction of labor)

**bisiliac diameter**   The distance between the iliac bones.

**bony dystocia, bony disproportion**   Cephalopelvic disproportion.

**brachial plexus**   A plexus of nerves that derives from the ventral rami of the fifth cervical through the first thoracic nerve roots. The fetal brachial plexus can be injured by overstretching or avulsion during delivery.

**Bracht method**    A technique for effecting vaginal breech delivery that simulates the natural mechanism of labor, involving supporting the fetus against gravity.

**Braxton Hicks contractions**    Uterine contractions that precede labor, observed most commonly in the third trimester of pregnancy. Named for John Braxton Hicks, 19th-century British obstetrician. (See false labor; prodromal labor)

**breech extraction**    Procedure for vaginal delivery of the fetus in breech presentation by introducing a hand into the uterus under anesthesia, identifying and grasping the fetal feet, and applying traction. It is much more hazardous than spontaneous or assisted breech delivery. (See Bracht method; breech presentation; assisted breech delivery)

**breech presentation**    Fetal presentation in which the buttocks or lower extremities are located in or over the maternal pelvis. Types include: frank breech if thighs are flexed and knees are extended over the abdomen and thorax; full or complete breech if thighs and knees are flexed; incomplete breech if foot or knee is down; single or double footling presentation if one or both feet are down, respectively; knee presentation if knee is down. (See complete breech; footling breech; frank breech; incomplete breech)

**bregma**    The portion of the fetal head where the arc of the coronal suture crosses the large fontanel; the brow.

**brow presentation**    A variant of cephalic presentation in which the fetal head is deflexed so that its brow (bregma) is lowermost in the pelvis.

**caput succedaneum**    The edema that develops in the subcutaneous tissue of the fetal scalp during labor. It results from venous or lymphatic stasis due to obstruction caused by pressure from the cervix or bony pelvis on the fetal scalp. Often shortened to "caput." Distinguishable from the more serious cephalhematoma (subperiosteal hematoma) by the limitation of cephalhematoma to the area of the cranial bone over which it occurs. (See cephalhematoma; subgaleal hemorrhage)

**cardinal movements**    Changes in the orientation of the fetal head within the maternal pelvis during labor and delivery. For a vertex presentation, these comprise engagement, descent, flexion, internal rotation, extension, restitution, external rotation and expulsion.

**caudad**    In the direction of the tail; opposite of cephalad or craniad.

**centrum tendineum (perinei)**    A condensation of dense connective tissue in the midline of the perineum to which attach the tendons of the superficial and deep transverse perinei, bulbospongiosus, external anal sphincter, and portions of the levator ani muscles. Also referred to as the perineal body. Its integrity is vital to the supportive function of the pelvic floor.

**cephalad**   In the direction of the head; craniad; opposite of caudad.

**cephalhematoma**   Subperiosteal collection of blood limited to the area of the cranial bone over which it occurs, as contrasted with the more benign and common caput succedaneum, which extends across suture lines on the skull of the newborn, or the much more serious subgaleal hematoma, which slowly develops as a boggy occipital mass after delivery, enlarging sometimes to cover the entire calvaria. Cephalhematoma and subgaleal hemorrhage are sometimes encountered as a complication of vacuum extraction or forceps delivery procedures. (See caput succadeneum; subgaleal hemorrhage)

**cephalic presentation**   Head-first fetal presentation. It is most often vertex presentation if the head is well flexed, but it may be sincipital, brow or face presentation instead, depending on the degree of deflexion. (See brow presentation; face presentation; sincipital presentation; vertex)

**cephalopelvic disproportion**   A situation encountered during labor in which the potential for traumatic vaginal delivery is high owing to a mismatch between the dimensions of the presenting part and the capacity of the pelvis. The probability of cephalopelvic disproportion is determined by integrating information from the labor curves pertaining to the course of labor and cephalopelvimetry. (See cephalopelvimetry; labor curves)

**cephalopelvimetry**   Method for evaluating the spatial relationship between the fetal presenting part and the maternal pelvis to determine if the pelvis can accommodate the fetus safely; a means for detecting probable cephalopelvic disproportion. (See cephalopelvic disproportion; Crichton maneuver; Müller-Hillis maneuver)

**cervical dilatation**   The opening of the cervix measured in centimeters; also the process of progressive opening of the cervix in the course of the first stage of labor. (See labor curves)

**cervical ripening**   Process by which the cervix is softened, effaced and perhaps dilated in preparation for spontaneous onset of labor or for making the cervix more favorable for induction of labor. It occurs spontaneously in most gravidas in late pregnancy, but it may involve administration of a ripening agent, such as a prostaglandin. (See priming, cervical)

**cesarean delivery**   Delivery by means of a major surgical procedure, in which the fetus is extracted by way of an incision made through the abdominal wall and the anterior uterus. The uterine incision can be transverse in the lower uterine segment (Kerr incision), vertical in the upper uterine segment (classical incision), or vertical in the lower segment (Kroenig incision). (See classical cesarean delivery; patient-request cesarean delivery)

**chorionicity**   Chorionic membrane status of twins in utero. If only one chorion encompasses both twins, they are clearly monozygotic (derived from a single ovum), whereas if each has its own chorion, they may be either monozygotic or dizygotic. (See zygosity)

**classical cesarean delivery**   Cesarean delivery carried out through a vertical incision in the upper uterine wall where the myometrium is thick. Although sometimes necessary, this approach is less preferable than a transverse cesarean incision made in the lower uterine segment.

**complete breech**   Breech presentation in which the fetal hips and knees are flexed so that buttocks and lower extremities are in or over the pelvic inlet.

**compound presentation**   A fetal malpresentation in which a limb is located alongside either the head or the breech in or over the pelvic inlet.

**conduction anesthesia**   Techniques in which local anesthetic agents are injected around nerves to inhibit impulse transmission. In obstetrics, they most commonly include epidural and spinal anesthesia. (See epidural block; neuraxial anesthesia)

**conduplicato corpora**   Delivery process for a transverse lie, in which the fetus is doubled on itself so that the head and the trunk come into the pelvis simultaneously; limited to very premature gestations.

**conjoined twins**   A severe congenital anomaly in which monozygotic twins are united as a consequence of incomplete separation of the dividing ovum during early embryogenesis. The types of union are designated according to the conjoined structures, such as craniopagus (joined at the head), thoracopagus (chest), omphalopagus (abdomen) or pygopagus (buttocks).

**cord prolapse**   Condition in which the umbilical cord descends alongside the fetus (occult prolapse) or in front of the fetus (overt prolapse), putting the fetus at risk of hypoxia from compression of the umbilical vessels. If the membranes rupture, a loop of cord may appear in the vagina or even outside the vaginal introitus.

**Crichton maneuver**   A means for determining the relation of the widest diameters of the fetal head to the pelvic inlet using suprapubic palpation (the fourth maneuver of Leopold) to assess how much of the head remains above the inlet; it helps to differentiate true descent from head molding. It is best done as a series of examinations over time during the fetal descent process. (See cephalopelvic disproportion; Leopold maneuvers)

**crowning**   State near the end of labor in which the lowermost part of the fetal head protrudes through the vulva as it descends, by the mechanism of extension, through the pelvic outlet.

**deceleration phase**   The terminal portion of the process of cervical dilatation during which the cervical rim retracts around the periphery of the fetal presenting part. In a term vertex presentation it begins when the cervix is 8 to 9 cm dilated.

**deflexion, fetal head**   Unfavorable attitude of the fetal head during its descent through the pelvis in labor, characterized by extension. Because the head is not optimally flexed, its presenting dimensions are relatively large. Small degrees of deflexion result in a sincipital presentation; larger degrees, a brow presentation; maximal extension, a face presentation. (See brow presentation; face presentation; sincipital presentation)

**descent, fetal**   Process by which the fetus traverses the birth canal in the course of labor. The mechanism by which the fetal head negotiates the pelvis during descent involves flexion, internal rotation, extension, restitution, and external rotation in sequence. (See birth canal; labor curves; mechanisms of labor)

**diagonal conjugate**   An approximate measure of the anteroposterior diameter of the inlet of the maternal pelvis obtained by vaginal examination, spanning the distance from the bottom of the symphysis pubis to the sacral promontory, if it can be reached. (See pelvimetry; sacral promontory)

**digital rotation**   Process by which an attempt is made to rotate the fetal head in a malposition to a more favorable position, using the fingertips against the edge of the parietal bone at the lambdoidal suture. It is not generally recommended because it is seldom effective, yet may be traumatic. (See malposition, fetal; manual rotation)

**dolichocephalic**   A descriptive adjective for a disproportionate fetal head in which the lateral diameter is narrowed relative to the anteroposterior dimension.

**dorsal lithotomy position**   Maternal position for conducting the delivery process, with the gravida on her back, buttocks at the edge of the table or bed, hips flexed and legs flexed and supported by assistants or fixed in stirrups. The term derives from its earlier use for doing lithotomy, the operation for removing bladder calculi.

**Dührssen incisions**   Radial incisions in the cervix used to free the trapped head of the fetus during a breech delivery. Usually made at 12, 8, and 4 o'clock positions. (See aftercoming head; entrapment, fetal head)

**dysfunctional labor**    Abnormal labor based on deviation from the limits of normal demonstrated by the patterns of cervical dilatation and fetal descent that evolve during the time the gravida is in labor. (See arrest of descent; arrest of dilatation; failure of descent; labor curves; prolonged deceleration phase)

**dystocia**    A general term encompassing any situation in which labor and delivery progress is slowed or stopped. (See cephalopelvic disproportion; dysfunctional labor; labor curves)

**ecbolic agent**    A drug that stimulates myometrial contractility; uterotonic. (See uterotonic agent)

**effacement, cervical**    Shortening of the cervical canal that occurs prior to or during labor. Usually expressed as a percent of the cervical length in the nonpregnant state, or as an estimate of the cervical length in centimeters.

**Elliot-type forceps**    A group of classic obstetric forceps designed for application to a round unmolded fetal head; the instruments have shared characteristics of overlapping shanks and rounded cephalic curve. (See forceps, obstetric; Simpson-type forceps)

**endopelvic fascia**    A continuous connective tissue network that invests the viscera of the pelvis and attaches them to the pelvic sidewall.

**engagement, fetal**    The entry of the fetal head into the maternal pelvis. Complete engagement occurs when the widest diameter of the fetal presenting part (the biparietal diameter for vertex presentations) has descended to or beyond the brim of the true pelvis. (See Crichton maneuver; station, fetal)

**entrapment, fetal head**    Complication encountered in vaginal breech delivery in which the fetal body is expelled, but the head is prevented from being delivered by an incompletely dilated cervix. It arises most often in the delivery of a premature fetus in breech presentation because the head is considerably larger than the body. (See Dührssen incisions; Piper forceps)

**epidural block**    A form of neuraxial anesthesia involving administration of a solution of a local anesthetic or narcotic agent into the peridural space. It is currently the most popular form of anesthesia for labor and delivery by virtue of its efficacy and relative safety. (See conduction anesthesia; neuraxial block)

**episiotomy**    Procedure for incising the perineum at delivery to create space for intravaginal manipulations or to prevent uncontrolled laceration of the perineum and surrounding structures during vaginal delivery.

**Erb palsy**   Injury to the upper trunk of the brachial plexus, involving the fifth, sixth, and sometimes seventh cervical nerve roots.

**extension, fetal head**   Unfavorable attitude of the fetal head during its descent through the pelvis in labor. Because the presenting fetal head dimensions are relatively large when extended, delivery may be more difficult and potentially traumatic. Sincipital presentation is associated with small degrees of extension; brow with more extension; face with most extreme extension. (See brow presentation; face presentation; sinicipital presentation)

**external cephalic version**   Procedure in which the breech or shoulder presentation is converted to a cephalic presentation by manipulating the fetus externally through the abdominal wall. (See breech presentation; transverse lie)

**external rotation**   The last component of the labor mechanism occurs after the fetal head has been delivered over the perineum and has aligned itself with the still-undelivered shoulders. As the shoulders undergo internal rotation with their descent through the pelvis, the head follows suit externally. (See mechanisms of labor)

**face presentation**   Malpresentation in which the fetal head is maximally extended so that the fetus's face is lowermost in the pelvis; mentum presentation. The referent site on the face for designating the fetal position is the chin (mentum). Although vaginal delivery is feasible and safe for many fetuses in face presentation, it is seldom done any longer. (See extension, fetal head)

**failure of descent**   A labor disorder in which descent of the presenting part has not yet begun by the time the labor has reached the deceleration phase or the onset of second stage labor. (See dysfunctional labor; dystocia; labor curves)

**failure to progress**   A nondescript term used to describe a period in which there is no progress in labor. Its use is not recommended because it encompasses a number of disorders, such as arrest of dilatation, arrest of descent and failure of descent, and it can also erroneously include the latent phase of normal labor. (See dysfunctional labor; dystocia; labor curves)

**false labor**   Condition of late pregnancy characterized by a period of uterine contractions, perceived by the gravida, but unassociated with cervical dilatation or fetal descent. The contractions are indistinguishable from those of true labor, but they eventually stop, making the diagnosis easy in hindsight. Sometimes, they continue without interruption into true labor, making the latent phase appear abnormally long. (See Braxton Hicks contractions; prodromal labor)

**false pelvis**   The part of the maternal pelvis above (i.e., cephalad to) the true inlet at the ileopectineal line. It has no bearing on the labor and delivery process.

**ferning**   Microscopic pattern of crystallization seen when amniotic fluid is dried on a glass slide. Ferning observed in a sample of fluid obtained from the vagina or cervical canal confirms that the membranes have ruptured.

**fetal lie**   Relation of the fetal axis to the longitudinal axis of the mother, including longitudinal, transverse, or oblique. (See brow presentation; face presentation; sincipital presentation; transverse lie; vertex)

**fetoscope**   A stethoscope designed to hear the fetal heart sounds through the maternal abdominal wall.

**first stage**   The portion of labor that extends from its onset to attainment of full cervical dilatation. Onset is often difficult to ascertain, but is generally considered to be when the gravida perceives regular uterine contractions. (See Braxton Hicks contractions; false labor; labor curves; latent phase)

**flat pelvis**   A type of female pelvis characterized by foreshortened anteroposterior and elongated transverse dimensions, wide forepelvis and subpubic angle, divergent sidewalls, blunt ischial spines and forward, straight sacrum with anterior angulation at the sacrococcygeal junction. Flat pelvis is associated with an occiput transverse labor mechanism and frequently requires cesarean delivery. (See Barton forceps; mechanism of labor; platypelloid pelvis)

**flexion point**   The portion of the fetal head to which the vacuum extractor cup should be applied. Also called the pivot point, it is in the sagittal plane about 2 cm anterior to the posterior fontanel. (See vacuum extractor)

**footling presentation**   Variant of breech presentation in which a lower extremity precedes the buttocks into the pelvis. Because the presenting part does not fill the pelvis, single or double footling presentation is more often associated with prolapsed cord than cephalic, frank or complete breech presentations. (See breech presentation; complete breech presentation; frank presentation; incomplete breech presentation)

**forceps, obstetric**   Instrument used for effecting operative vaginal delivery. The wide variety of forceps that are available for clinical use fall into two main categories: classic varieties (Elliot and Simpson types) and special forceps (Kielland, Barton, and Piper, among others). (See Elliot-type forceps; Barton forceps; Kielland forceps; Piper forceps; Simpson-type forceps)

**forepelvis**   Anterior segment of the pelvic inlet located between the superior rami of the pubic bones. It is characteristically rounded in the gynecoid pelvis, wide in the flat pelvis, and narrow in both android and anthropoid pelves.

**forewaters**    An accumulation of amniotic fluid palpable on vaginal examination between the fetal membranes and the lowermost portion of the fetal presenting part.

**fossa navicularis**    A depression just external to the hymeneal ring at the posterior junction of the labia minora, overlying fibers of the bulbospongiosus muscle. The shelf-like area of the fossa should be reconstructed during episiotomy or laceration repair. (See episiotomy)

**fourth stage**    The initial hours after delivery of the placenta. During this time parent–infant bonding usually occurs. Surveillance for the development of postpartum hemorrhage is important during this period.

**frank breech presentation**    The most common variant of breech presentation in which the fetal hips are flexed and knees extended so that the legs are straight up against the abdomen and the thorax, serving to splint the vertebral column. (See breech presentation; complete breech presentation; footling breech presentation; incomplete breech presentation)

**fundal height**    Measure of uterine size obtained by means of a tape measure applied from the top of the symphysis pubis to the top of the uterus. It is useful, when used serially over time, as an indicator of fetal growth. It is thus an alert to possible fetal growth restriction, fetal macrosomia, multiple pregnancy, and misdating of gestational age. (See fundus; growth restriction, fetal; multiple pregnancy; uteroplacental insufficiency)

**fundal pressure**    External force applied to the top of the uterus to impress the fetus into the pelvis. It can be appropriate to use gentle fundal pressure briefly to aid in determining the likelihood of cephalopelvic disproportion, but not for supplementing maternal bearing-down efforts to effect delivery because doing so is potentially traumatic. (See Müller-Hillis maneuver)

**fundus**    A term commonly applied to refer to the upper external extremity of the uterus, as distinguished from the uterine corpus and cervix. More correctly, the uterine fundus is the uppermost portion of the uterine cavity.

**funnel pelvis**    Characteristic shape of the android pelvis in which the dimensions at the cephalad end of the pelvis (inlet or superior strait) are greater than those in the middle (midplane or midcavity), which in turn are greater than those at the caudad end (outlet or inferior strait). (See android pelvis)

**glabella**   The prominence of the frontal bone palpable just above the root of the nose.

**gluteal cleft**   Indentation between the buttocks. (See natal cleft)

**gravid**   Pregnant (adjective).

**gravida**   A pregnant woman (noun). (See multigravida; nulligravida)

**gravidity**   A measure of the number of pregnancies a woman has had, including the current one.

**growth discordance, fetal**   Discrepancy in the size of twins, based on estimates of fetal weight obtained by ultrasonographic measurements. Considered clinically relevant when there is greater than 25% difference (calculated as the weight difference divided by the weight of the larger fetus, times 100) because of the large error in weight estimates. A useful indicator of twin-twin transfusion syndrome. (See stuck twin; twin-twin transfusion syndrome; weight discordance, fetal)

**growth restriction, fetal**   Failure of the fetus to grow according to expectations for gestational age based on population-based data; an indicator of possible uteroplacental insufficiency. Previously called intrauterine growth retardation. (See uteroplacental insufficiency)

**gynecoid pelvis**   Most common variant of pelvic architecture in gravidas. It is characterized by a rounded inlet, equal anteroposterior and transverse dimensions, parallel sidewalls, average forepelvis, ischial spines and subpubic arch. It is associated with an occiput anterior mechanism in labor. (See android pelvis; anthropoid pelvis; flat pelvis; mechanisms of labor; platypelloid pelvis)

**HELLP syndrome**   A severe variant of pregnancy-induced hypertension, typically with some combination of hemolysis, elevated liver enzyme levels, and low platelet count. Given its potentially serious impact on mother and fetus, it is often an indication for prompt delivery.

**high forceps**   A delivery procedure in which obstetric forceps are applied to a fetal head that is not engaged in the pelvis, specifically before the biparietal diameter of the fetal head has descended to or below the pelvic inlet. Because of the high risks associated with its use, high forceps operations are never appropriate. (See low forceps; midforceps; outlet forceps)

**high-order multifetal pregnancy**   A pregnancy in which there are three or more fetuses. (See multiple pregnancy)

**hydramnios**   Excessive volume of amniotic fluid; synonymous with polyhydramnios. (See amnioreduction; polyhydramnios)

**hydrops, fetal**   A condition of extreme fetal edema or anasarca associated with fetal isoimmunization, aneuploidy, certain infections, and other etiologies.

**hypercontractility, uterine**   Uterine hyperactivity associated with several identifiable contraction patterns, including those that are too long (uterine tetany), those that occur too frequently (uterine tachysystole), those that do not relax between them (uterine polysystole), those that are coupled (uterine coupling), and those associated with increased basal tonus (hypertonus). The adverse fetal effect of hypercontractility results from inadequate reoxygenation of the intervillous space to maintain fetal well-being. Its causes include exogenous oxytocin and abruptio placentae, among others. (See augmentation of labor; hyperstimulation, uterine; oxytocin; prostaglandins)

**hyperextension, fetal head**   Marked deflexion of the aftercoming head of a fetus in a breech presentation causing posterior angulation of the vertebral column at the neck, exposing the fetus to potentially serious risk of spinal cord injury if vaginal delivery is attempted. Hyperextension in a breech presentation constitutes a strong indication for cesarean delivery.

**hyperstimulation, uterine**   Uterine hypercontractility resulting from administration of a uterotonic agent, such as oxytocin or prostaglandin. (See ecbolic agent; hypercontractility, uterine; oxytocin; prostaglandins; uterotonic agent)

**hypertonus, uterine**   A form of uterine hypercontractility in which the basal tonus of the uterus is increased above 15 mmHg. (See hypercontractility, uterine; hyperstimulation, uterine)

**hysterotomy**   Any operative procedure in which the uterus is incised. In clinical usage, it usually refers to surgery involving incision in the fundal aspect of the gravid uterus.

**incomplete breech**   A type of breech presentation in which one or both limbs present in advance of the buttocks. (See breech presentation; complete breech presentation; footling presentation; frank breech presentation)

**induction, labor**   Process by which labor is initiated artificially through mechanical or pharmacologic means. (See amniotomy; ecbolic agent; prostaglandins; stripping membranes; uterotonic agent)

**inferior strait of pelvis**   Pelvic outlet.

**instrumental delivery**   Procedure for effecting delivery involving use of forceps or vacuum extractor.

**internal podalic version**   Procedure for converting a fetus in transverse or oblique lie to a double footling breech presentation by manual manipulation. It is undertaken in the second stage of labor under anesthesia. It involves introducing a hand through the vagina high into the uterus, identifying and grasping the fetal feet, and applying traction. It is often followed by breech extraction, although allowing labor to proceed is an acceptable option. (See breech extraction; external cephalic version; transverse lie; version)

**intrauterine pressure transducer**   Device for objectively and accurately measuring the pattern of uterine contractile pressure. The information on contractility is obtained by a strain gauge placed within the uterine cavity by way of the vagina and the cervix. (See hypercontractility, uterine; hyperstimulation, uterine)

**introitus, vaginal**   The entrance to the vagina.

**inversion, uterine**   A complication encountered after delivery in which the fundus of the uterus collapses into the uterine cavity, thus turning the uterus inside-out. The inversion may involve just the fundus, or, in extreme cases, the entire uterus.

**Kielland forceps**   An obstetric forceps designed for application to a fetal head arrested in occiput posterior position in an anthropoid pelvis. It is a long, straight, lightweight instrument with a negligible pelvic curve, overlapping shanks and a sliding lock. Also useful for rotation of occiput transverse positions. It is seldom used today because difficult and potentially traumatic forceps operations have been largely replaced by cesarean delivery. (See anthropoid pelvis; forceps, obstetric)

**labor curves**   Graphic representation of the serial changes in cervical dilatation and fetal station as a function of time during labor.

**laminaria**   Hydrophilic rods, composed of a form of seaweed that absorbs fluid so they expand. When placed in the cervical canal, they serve to dilate the cervix slowly over time without injury.

**latent phase**   The portion of labor that extends from its onset to the beginning of the active phase. (See labor curves; prolonged latent phase)

**Leopold maneuvers**   A sequence of four kinds of abdominal examination used to identify the fetal presentation and position, the degree of engagement, and the flexion or extension of the fetal head.

**linea alba**   A narrow band of dense connective tissue in the midline of the abdominal wall. It separates the two bellies of the rectus abdominal muscle.

**low forceps**   A procedure in which a forceps instrument is applied to a fetal head that is at or below station +2 and no more than 45 degrees from a direct occiput anterior or posterior position. (See forceps, obstetric; high forceps; midforceps; outlet forceps)

**macrosomia, fetal**   A fetus of unusually large size for its gestational age, either based on population-based data, e.g., heavier than the 10th percentile for age, or arbitrarily-defined limits, such as 4000 g or 4500 g at term.

**malposition, fetal**   Abnormal fetal position, including any position that is not direct occiput anterior or within 45 degrees of direct occiput anterior.

**manual rotation**   Procedure for rotating a fetal head in a malposition, such as occiput transverse or occiput posterior, to the more favorable occiput anterior by using a hand placed intravaginally to grasp both sides of the head and apply rotational torque. Not recommended because it seldom achieves its objective and can be traumatic. (See digital rotation; malposition, fetal)

**Mauriceau-Smellie-Veit maneuver**   A technique to aid emergence of the fetal head during vaginal breech delivery. The attendant flexes the head by exerting pressure on the malar eminences or the fetal mandible. (See aftercoming head; breech delivery; hyperextension, fetal head)

**McRoberts maneuver, position**   A technique used to resolve shoulder dystocia in which the mother's hips and knees are acutely flexed. (See shoulder dystocia)

**mechanisms of labor**   The sequence of movements the fetus undergoes in accommodating itself passively to the birth canal during descent and delivery, including engagement, flexion, internal rotation, extension on the pelvic floor, and restitution, or external rotation. (See cardinal movements; deflexion, fetal head; descent, fetal)

**meningomyelocele**   Congenital fetal anomaly in which there is a defect in the vertebral column that permits the spinal cord and its investing membranes to protrude.

**mentum**   The chin, a reference point for designating the fetal position of a fetus in face presentation. (See face presentation)

**metroplasty**   Surgical procedure for correcting an anatomic anomaly of the uterus, such as uterus didelphys (double uterus). It usually consists of a transverse incision across the top of the uterus, excision of a segment of the uterine wall, and reconstruction of the uterus so it has a single unified cavity. The incision is vulnerable to rupture in a future pregnancy.

**midforceps**   Operative vaginal delivery procedure in which a forceps instrument is applied to a fetal head that is above station +2 or more than 45 degrees off direct occiput anterior or posterior position. It is associated with a higher risk to mother and fetus than low or outlet forceps; it is, therefore, not recommended except under special circumstances that minimize potential harm. (See forceps, obstetric; high forceps; low forceps; outlet forceps)

**midpelvis**   The midcavitary plane, centered on the plane of the ischial spines. (See birth canal; inferior strait; superior strait)

**moldability, fetal head** Capacity of the fetal head to be remodeled (i.e., deformed) by the forces of labor. It is dependent on the intensity of those forces, the pliability of the skull bones (as related to fetal maturity and calcium deposition), the elasticity of the connective tissue between the cranial plates, and the constraints of the bony pelvis. (See molding, fetal head)

**molding, fetal head** Changes in the shape of the fetal head during labor caused by gradual deformation and overlapping of the cranial bones.

**Montevideo unit** A quantitative assessment of uterine contractile activity during labor, called "uterine work." It is determined by summing the net (peak minus baseline tonus) contraction pressure amplitudes in a 10-minute window, based on continuous evaluation by an internal strain gauge. (See intrauterine pressure transducer)

**Müller–Hillis maneuver** A technique of cephalopelvimetry that helps to identify the probability of cephalopelvic disproportion. In the second stage or late first stage, at the height of a contraction, firm pressure is placed on the uterine fundus. A vaginal examining hand determines the degree of rotation and descent that occurs during the contraction.

**multigravida** A woman who has been pregnant two or more times. (See gravida, nulligravida, primigravida)

**multipara** A woman who has had two or more births of babies with weights over 500 g. (See nullipara; primipara)

**multiparous** Relating to a multipara (adjective).

**multiple gestation** Pregnancy carrying two or more fetuses. (See high-order multifetal pregnancy)

**myomectomy** Surgical procedure in which leiomyomata uteri are removed, leaving a functional uterus in situ.

**natal cleft** The furrow between the buttocks; gluteal cleft.

**neuraxial anesthesia, block** Conduction anesthesia involving the spinal cord or nerve roots. In obstetrics, it usually refers to spinal (subarachnoid) or epidural anesthetic techniques. (See conduction anesthesia; epidural anesthesia)

**nuchal arm** A complication of breech delivery in which the shoulder is extended and the elbow flexed with the forearm located posteriorly along the fetal neck. Nuchal arms usually obstruct the delivery of the aftercoming head. They must, therefore, be corrected expeditiously before vaginal breech delivery can be completed safely. (See aftercoming head; breech presentation; assisted breech delivery; breech extraction)

**nulligravida**    A woman who has never been pregnant. (See gravida; multigravida; primigravida)

**nullipara**    A woman who has had no previous delivery of a fetus weighing more than 500 g. (See multipara; primipara)

**nulliparous**    Relating to a nullipara (adjective).

**oblique lie**    A variant of transverse lie (shoulder presentation) in which the fetal body lies at an oblique angle to the mother's axis. Both are managed in about the same way. (See transverse lie)

**obstructed labor**    Any constellation of conditions that makes safe vaginal delivery unlikely because the fetus is not able to be accommodated safely by the maternal pelvis. Causes include cephalopelvic disproportion, fetal malpresentations, and maternal or fetal masses. (See dysfunctional labor; bony dystocia; disproportion)

**omphalocele**    A congenital malformation in which abdominal viscera herniate through the abdominal wall at the base of the umbilical cord.

**outlet forceps**    Instrumental operation in which forceps is applied to a fetal head that has reached the pelvic floor or perineum and is within 45 degrees of the direct occiput anterior or posterior position. (See forceps, obstetric; high forceps; low forceps; midforceps)

**outlet strait of pelvis**    The inferior strait, the lowermost aspects of the birth canal bounded by the inferior pubic rami, coccyx and perineum.

**oxytocin**    A uterotonic hormone stored in and released from the posterior pituitary gland. Synthesized oxytocin is available for pharmacologic administration via dilute intravenous solution by controlled pump to induce or augment labor as well as for managing postpartum atony. (See augmentation of labor; hypercontractility, uterine; hyperstimulation, uterine; induction of labor)

**paradigm**    Flow diagram to illustrate steps in decision-making; algorithm, decision tree.

**parametrium, parametria**    Connective tissue found lateral to the uterine cervix and corpus, containing blood vessels and lymphatics.

**parity**    A measure of the number of deliveries a woman has had.

**parous**    Relating to parity (adjective).

**parturient**    A woman in labor.

**parturition**    The process of labor and delivery; childbirth.

**patient-request cesarean**    Elective cesarean delivery undertaken at the request of the gravida.

**pelvic division of labor**   That part of the labor process during which most fetal descent usually occurs, specifically the deceleration phase and the second stage.

**pelvic floor**   A complex musculofascial barrier between the pelvic cavity and the perineum. The pelvic floor includes the levator ani, coccygeus, deep transverse perinei, and urethral sphincter muscles and their supporting fasciae. Its structures support the pelvic viscera and contribute to continence.

**pelvimetry**   Clinical method for evaluating the anatomical architecture and capacity of the pelvis. It provides information of value in regard to the characteristics of the pelvis to inform caregivers about the probable mechanism of labor and determines whether an average fetus will be likely to encounter problems negotiating the pelvis safely during labor and delivery. (See cephalopelvimentry; Müller-Hillis maneuver)

**Pfannenstiel incision**   A suprapubic incision for surgical access to the abdominal cavity. It consists of a transverse incision through skin, subcutaneous fat and fascia, and anterior rectus sheath, plus a vertical incision through the linea alba between the rectus muscles and the peritoneum. It yields a strong cosmetically-acceptable wound with a low probability of dehiscence.

**phase of maximum slope**   The linear portion of the active phase of the first stage of labor between the acceleration phase and the deceleration phase. Its slope (rate of dilatation in centimeters per hour) is a utilitarian clinical indicator as to whether progress of cervical dilatation is normal or not. (See acceleration phase; active phase; deceleration phase; labor curves)

**Piper forceps**   An obstetric forceps designed for application to the aftercoming fetal head in a vaginal breech delivery. It is a long instrument with separated shanks and backward-curving handles specifically made to be applied from beneath the already-delivered fetal body. (See aftercoming head; breech presentation; assisted breech delivery; breech extraction)

**placenta previa**   Abnormal placentation in which the placenta implants at or over the internal os of the cervix. Cesarean delivery is necessary for managing this condition.

**platypelloid pelvis**   Flat pelvis; a pelvis that is elongated transversely and foreshortened in the anteroposterior diameter. It is associated with the occiput transverse mechanism in labor. (See android pelvis; anthropoid pelvis; Barton forceps; flat pelvis; gynecoid pelvis)

**polyhydramnios**   Hydramnios; excessive amniotic fluid volume. (See amnioreduction; hydramnios)

**polysystole, uterine**   A form of uterine hypercontractility in which uterine contractions fail to relax completely before the next contraction begins. It is often associated with fetal hypoxia. (See hypercontractility, uterine; hyperstimulation, uterine; oxytocin; prostaglandins)

**position, fetal**   Designation of the relation of a fetal referent point (occiput for vertex, bregma for brow, mentum for face, sacrum for breech, and acromion for shoulder presentation) to the maternal pelvis (right, left, anterior, posterior). (See brow presentation; face presentation; presenting part, fetal; shoulder presentation; transverse lie)

**posterior commissure**   The portion of the introitus where the labia majora meet posteriorly in the midline. Also called the posterior labial commissure.

**postterm pregnancy**   Gestational duration that exceeds 42 completed weeks from the last menstrual period.

**Poupart's ligament**   The inguinal ligament. Extends from the anterior superior iliac spine to the pubic tubercle.

**precipitate descent**   A labor dysfunction in which fetal descent in the second stage that exceeds 5 stations (cm)/h in a nullipara or 10 stations (cm)/h in a multipara. (See dysfunctional labor; descent, fetal; hypercontractility, uterine; hyperstimulation, uterine; oxytocin; prostaglandins; station, fetal)

**precipitate dilatation**   A labor dysfunction in which cervical dilatation in the active phase exceeds 5 stations (cm)/h in a nullipara or 10 stations (cm)/h in a multipara. (See dysfunctional labor; descent, fetal; hypercontractility, uterine; hyperstimulation, uterine; oxytocin; prostaglandins; station, fetal)

**presenting part, fetal**   The portion of the fetus that is lowermost in or over the inlet of the maternal pelvis. (See breech presentation; brow presentation; face presentation; shoulder presentation; transverse lie; vertex presentation)

**primigravida**   A woman who is pregnant for the first time. (See gravida; multigravida; nulligravida)

**priming, cervical**   Process by which the unripe cervix is made more favorable for labor induction, usually accomplished either by mechanical means or by the administration of prostaglandins. (See cervical ripening; induction of labor; prostaglandins)

**primipara**   A woman who has had one pregnancy that resulted in the birth of a baby weighing more than 500 g. (See multipara; nullipara)

**prodromal labor**  A stage preceding actual labor. During the prodromal period, Braxton Hicks contractions may become more prominent, the cervical mucus plug may be lost, and some ripening of the cervix may occur. (See Braxton Hicks contractions; false labor)

**prolonged deceleration phase**  A labor dysfunction in which the duration of the deceleration phase exceeds 3 h in a nullipara or 1 h in a multipara. (See deceleration phase; dysfunctional labor; labor curves)

**prolonged latent phase**  A labor dysfunction in which the latent phase duration exceeds 20 h in a nullipara or 14 h in a multipara. (See dysfunctional labor; latent phase; labor curves)

**promontory, sacral**  The anterior prominence of the first sacral vertebral body projecting into the pelvis at the level of the superior strait. It is a landmark for measuring the true conjugate, the anteroposterior diameter of the pelvic inlet. (See obstetric conjugate; true conjugate)

**prostaglandins**  A variety of prostanoic acids with several functions, including vasoconstriction, vasodilation and stimulation of bowel, bronchus and uterus. In obstetrics, some prostaglandins act to change the characteristics of the cervix so it becomes more amenable to induction of labor. Their uterotonic action also sometimes initiates labor. (See cervical ripening; hypercontractility, uterine; hyperstimulation, uterine; induction of labor; oxytocin; priming cervical)

**protracted active phase**  Disorder of the active phase of cervical dilatation in which dilatation progresses linearly at a rate below normal (<1.2 cm/h in nulliparas; <1.5 cm/h in multiparas). (See active phase; dysfunctional labor; labor curves)

**protracted descent**  Disorder of the second stage (often beginning in the deceleration phase of the first stage, but seldom diagnosed then) in which fetal descent progresses actively at a rate below the normal range (<1.0 stations (cm)/h in nulliparas; <2.0 stations (cm)/h in multiparas). (See deceleration phase; descent, fetal; dysfunctional labor; labor curves; second stage)

**psychoprophylactic technique**  A program of education, breathing exercises, and psychological and physical conditioning used to prepare a gravida to experience her labor and delivery with minimal or no analgesia or anesthesia.

**restitution, fetal head**  Spontaneous rotation of the fetal head resulting from the head realigning with the shoulders immediately after it is delivered over the perineum. (See external rotation; mechanisms of labor)

**retinaculum uteri**   The aggregate of musculofascial structures that anchor the uterus in the pelvis. It includes the cardinal, round, uterosacral, and pubo-vesico-uterine ligaments.

**second stage**   The portion of labor between full cervical dilatation and delivery of the fetus during which most fetal descent occurs. (See descent, fetal)

**secundines**   The placenta and the fetal membranes.

**selective fetocide**   Method for reducing the number of fetuses in high-order multifetal pregnancy to improve morbidity and mortality outcomes for the remaining fetuses. It usually involves transabdominal injection of potassium chloride into the fetal heart. (See high-order multifetal pregnancy)

**shoulder dystocia**   A situation in which the shoulders fail to deliver spontaneously after delivery of the fetal head. (See bisacromial diameter; McRoberts maneuver; position; suprapubic pressure; symphysiotomy; Woods maneuver; Zavanelli maneuver)

**shoulder presentation**   Transverse lie; a malpresentation in which the long axis of the fetus is perpendicular to the long axis of the mother. The acromial process is the referent point for determining the fetal position. If the malpresentation cannot be corrected by version, cesarean section is necessary for safe delivery of a fetus. Oblique lie is a variant of shoulder presentation. (See external cephalic version; oblique lie; transverse lie; version)

**Simpson-type forceps**   A group of classic obstetric forceps designed for application to an elongated molded fetal head; the instruments all have separated shanks and a tapered cephalic curve. (See Barton forceps; Elliot-type forceps; Kielland forceps; molding, fetal head)

**sinciput**   The area of the fetal head lying anterior to the large (anterior) fontanel. (See bregma; mentum; sincipital presentation; vertex)

**sincipital presentation**   A minor malpresentation in which the low-ermost presenting part of the fetal head is the sinciput. It is considered unstable because it will eventually convert spontaneously either to a vertex presentation or to a brow presentation; military attitude. (See brow presentation; cephalic presentation; face presentation; sinciput; unstable lie; vertex presentation)

**station, fetal**   A measure of the level to which the most dependent aspect of the fetal presenting part has descended in the birth canal. Stations are designated by centimeters above and below the plane of the ischial spines, which is station 0. The term "station -1" indicates the forward leading edge of the presenting part is 1 cm cephalad to this level; "station +2" means it is 2 cm caudad. (See caudad; cephalad; descent, fetal; labor curves)

**stripping membranes**    Procedure in which the chorioamniotic membranes are separated from their attachment to the decidua by a sweeping movement of the intracervical fingers. It is done to induce labor at or near term. (See induction of labor)

**stuck twin**    Term used to describe the donor twin in severe twin-twin transfusion syndrome affecting diamniotic (but monozygotic) twins. Because diminishing amniotic fluid results in extreme oligohydramnios (anhydramnios), the fetus is tightly constrained by the membranes, making it appear to be tightly adherent (i.e., stuck) to the inside of the uterine wall. (See chorionicity; multiple pregnancy; oligohydramnios; twin-twin transfusion syndrome; zygosity)

**succenturiate lobe, placental**    Supernumerary placental segment separate from the main placental mass, but connected to it by umbilical vessels that run between the amnion and the chorion. It is of importance because it may not be recognized at delivery, and thus left behind to expose the gravida to the risks of later infection and hemorrhage.

**superior strait**    The pelvic inlet. (See false pelvis; inferior strait; midpelvis)

**supine hypotension syndrome**    A condition in which a gravida experiences dizziness and syncope when she is supine. It occurs as the consequence of aortocaval compression from the gravid uterus, which reduces venous return to the heart and cardiac output in turn. It may reduce uterine blood flow and placental perfusion, causing fetal hypoxia. (See aortocaval compression)

**suprapubic pressure**    Manual force applied to the lower abdomen just above the superior rami of the pubis. It is used primarily for attempting to correct impaction of the anterior shoulder in cases of shoulder dystocia, so as to try to reduce the diameter of the fetal shoulder girdle by flexing it with pressure directed against the shoulder in the direction of the fetal chest. (See bisacromial diameter; shoulder dystocia)

**symphysiotomy**    Surgical division of the symphysis pubis during delivery for management of severe shoulder dystocia, rarely used. (See shoulder dystocia)

**symphysis pubis**    The fibrocartilaginous joint in the anterior midline of the pelvis where the left and right pubic bones meet. It softens under the influence of pregnancy hormones and becomes flexible and distensible. Diastasis (separation) of the joint, which may occur during the prenatal course or in a traumatic or excessively rapid vaginal delivery, can be painful and even crippling. (See diagonal conjugate; true conjugate)

**subgaleal hemorrhage**   Bleeding into the subgaleal space between the cranial periosteum and the scalp galea aponeurosis. It is encountered, albeit infrequently, as a complication of vacuum extraction or traumatic delivery. It results from rupture of the emissary veins that course between the dural sinuses and the scalp veins. A boggy occipital mass usually develops gradually in the first several days after delivery and spreads over the entire roof of the skull (calvaria). The presence of such an enlarging mass serves to alert care providers to its presence. The subgaleal space can accommodate as much as half the newborn baby's blood volume, causing hypovolemic shock. (See caput succedaneum; cephalhematoma)

**sulcus, vaginal**   In obstetrics this term refers to the lateral fornices of the vagina. A sulcus laceration is one that generally extends longitudinally along the posterolateral wall of the vagina. It can be deep and the source of considerable hemorrhage.

**synclitism**   The fetomaternal spatial relationship by which the planes of the fetal head remain parallel with the planes of the birth canal over the entire course of fetal descent in labor and delivery. (See asynclitism)

**tachysystole, uterine**   A form of hypercontractility in which uterine contractions occur in rapid succession. It is defined as a pattern of contractions that recur more frequently than every 2 minutes. More pathophysiologically, contractions are so close together that there may not be enough time for the intervillous space to be reoxygenated by maternal uterine blood flow, leaving the fetus hypoxic. (See hypercontractility, uterine; hyperstimulation, uterine; intervillous space; oxytocin; prostaglandins)

**tetany, uterine**   A type of hypercontractility characterized by excessively long uterine contractions, lasting longer than 90 seconds. Even a well-oxygenated healthy fetus may experience hypoxia as the intervillous space becomes deoxygenated over this length of time. (See hypercontractility, uterine; hyperstimulation, uterine; intervillous space; oxytocin; prostaglandins)

**therapeutic rest regimen**   Treatment program for managing the labor disorder of prolonged latent phase by administering narcotic analgesia, such as meperidine or morphine, to stop uterine contractions temporarily and provide an interval of rest for the gravida. When she awakens, she will be out of labor, in the active phase of labor, or continuing to have ineffective latent phase uterine contractions. (See dysfunctional labor; labor curves; latent phase)

**third stage**   The portion of labor between delivery of the fetus and delivery of the placenta.

**tocodynamometer**    External electromechanical device for assessing uterine contractions. It actually records changes in the curvature of the abdominal wall, so it is unable to measure either basal tonus or contraction amplitude. (See hypercontractility, uterine; hyperstimulation, uterine)

**tocolytic drug**    A medication used to reduce uterine contractility. (See ecbolic agent; hypercontractility, uterine; hyperstimulation, uterine; oxytocin; prostaglandins; uterotonic agent)

**tragus**    A projection of the ear cartilage just anterior to the opening of the external ear canal. Use as a landmark to identify the fetal ear and its orientation. It is useful when fetal head position cannot be verified by palpation of the cranial bones.

**transversalis fascia**    Connective tissue layer in the abdominal wall lying between the parietal peritoneum and the overlying muscles of the abdominal wall with their investing fasciae.

**transverse lie**    Shoulder or oblique fetal presentation.

**Trendelenburg position**    Supine position in which the patient's head is lower than her pelvis. It is useful to facilitate transabdominal pelvic surgery. It allows the bowel to be displaced cephalad out of the operative field and thereby improve exposure.

**trial forceps**    A delivery procedure in which obstetric forceps are applied in an attempt to effect vaginal delivery even though the capacity of the pelvis. To accommodate the fetus safely the fetus is unclear. Because it is potentially hazardous, it is not recommended except under limited circumstances and in skillful hands. (See cephalopelvic disproportion; forceps, obstetric)

**trial of labor**    Process by which labor is allowed to proceed, either spontaneously or under the influence of a uterotonic agent, to determine if progressive cervical dilatation and fetal descent can occur. It must be undertaken only by knowledgeable personnel who are carefully monitoring progress to ensure against harm. (See cephalopelvic disproportion; cephalopelvimetry; dysfunctional labor; labor curves)

**true conjugate**    The anteroposterior diameter of the true inlet, measuring from the back of the symphysis pubis to the sacral promontory. It is not available by direct clinical evaluation, but estimated instead by subtracting 1.5 cm from the obstetric conjugate, which can be obtained by vaginal examination, measuring from the bottom of the symphysis pubis to the sacral promontory. (See pelvimetry; obstetric conjugate)

**twin-twin transfusion syndrome**    Condition affecting twin monozygotic pregnancies in which a placental anastomosis connecting the vasculature of the twins permits one of them to pump blood (the donor twin) into the circulation of the other (the recipient twin). The donor may thus become anemic and underdeveloped with oligohydramnios; the recipient may grow large and polycythemic with hydramnios. The syndrome can be injurious to both twins. (See chorionicity; hydramnios; multiple pregnancy; oligohydramnios; zygosity)

**unstable presentation or lie**  Sincipital and brow presentations are considered unstable because in each the head is likely to convert to another presentation during labor. Sincipital presentation may spontaneously convert to vertex or brow presentation; brow to vertex or face. Similarly, transverse or oblique lies are unstable because they often convert to a longitudinal lie, becoming a breech or cephalic presentation. (See brow presentation; oblique lie; sincipital presentation; transverse lie)

**uterotonic agent**  A drug that stimulates myometrial contractility; ecbolic. (See ecbolic agent; hypercontractility, uterine; hyperstimulation, uterine; oxytocin; prostaglandins; uterotonic agent)

**vacuum extractor**  An instrument for effecting vaginal delivery by applying traction to the fetal head. It consists of a metal or plastic cup attached to the fetal scalp by means of negative pressure (vacuum); ventouse. Scalp and subcutaneous tissue are drawn into the cup to form a "chignon" for traction purposes. While the vacuum extractor is generally safer than forceps, possible complications associated with its use include cephalhematoma (subperiosteal hematoma) and even more serious subgaleal hemorrhage (bleeding into the potential space between the skull periosteum and the scalp galea aponeurosis). It is important to be knowledgeable about when to use the vacuum extractor and to be skillful and gentle in its use. (See cephalhematoma; flexion point; forceps, obstetric; subgaleal hemorrhage)

**Valsalva maneuver**  Bearing-down or forced expiratory effort produced by closing the glottis and pushing with diaphragmatic and abdominal muscles. It is used to complement uterine contractile forces in second stage labor to facilitate vaginal delivery. Distention of the vagina and perineum by the descending fetus in second stage of labor reflexively stimulates spontaneous bearing-down efforts in the gravida if she does not have the reflex inhibited by neuraxial block anesthesia. If the reflex is blocked, the gravida has to be taught to bear down effectively. (See descent, fetal; neuraxial anesthesia; second stage)

**vanishing twin**  Term applied to the death in utero of one member of a twin pair. It occurs commonly in the first trimester of twin gestations, and is often undetected unless early ultrasonographic imaging has previously diagnosed the multiple pregnancy. Generally, an innocuous occurrence, other than its emotional impact on the mother. (See multiple pregnancy)

**vasa previa**   Condition in which one of the umbilical vessels courses in the fetal membranes over the internal os of the cervix. It results when the umbilical cord implants into the membranes (velamentous insertion) instead of the chorionic plate of the placenta. Vasa previa may result in fetal hemorrhage with death from exsanguination if the membranes should rupture and lacerate the affected vessel. (See velamentous insertion of umbilical cord)

**vectis**   An instrument (usually one forceps blade) used to aid the delivery of the fetal head at cesarean delivery. (See forceps, obstetric)

**velamentous insertion of umbilical cord**   Anomalous insertion of the umbilical cord, with its umbilical vein and arteries, into the chorioamniotic membranes at a distance from the edge of the placenta. It is generally of no clinical concern unless one of the vessels crosses the internal os of the cervix, forming a vasa previa, which exposes the fetus to the risk of serious hemorrhage in the event the membranes rupture and lacerate the umbilical vessel. (See vasa previa)

**version, fetal**   Event that occurs spontaneously or as a result of manipulations in which a fetal malpresentation is corrected. External cephalic version (of a breech to a vertex presentation by external maneuvers) and internal podalic version (of a transverse lie to a breech presentation by internal manipulation) are examples of operative procedures to effect version. External version to correct breech presentation is commonly practiced to reduce the need for cesarean delivery. Internal version is seldom done any longer because it carries serious risks. (See breech presentation; external cephalic version; internal podalic version; shoulder presentation; transverse lie)

**vertex**   The area of the fetal head that lies between the two fontanels. (See vertex presentation)

**vertex presentation**   The most common variant of cephalic presentation in which the fetal head is maximally flexed so that the vertex is lowermost in the maternal pelvis, optimal for safe vaginal delivery. (See cephalic presentation; vertex)

**water intoxication**   A serious condition of profound hyponatremia with encephalopathy, manifested by confusion, loss of consciousness, and convulsions. It results from the antidiuretic hormone-like effects of infusion of excessive oxytocin. (See oxytocin)

**weight discordance, fetal**   Discrepant fetal growth between twins, often signifying the presence of the twin-twin transfusion syndrome. (See growth discordance, fetal; multiple pregnancy; twin-twin transfusion syndrome)

**Woods maneuver**  A technique to resolve shoulder dystocia in which the fetus is rotated 180 degrees so that the shoulder originally found posteriorly at or above the sacrum is grasped by the intravaginal hand and moved to an anterior position in the pelvis at the symphysis pubis. Also referred to as a screw or corkscrew maneuver. (See shoulder dystocia)

**Zavanelli maneuver**  A technique to resolve shoulder dystocia in which the fetal head, which has already delivered, is replaced into the vagina, and cesarean delivery is then done. Usually used as a last resort when conventional methods are unavailing. (See shoulder dystocia)

**zygosity**  Status of twins based on whether they are derived from fertilization of one ovum (monozygotic) or two ova (dizygotic). Zygosity is determined by studies of gender and characteristics of their placentas and membranes. Further clarification may be necessary, including assessment of blood type and DNA profile. (See chorionicity; multiple pregnancy)

# Index

---

*Labor and Delivery Care: A Practical Guide*, First Edition. Wayne R. Cohen and
Emanuel A. Friedman. © 2011 John Wiley & Sons, Ltd.
Published 2011 by John Wiley & Sons, Ltd